The Patient's Guide to Medical Tests

By Faculty Members at
The Yale University School of Medicine

Barry L. Zaret, MD
Senior Editor

Peter Jatlow, MD and Lee D. Katz, MD
Associate Editors

Genell J. Subak-Sharpe
Editorial Director

Diane Goetz
Managing Editor

Houghton Mifflin Company
Boston New York

Library of Congress Cataloging-in-Publication Data

The patient's guide to medical tests / by faculty members at the Yale University School of Medicine : Barry L. Zaret, senior editor . . . [et al.]

p. cm.

Includes index.

ISBN 0-395-76536-6

1. Diagnosis. 2. Medicine, Popular. I. Zaret, Barry L.

RC71.P38 1997

616.07'5—dc21 96-53904

CIP

Printed in the United States of America

RRD 10 9 8 7 6 5 4 3 2

Acknowledgments

As would be expected, putting together a book of this scope inevitably involves enlisting the help of scores of dedicated people. While it is impossible to cite all of the people who have made this book possible, there are some whose efforts deserve special mention.

Above all, we are indebted to the dozens of Yale officials, physicians, researchers, and other staff members who have made this book possible. In addition to the faculty members who contributed chapters in their areas of medical specialty, we would like to thank a number of physicians, nurses, technicians, and other professionals who gave their time to be interviewed. These include Kevin Anderson, MD; Raymond Bahado-Singh, MD; James Birgulto; Elizabeth Canning, RN; John Chaloupka, MD; Eugene Cornelius, MD; Patricia Creem, RN; Anne Curtis, MD; Cynthia Dabbraccio, RN; Virginia DeFilippo; Miriam S. DiMaio; Steven Fischer, MD; Morton Glickman, MD; Jonathan Goldstein, MD; John Hayslett, MD; Paul Hoffer, MD; Gabor Huszar, MD; Carol Lee, MD; George Letsou, MD; Eileen Levine, RN; John Orloff, MD; Jeffrey Pollak, MD; Carol Powell; Zachery Rattner, MD; Patrick Ruwe; Geri R. Spollett; Mark Topazian, MD; Barbara Ward, MD; Joseph Zelson, MD; and Tony Zreik.

A team of skilled medical writers and editors have worked diligently to make the manuscript readable and understandable. They include Catherine Caruthers, Carl Lowe, Claudia B. Scalzi, and Luba Vikhanski. Philip Bashe interviewed dozens of patients, physicians, technicians, and others for their special insight into what really happens during a test. Nicole Freeland has pitched in to check facts, help with editing, and keep track of the myriad details to get the final manuscript in shape. From Dr. Zaret's office, Astrid Swanson has been invaluable in helping keep track of manuscripts and seeing to other details.

We also want to thank Frances Tenenbaum, our editor at Houghton Mifflin, for her patience and insightful handling of this book. The copy editor, Brian Jones, has done a marvelous job catching all those inconsistencies that somehow creep into this kind of manuscript.

We also acknowledge the talent and diligence of our illustrators, Wendolyn B. Hill of Yale's Department of Biomedical Communications, and Briar Lee Mitchell.

Finally, we want to thank the many spouses who have done everything from critiquing chapters to babysitting.

The Editors

Contributors

Kevin R. Anderson, MD
Assistant Professor of Surgery (Urology)

Margaret J. Bia, MD
Professor of Medicine
Director, Transplant Nephrology

Lawrence M. Brass, MD
Professor of Neurology

Florence Comite, MD
Associate Professor, Internal Medicine,
Pediatrics, Obstetrics and Gynecology

Leo M. Cooney Jr, MD
Humana Foundation Professor of Geriatric Medicine
Chief, Section of General Internal Medicine

Joshua Copel, MD
Professor, Obstetrics and Gynecology
Section Head, Maternal-Fetal Medicine

José C. Costa, MD
Professor of Pathology and Biology

Joseph E. Craft, MD
Associate Professor of Medicine
Chief, Section of Rheumatology

Robert M. Donaldson Jr, MD
David Paige Smith Professor of Medicine

Thomas P. Duffy, MD
Professor of Medicine (Hematology)

Jack A. Elias, MD
Professor of Medicine
Chief of Pulmonary and Critical Care Medicine

Gerald Friedland, MD
Professor of Medicine
Director, AIDS Program

Craig D. Friedman, MD
Associate Professor, Otolaryngology, Facial Plastic Surgery

Richard J. Gusberg, MD
Professor of Surgery and Chief, Section of Vascular Surgery

Janet B. Henrich, MD
Associate Professor of Medicine and of Obstetrics and Gynecology
Director, Women's Health Program & The National Center of Excellence in Women's Health

Angela R. Holder, LLM
Clinical Professor of Pediatrics (Law)

Ralph I. Horwitz, MD
Harold H. Hines Jr. Professor of Medicine and Epidemiology
Chairman, Department of Internal Medicine

Peter Jatlow, MD
Professor and Chairman, Department of Laboratory Medicine
Professor of Psychiatry

Peter Jokl, MD
Professor of Orthopedics and Rehabilitation
Chief, Section of Sports Medicine

Fred S. Kantor, MD
Paul B. Beeson Professor of Medicine

Lee D. Katz, MD
Associate Professor of Diagnostic Radiology,
Internal Medicine, and Orthopedic Surgery

Maurice J. Mahoney, MD, JD
Professor of Genetics, Pediatrics, and Obstetrics and Gynecology

David L. Olive, MD
Professor of Obstetrics and Gynecology
Chief of Reproductive Endocrinology and Infertility

Vincent Quagliarello, MD
Associate Professor of Medicine
Clinical Director, Infectious Diseases

Petrie M. Rainey, MD, PhD
Associate Professor of Laboratory Medicine

Michael O. Rigsby, MD
Assistant Professor of Medicine (Infectious Diseases)

Richard Robbins, MD
Formerly Associate Professor of Medicine (Neuroendrocrinology), Yale
Now Professor of Medicine, Cornell University Medical College
Chief of Endocrinology, Memorial Sloan-Kettering
Cancer Center, New York

David J. Schonfeld, MD
Associate Professor of Pediatrics and Child Study

Peter E. Schwartz, MD
Professor of Obstetrics and Gynecology
Director of Gynecologic Oncology

John F. Setaro, MD
Assistant Professor of Medicine
Section of Cardiovascular Medicine
Director, Cardiovascular Disease Prevention Center

Phillip E. Shapiro, MD
Associate Clinical Professor of Dermatology

Robert S. Sherwin, MD
C. N. H. Long Professor of Medicine

Kathleen M. Stoessel, MD
Associate Professor of Ophthalmology

Lynn Tanoue, MD
Assistant Professor of Medicine

Joseph B. Warshaw, MD
Professor and Chairman, Pediatrics
Deputy Dean of Clinical Affairs, School of Medicine

Robert M. Weiss, MD
Professor and Chief, Section of Urology

Barry L. Zaret, MD
Robert W. Berliner Professor of Medicine
Chief, Section of Cardiovascular Medicine
Associate Chairman of Clinical Affairs,
Department of Internal Medicine
Professor of Diagnostic Radiology

Contents

Introduction

Modern diagnostic testing may date back as far as 1612, the year the Italian physician Sanctorius developed a thermometer to measure body temperature. Although Sanctorius's elaborate device (a graduated coil filled with glass beads and partially immersed in water) has been replaced by electronic instant-read models, temperature taking remains one of the most basic and routine of diagnostic tests.

Like the thermometer, the technology involved in diagnostic tests continues to evolve, becoming ever more sophisticated. Imaging becomes more and more comprehensive and precise. Endoscopy and the miniaturization of instruments have revolutionized not only diagnosis but also surgery. The automation of laboratory procedures means that tests can be done rapidly, in large volume, and with very small or "micro" amounts of specimens.

Computers have had a major influence on testing as well. They can produce graphic representations of information gleaned from other tests; take conventional computed tomography (CT) and magnetic resonance imaging (MRI) scans and build three-dimensional images; and allow for greater accuracy of test results, making reporting and tracking easier.

THE SWINGING PENDULUM

The incredible advances in medical technology of the last few decades are reflected in an ever growing number of costly tests and procedures. Indeed, tests and procedures are the fastest growing—and most costly—area of medicine. On the one hand, regulators charge that vast numbers of tests and procedures are unnecessary, and that many are actually performed to make money. Numerous studies show that patients who are well insured are more likely to undergo a battery of tests than those who are in a managed-care group or are uninsured.

On the other hand, there are patients who are told to wait or are urged to settle for a less-costly alternative. Should these patients be asked to forgo an expensive test, even if it is likely to alter the course of treatment? Which side in this argument is right? And how can individuals decide what is best for them? Such questions are at the root of today's often acrimonious debate over how to rein in health care costs without denying essential medical care.

As this debate continues, it is increasingly vital that each person take charge of making sure he or she gets the appropriate health care. Today, more than 70 million Americans are in some type of HMO (health maintenance organization) or other managed-care plan. Under these plans, a primary (gatekeeper) doctor often has a vested interest in keeping costs down. In theory, this sounds good. But what happens if you develop an illness that is costly or difficult to treat? In some instances, patients do get appropriate referrals and the best of care; but a growing number of real-life examples indicate that, quite often, patients must be prepared to fight the system. An uninformed patient is more likely to bow to authority figures and end up being denied needed treatment at an early stage when it is more likely to be effective and, ironically, less costly. The purpose of this book is to help you to become a better-informed health care consumer.

TYPES OF DIAGNOSTIC TESTS

Generally, tests fall into one of the following five categories:

1. *Biochemical analysis* of body fluids, including urine, blood, sweat, cerebrospinal fluid, and saliva. The presence or absence of various chemical compounds, such as hormones, proteins, enzymes, and minerals, or their presence in abnormally high or low levels, may indicate organ damage or disease.

2. *Imaging*, including X-rays, ultrasound, CT scanning, radioisotope scanning, and MRI. These noninvasive imaging methods allow doctors to see inside the body. Some are better for showing hard structures, such as bones; others, for soft tissue or hollow organs. Imaging not only aids in diagnosis but also facilitates treatment by allowing surgeons to "see" in advance the conditions they will find once the body is opened. This advance planning shortens the time that the patient will be under anesthesia and therefore lowers the risk of surgery.

3. *Endoscopy,* a diagnostic technique that uses a tube to view directly the interior of hollow organs such as the stomach, lungs, or uterus. Flexible fiber-optic tubes have largely replaced larger and more uncomfortable rigid tubes, reducing discomfort to the patient. Moreover, miniature tools can be introduced through the tube to take biopsy samples, remove stones, or open blockages.

4. *Biopsy*, in which a small sample of tissue is examined under a microscope. Biopsy samples are removed from the body by scraping, surgery, or endoscopy, or with a needle. The appearance of abnormal cells in the sample helps clarify diagnoses.
5. *Genetic analysis of cells* detects genetic defects responsible for certain inherited disorders. These cells can be obtained from the blood, skin, or bone marrow of children and adults, or prenatally, from the placenta, amniotic fluid, or chorionic villi.

How Doctors Use Diagnostic Tests

As a rule, doctors order or perform the simplest, least-expensive, and least-invasive tests first. Sometimes a single test, when taken together with a physical examination and the patient's symptoms, can be enough for a diagnosis. In other cases, the first round of tests only rules out various conditions but may not point to a single diagnosis. More specific, and sometimes more invasive, tests must be ordered until the diagnosis is certain.

Once a diagnosis has been made, there are still two reasons more tests may be ordered. The first is to help determine the best method of treatment. For example, a biopsy may determine that the patient has cancer, but many other tests are necessary to determine the best approaches to treatment. The second reason, and actually the one that accounts for the largest volume of tests, is to monitor therapy—to be sure that the drugs, radiation, physical therapy, or other form of treatment is being used in an appropriate amount and is performing effectively.

WHAT YOU CAN DO YOURSELF

Patients are being asked to play a more active role in their own health care, and this extends to medical tests. Home medical testing now makes it possible for people to anticipate health problems and seek treatment in good time. Of course, home tests are not intended to take the place of a doctor's examination. When tests are properly used, however, the results can save the doctor's time and help to guide decisions on care.

Home-testing equipment—which was limited to thermometers just a few years ago—now allows computer-controlled evaluation of heart rate, blood pressure, and blood glucose levels. Chemical-based tests provide for simple dipstick testing of blood and urine or sophisticated methods of confirming pregnancy. Home-testing products are widely available at pharmacies, supermarkets, and health and food stores, as well as by mail order. Some tests need no equipment at all.

The US Food and Drug Administration (FDA) recommends the following precautions for the safe use of home tests and all medical self-care products:

1. Check the expiration date for tests containing chemicals. Don't buy a kit unless you intend to use it before the expiration date.
2. Follow storage instructions. Keep containers tightly sealed, out of children's reach, and away from light, moisture, and extremes of temperature.
3. Read the instructions to make sure you understand the test and how to use it. Follow the steps in order, and use a clock or watch if the test must be timed.
4. Note special precautions, such as avoiding certain foods or drugs before testing. Take the test at the recommended time.
5. If you are color-blind, ask someone else to help you interpret the results of tests that use color indicators.
6. If the test requires urine, collect the specimen in a clean, dry container; traces of soap, sugar, or other residues can cause faulty results.
7. Know what action to take if the results are positive, negative, or unclear.
8. If you have questions about a test or its results, consult a pharmacist or other health care professional. Check the package for a telephone number to call for further information. (See the appendix for descriptions of some of the most common home medical tests.)

HOW TO USE THIS BOOK

This book is divided into two parts. Part I includes information important to all readers, regardless of which tests they may be facing. Educated consumers should know about their rights in receiving or refusing medical care and about the process of informed consent. These issues are covered in chapter 1. Likewise, virtually every consumer, even those who are in good health, will face screening tests at some point in life. Chapter 2 discusses the pros and cons of popular screening tests and details those that may not be worthwhile. Chapters 3 and 4 then give general overviews of imaging and laboratory tests, respectively, which together comprise the bulk of diagnostic tests.

Part II contains chapters organized by organs, organ systems, or major diseases or groups of diseases, or by the consumers (women, or infants and children) who are subject to testing. Each of the chapters in Part II consists of three main sections:

1. An introduction explaining the normal workings of the organ or organ system involved and summarizing pertinent disorders and their symptoms.

2. A description of the diagnostic process: how a doctor goes about collecting information by performing a physical examination, taking a careful patient history and, if necessary, ordering diagnostic tests.

3. Detailed descriptions of the major relevant diagnostic tests.

In compiling the lists of tests and preparing their descriptions, we talked not only with the doctors who order and interpret tests, but also with the nurses and technicians who perform them and the laboratory scientists who analyze them. Since doctors are not always involved in actually performing the tests, we thought it was important to question those who are, about what patients need to know—their most important questions and concerns.

For each test described, we summarize the following general information in a table for easy reference: where the test is done and by whom, how long it takes and when the results will be ready, a realistic view of any pain or discomfort involved, special equipment needed, the potential risks or complications of the procedure, and its average cost.

A few explanations of these summarized factors are necessary. Procedures vary from region to region and from doctor to doctor, and they are constantly changing. For example, as doctors and technicians perform certain tests more frequently, they become more skilled in their use and the risk to the patient declines. While these tests may have originally required the patient to be admitted to the hospital as a safety precaution, they can now be done on an outpatient basis.

In the general information tables, under the heading How Long It Takes, we have given the time the patient is involved. It may take a doctor or nurse only a few seconds to take a sample of mucus or other secretion when an infection is suspected, but it may take weeks in the laboratory to grow a culture of the infectious agent. Thus, we have another column, under the heading Results Ready When that indicates how long the patient may have to wait to receive an answer.

The section on average costs is coded: $ is low cost, generally less than $100; $$ are moderately expensive, ranging from $100 to $500; $$$ are high-cost tests of $500 or more. It also should be noted that costs vary dramatically from region to region and may depend on whether the test is performed in a doctor's office, commercial laboratory, or hospital. With simple tests, such as blood tests, the cost for taking the sample may or may not be included in the doctor's fee, although the analysis will usually be billed separately. And, of course, fees are subject to change. We have tried to give an average price range as a guideline, but you may find local fees to be higher or lower.

Following the general information table for each test described, we provide further information, description, and explanation under a standard series of subheads.

- *Other names.*
- *Purpose.* The main uses of the test. If you are faced with a test that does not seem to fit one of these uses, you may want to ask your doctor why it is being done.
- *How it works.* A brief description of the technology that makes the test possible.
- *Preparation.* Advance preparation may include fasting, avoiding certain foods, or discontinuing medication.
- *Test procedure.* A step-by-step description.
- *Special precautions.*
- *Variations.*
- *After the test.* What normal reactions to expect (eg, moderate pain, cramping, or light bleeding), and any warning signs of complications (eg, fever, swelling, heavy bleeding, or intense pain) you should look for in the days following the test.
- *Factors affecting results.* These are generally factors within your control (eg, following a restricted diet before the test) or ones that must be taken into consideration when interpreting the results (eg, your age or sex). Of course, factors such as the experience of the person performing the test or the reliability of the lab analyzing the results can also affect the results, but are generally beyond the patient's control.
- *Interpretation.*
- *Advantages.*
- *Disadvantages.*
- *The next step.* Some of the possible next steps in the diagnostic process.

Although the information on individual tests is up to date as of this writing, it should be noted that new tests are being developed and introduced constantly and older ones are being refined. If your doctor recommends a test that is not in this book, it may be that it was developed after publication. Ask your doctor if he or she is recommending a new test and, if so, what you should expect. Also, there are thousands of different tests; only the more common are included in this book. So it may be that a test your doctor is recommending has been in use for some time, but it is done only rarely. Again, don't hesitate to ask for the kind of information that is provided for the tests included in this book.

I GENERAL OVERVIEW

Angela R. Holder, LLM

1 Patients' Rights and Informed Consent

When you are ill, it's natural to want to know what's wrong so you can be treated promptly and properly. In these circumstances, it's easy to agree readily to any diagnostic tests and treatment your physician proposes so that you can start on the road to recovery. Even so, it is your right to know exactly what your doctor plans at each step of the way.

WHAT IS INFORMED CONSENT?

As a competent adult, you have the right to have any proposed medical procedure fully explained so that you can make an informed decision about it. It is your body, and you have the right to either approve or refuse any diagnostic test or treatment. As an Ohio court said in a famous 1973 informed consent case, *Congrove v Holmes*, "The informed consent doctrine is based on the proposition that every competent person is the final arbiter of whether or not he gets cut, by whom he gets cut, and where he gets cut."

"Informing" means that your physician or other health care provider must explain what will be done during the procedure *in language you can understand*. For example, if the procedure involves drawing a number of blood samples, you have the right to know how many times you will be stuck.

Most experts in this area of law also believe that a patient has the right to know why the test or treatment is being proposed. In other words, you have the right to know the suspected or confirmed diagnosis. Until about 20 years ago, many physicians were reluctant to tell people that they had cancer. It's hard to imagine how these physicians convinced their patients to undergo chemotherapy or radiation without telling them why the treatment was necessary. Since you cannot reasonably decide whether to undergo a test or treatment without knowing why it is being recommended, you have a right to insist that the reasons be clearly explained.

The physician must also explain the risks of any test or procedure, no matter how unlikely they may be. Any risks, from the relatively minor (such as itching at an injection site) to the extremely serious (blindness, paralysis, or death) must be mentioned. However, obvious risks, such as the possibility of a bruise after blood is drawn, need not be covered when your practitioner is describing the risks of a test.

You must also be told what the expected benefits of a procedure are. If, for example, a complex, painful, or expensive test is proposed, you have the right to know whether, if the results are positive, the condition can be treated and by what means. If the diagnostic test, regardless of its result, would not affect the course of your treatment, ask why you should assume the risk or the expense for little or no benefit.

Always ask your physician the following questions:

- What are the benefits of the test?
- What are the risks?
- Is the test merely "routine"?

Sometimes "routine" tests are ordered simply because "they always are." In such cases, you should feel free to decline, since you or your insurance company will have to pay for these tests (and, increasingly, insurance companies are refusing to pay).

Some other questions you might want to ask include:

- *Is your condition self-limiting?* That is, will it improve if you leave it alone and simply forgo the test or treatment? If you will get well in time regardless of what treatment you do or don't receive (even if treatment might restore your health faster), you have the right to know that.
- *Are alternatives available?* You also have the right to know of alternative tests or treatments that achieve the same result. For example, would an X-ray provide the same information as a magnetic resonance image (MRI)? If so, the X-ray is likely to be considerably less expensive.
- *Is the test for research purposes?* A physician who wishes to verify that a new diagnostic test works as well as the standard one may ask patients suspected of having the disorder to have the new test in addition to the standard one. Any intervention designed for research purposes—to generate knowledge, not to provide therapeutic benefit for the patient—must be presented as such. You are absolutely free to refuse, on any grounds, to participate in a research study.

REFUSAL OF TESTS OR TREATMENT

If a physician urges you to have a diagnostic test, you, as a competent adult, may refuse it. Before doing so, however, it is important to understand why the physician believes the test is necessary and what may be the possible consequences of having an undiagnosed problem. If you are refusing because you are afraid (either of the risks of the test or of finding out the diagnosis), discuss your fears with your physician. He or she may be able to offer an acceptable alternative or help allay your concerns.

Whatever your reasons, you may legally refuse any diagnostic test or procedure, but be sure to talk about your decision with your doctor so that you have a clear understanding of the implications of your choice.

PATIENT TIPS

- Don't refuse a test because you can't afford it without discussing it with your doctor. Financial arrangements can sometimes be made.
- If you are refusing a test or procedure on religious grounds, discuss your concerns with your doctor so that you can agree on a suitable alternative.

GIVING YOUR CONSENT

Once a medical test or procedure has been fully explained to you, you will be asked to sign a consent form stating that its purpose, potential benefits, and possible hazards and inconveniences have been explained to your satisfaction (see figure 1.1). The doctor will also sign the form and may add comments.

If you have to give permission for a child or relative by telephone, the doctor must file a form stating that the test or procedure you are authorizing has been fully explained to you (see figure 1.2). In this case, the phone call will be monitored by a third party, who will also sign the doctor's form.

In the event that neither you nor another family member can be reached in an emergency to give consent for a minor child or incapacitated adult, the responsible physician must fill out an emergency authorization form and have it signed by a hospital administrator (see figure 1.3). The doctor must note on the patient's chart exactly what steps were taken to attempt to contact a family member and why it was necessary to proceed without permission.

Court-Ordered Treatment for Communicable Diseases

Persons suspected of having certain contagious diseases (such as tuberculosis) can be compelled to accept testing or treatment. If a person refuses to be tested and the risk to the public's health is considered

Date: ______________, 19____ Time__________ A.M. / P.M.

The general purpose, potential benefits, possible hazards and inconveniences of ______________________________
____
Specify Operation or Special Proceduce

have been explained to my satisfaction by Dr. ______________________ and alternatives have been discussed.

I hereby consent to the performance of the operation or special procedure named above, under his or her direction with whatever anesthesia, treatment, dressing, medication or transfusion is necessary upon ______________________
myself or name of patient

I also authorize the Hospital to preserve for diagnostic, scientific or teaching purpose or otherwise dispose of the tissue or parts removed as a result of the procedure authorized above.

I further authorize my physician to do whatever may be necessary in the event that any unforseen conditions arise during the course of the operation or procedure.

Signed ______________________________
(Patient or person authorized to consent for patient)

PHYSICIAN'S NOTE

I have informed ______________________ of the general purpose, potential benefits, possible hazards and
(Patient or Relative or Guardian)
inconveniences of the above procedure to be performed under my direction and alternative methods of treatment have been discussed.

ADDITIONAL PHYSICIAN COMMENTS: ____
____

FIGURE 1.1 This is a sample of the permission form used at Yale–New Haven Hospital for an operation or other special procedure.

Date: ______________, 19____ Time__________ A.M. / P.M.

I have spoken by telephone with ____,

the ______________________ of ______________________________ and have explained the
Relationship / Name of Patient

general purpose, potential benefits, alternate procedures and possible hazards and inconveniences of the following operation or special procedure: ____
SPECIFY

I have obtained permission from this person, to perform the operation or special procedure named above with whatever anesthesia, treatment, dressing, medication or transfusion is necessary. I have also obtained permission for the Hospital to preserve for diagnostic, scientific or teaching purposes or otherwise dispose of the tissue or parts removed as a result of the procedure authorized above.

I futher obtained permission to do whatever may be necessary in the event that any unforeseen conditions arise during the course of the operation or procedure.

Signature: ______________________________
Responsible Physician

Witness' Signature ____
Person Who Monitors Telephone Conversation

FIGURE 1.2 This is a form that is used at Yale–New Haven Hospital when permission is obtained by telephone.

Date: ______________, 19____ Time__________ A.M. P.M.

We have been unsuccessful in our attempts to contact ______________________________
(Name of relative or guardian)

the ______________________________ of ______________________________
(Relationship of Patient) (Name of Patient)

Signature: ______________________________
(NAME AND TITLE)

I believe it is essential to perform the following operation or procedure ______________________________
(Specify operation or procedure)

______________________ without further delay.

Signature: ______________________________
(Responsible Physician)

NOTE: The physician is required to make a full note on the chart indicating the necessity to proceed and what steps were taken to contact the patient's next of kin.

FIGURE 1.3 This is a sample of an emergency authorization form, which is used at Yale–New Haven Hospital when permission cannot be obtained in person or by telephone.

great—as in the case of tuberculosis, which can be spread by casual contact—a doctor or hospital may obtain a court order to test and, if necessary, to treat the person.

Minor Patients

Parental consent for diagnostic tests and therapy is necessary for preadolescent children, except in an emergency. (The laws regarding adolescents are discussed below.) For example, if a first grader becomes seriously ill at school and her parents cannot be located immediately, the emergency room physician can diagnose and treat the problem.

In most cases, parents have the right to make medical decisions about their children. Nevertheless, failure to obtain any medical care at all for an obviously ill child may constitute child neglect under the child abuse and neglect laws that exist in all states. It is, however, entirely up to the parents to decide who should care for their child. If one physician believes that the treatment advocated by another will be ineffective in combating the child's problem, the courts will not intervene. All that is required of parents to avoid being convicted of child neglect, or having the treatment given under court order, is that their child be in the care of a physician and that they and the physician agree on the course of treatment.

Minors living away from home who are self-supporting, married, or in the military have the right to consent to medical care for themselves. College students under 18 normally fall into this category of "emancipated minors" even if their parents are paying the cost of college.

Today, even dependent adolescents have much more authority to make medical decisions for themselves than did teenagers in previous generations. In the early 1960s, thousands of teenagers with venereal disease refused to see a doctor for fear that their parents would find out. To combat this public health problem, all states now permit physicians to diagnose and treat minors for sexually transmitted diseases without parental consent. Some states, in fact, prohibit informing or even billing parents in order to keep treatment confidential. For the same reason, almost all states allow treatment for alcohol or drug dependency without parental knowledge.

About half the states permit teenagers who have reached a certain age to consent to any type of treatment, including diagnostic testing. Even in states without such statutes, however, no physician has been held liable in the past 40 years for diagnosing or treating an adolescent without parental knowledge as long as the young person was sufficiently mature to give the same level of informed consent as an adult would. This is known as the "mature minor" rule.

Adults Who Cannot Consent

There are times when an adult is temporarily or permanently incapable of making decisions about medical procedures: an unconscious accident victim, an elderly patient too confused to understand the implications of medical advice, or a patient just too sick to take in what the physician is saying.

In an emergency, a physician doesn't have to wait until an unconscious patient's family is contacted in order to evaluate and treat the patient's injuries. Even if family members are located, it isn't likely that they can refuse emergency diagnostic tests to evaluate the unconscious patient's condition. Although families can, in many circumstances, decide to let a dying patient "go in peace," they need to know the diagnosis, the therapeutic options, and the prediction for recovery before they can make that decision.

If a conscious patient is unable to make an informed decision for whatever reason, the family may usually do so on the patient's behalf. Who can give formal consent, that is, sign consent forms? In order according to their availability, it is usually a spouse, an adult child, the patient's parent, or a brother or sister.

In some cases a court will appoint a guardian or conservator to protect the property interests of and make decisions for an incompetent person. If there is a dispute between the guardian and a family member present, the physician will usually ask the

PATIENT TIPS

- Although it is difficult to contemplate, there may come a time when you are incapable of making your own decisions. You owe it to your family or close friends who may have to make decisions on your behalf to discuss your wishes now. Appoint a health care proxy and an alternate, and be as specific as you can about how you wish to be treated.
- If you wish to be an organ donor, sign a donor card or your driver's license and discuss your wishes with your family—who will make the ultimate decision, even if you have signed a card.

hospital's lawyer to help resolve the dispute, perhaps by seeking a court order.

A patient with a mental illness, even one who has been involuntarily committed to a mental hospital, doesn't lose the right to make medical decisions as long as the mental illness doesn't directly affect the patient's understanding of the medical problem and ability to consent to or refuse treatment.

MEDICAL TESTING FOR NONMEDICAL REASONS

Someone other than a patient may occasionally request a diagnostic test for a reason other than medical treatment. For example, a police officer accompanying an unconscious accident victim to the emergency room may ask for a blood alcohol test to find out if the patient was driving under the influence of alcohol. Or an employer may demand that an employee be tested for drug use.

If the patient cannot consent to diagnostic tests *necessary for treatment*, the tests may be performed anyway. For example, the unconscious accident victim may need emergency surgery. To operate safely, the anesthesiologist and surgeon will usually require a blood alcohol test to find out if the patient is intoxicated, or the doctor may order the test to determine if the patient is unconscious from an undetected head injury or has simply passed out from too much alcohol. The result of that test, however, may not be released to the police without either the patient's consent or a court order. In other words, the test may not be done without a medical reason, no matter how much pressure is applied by law enforcement officers.

The patient's constitutional rights are violated if diagnostic information is inappropriately disclosed to the police or a prosecuting attorney. In most states this means that the result of the blood alcohol test cannot be used in evidence if the patient is later charged with drunk driving. In all states, the patient will likely be able to sue successfully the physician who released the information. Once a person is restored to consciousness or competence, that person may refuse to disclose his or her medical records to the police. In that event, the ability of the police to obtain blood alcohol tests by court order varies from state to state; only a local attorney can give valid advice on the issue.

Similarly, the right of an employee to refuse testing for drug use varies among the states, and a local lawyer is best qualified to advise on these rights as well.

Schools cannot require that students be tested for illegal substances without parental knowledge and consent. If such testing is done without the parent's permission, whether a student found to have used these substances can be expelled or otherwise disciplined by school authorities depends on the law of the particular state.

MANDATORY REPORTING OF TEST RESULTS

A number of diseases, ranging from measles to tuberculosis to AIDS, are reportable to state health departments. The information is used primarily for record keeping, to track outbreaks of infectious diseases, and to plan quarantines if necessary.

All states require reporting of sexually transmitted diseases. In many states, a positive HIV test (see below) must be reported to the state department of health; in other states, only actual illness with AIDS must be reported.

HIV TESTING

A positive HIV test or a diagnosis of AIDS itself can have far-reaching social and legal, as well as medical, consequences. For these reasons the results are kept confidential. For example, a positive HIV test may affect employability, insurability (if the insurance carrier cancels a policy when it audits the medical records of a doctor visit or hospitalization), and the right to attend school or college or to travel. AIDS patients have been evicted from their homes in many areas of the country. In most states it is illegal to test a person for HIV without obtaining informed consent and providing pretest counseling about the consequences of a positive result. In these states the patient is usually required to sign a state-supplied consent form that details all the social and legal consequences of a positive test result.

In many states efforts are under way to permit HIV testing of hospitalized patients without their consent (and presumably without their knowledge) as part of the battery of tests usually performed on admission. At present, however, this is not permitted. The rights of HIV-infected persons vary widely in different states. If you are considering being tested or have received a positive result, you may wish to contact a knowledgeable local lawyer for advice.

Ralph I. Horwitz, MD

2 The Role of Screening: Tests for People Without Symptoms

The case of Osborne M., a 51-year-old electrical engineer, father of two and grandfather of one:

> *Both sides of my family have seen a lot of cancer. I was particularly concerned about colon cancer because two uncles had had it and one had died from it. At my annual physical, I asked my doctor about having a sigmoidoscopy, an exam in which a flexible viewing tube is passed through the rectum into the colon to check for tumors or other potentially cancerous growths. Being fairly health conscious, I knew that sigmoidoscopy is recommended every three to five years for people aged 50 and over, even if they don't have symptoms.*
>
> *Because of my family history, my doctor recommended a colonoscopy instead. He explained that it's usually recommended for people who have a higher-than-average risk of cancer.*
>
> *I was anxious about having the test, but they gave me a sedative beforehand, and it went very smoothly. It really wasn't tough at all. In fact, I got to watch everything on a monitor, which was very interesting.*

The Tests Both sigmoidoscopy and colonoscopy involve the passing of a flexible viewing tube through the rectum into the colon. A sigmoidoscope is about 23 inches long and reaches about midway into the colon. It is recommended for people at average risk of colon cancer. A colonoscope is twice as long, covering the entire organ, and is recommended for people at increased risk.

The Outcome Much to Osborne's relief, the colonoscopy showed nothing abnormal. Since his doctor explained that polyps that eventually turn cancerous take about five years to do so, he plans to repeat the test every three to five years, in the hopes that any polyp discovered can be removed before it becomes malignant.

SCREENING FOR UNDETECTED DISEASES

Screening tests are intended to detect potential health problems in people who have no signs or symptoms of disease. The goal is to help people stay healthier and live longer by sounding an early warning. For example, people with diagnosed high blood pressure may significantly reduce their risk of heart disease and stroke if they can lower their blood pressure by losing weight, exercising more, modifying their diet, or taking appropriate medication.

About 20 years ago, doctors were encouraged to screen patients for a number of disorders in the hope that sickness and premature death could be reduced or prevented. Since then, the number of screening tests has increased, but the attitude toward screening has changed. In the past decade, experts have voiced concern that some screening tests may do more harm than good, or may cost more than they save. These experts have stressed the need for evidence to support intuitive assumptions about the benefits of screening: Is there proof that the available tests accurately identify the disease? Have studies demonstrated that screening for a particular disorder has reduced suffering and deaths?

This requirement for evidence has produced major changes in the list of recommended screening procedures. For example, screening for gout or diabetes is no longer recommended, while breast cancer screening has increased. For many disorders, however, doctors still disagree about the usefulness of screening procedures.

WHEN IS SCREENING BENEFICIAL?

Screening is effective only if the test detects the abnormality in the majority of cases and produces few ambiguous results. For example, blood pressure measurement with a cuff (sphygmomanometer), when properly performed, is generally highly accurate and strongly recommended as a screening method for hypertension, for high blood pressure. In contrast, there is no universally accepted screening test for ovarian cancer in women who have no symptoms. (However, a reliable test can confirm ovarian cancer in women who do have symptoms.)

Prenatal screening for certain genetic disorders is both effective and beneficial (see chapter 24).

Some of the most effective screening tests are described below.

Pap smears. This simple test detects early cancers or abnormalities in the cervix that precede the development of cancer. Regular use of Pap smears in the United States, Canada, and several European countries has dramatically increased the number of cancers detected early, and is believed by many to have increased life expectancy for women.

Phenylketonuria (PKU) testing for newborns. Babies born with this disorder have a metabolic abnormality that can lead to severe, irreversible mental retardation unless they are kept on a special diet that excludes phenylalanine, a natural component of many high-protein foods. However, when dietary restrictions are introduced early, 95% of the children grow up with normal or near-normal intelligence.

Vision and hearing exams. Beneficial throughout life for identifying correctable deficiencies, these are especially useful for older adults, who are more prone to develop degenerative disorders.

In contrast, screening tests for the following diseases offer few benefits.

Diabetes. Early detection of diabetes does not seem to alter the course of the disease.

Sickle-cell anemia. While this blood disorder is easy to detect, it is difficult to treat. Doctors recommend screening only in high-risk individuals and in special situations—for example, before surgery, because anesthesia poses a risk to people who have the anemia and, to a lesser degree, to those with sickle-cell trait.

In addition, the usefulness of some screening procedures is not always as clear-cut as the examples offered above. Regarding these tests, experts differ on whether to wait for more definitive proof or to screen on the belief that doing so may be beneficial. Controlled tests to resolve such debates are often costly, time-consuming, and difficult to perform. For many common disorders or risk factors for disease, such large-scale studies have not been performed. One prominent example is blood levels of cholesterol, an indication of risk of coronary heart disease. Some experts say all adults and even children should be screened for their cholesterol levels, while others believe there is nothing to gain from looking at cholesterol levels before middle age. (For details on the cholesterol testing debate, see the discussion of coronary heart disease below.)

THE RISKS OF SCREENING

Some screening tests carry certain risks, so the potential benefits of the test must be weighed for each patient. Invasive screening tests (those in which an instrument is introduced into the body) carry more risk than noninvasive tests. For example, sigmoidoscopy, a test in which the doctor inserts a viewing instrument into the rectum to inspect the bowels, can detect tumors but involves a small risk of puncturing the colon or rectum.

False Results

Even the most reliable test can occasionally be wrong. False-negative results—those that show no abnormality when in fact one exists—can lull an individual into a false sense of security that may prevent him or her from seeking medical help when symptoms do appear. A more common problem, however, is false-positive results—those that show an abnormality in the absence of the disease. For example, exercise stress tests often produce false-positive results, indicating possible heart disease, when they are performed on women who have no symptoms. For this reason, these tests are not recommended as a screening test for asymptomatic women. (Doctors don't know why these false-positives occur, and they note that this doesn't happen as often with men, even asymptomatic men, nor with women who do have symptoms.) Prostate-specific antigen (PSA), sometimes used to screen for prostate cancer, can produce both false-positive and false-negative results (see below).

Even when a test detects a genuine abnormality, in some cases there is a risk that treatment may be worse than the problem that is revealed. One example is the questionable value of using a cholesterol-lowering drug, which may have serious side effects, in people with only slightly elevated cholesterol levels.

Finally, screening may have an adverse psychological effect. In one study, when researchers measured blood pressure in a group of Canadian steelworkers, the rate of absenteeism increased threefold among the workers who were told that their blood pressure was abnormally high. This is called the "labeling" effect—a pattern in which people start acting sick and treating themselves as more fragile once they are "labeled" as having a medical problem.

EARLY DETECTION REVISITED

Timely diagnosis is often crucial for effective treatment. But does this mean that everyone should be screened for disorders such as cancer, which tend to produce symptoms only by the time they are well advanced? Surprisingly, for many cancers, early detection does *not* increase survival rates. Doctors believe that for some tumors, early detection while the tumor is small doesn't lead to better outcomes, but simply delivers the bad news earlier.

Early detection sometimes fails because tests cannot reveal the problem early enough. For example, chest X-rays and sputum cultures are inadequate for detecting lung cancer at an early stage. For this reason, research is now focusing on developing tests to detect substances released into the blood when a cancer first appears. Although such tests are promising, most are still not completely reliable. For example, measuring the blood concentration of prostate-specific antigen (PSA) has been suggested as a screening test for prostate cancer because this chemical is often released in significant amounts by malignant prostate tumors. However, a noncancerous prostate may release a great deal of PSA simply because it is enlarged. Conversely, some men with prostate cancers have normal PSA levels.

CONTROVERSY OVER GUIDELINES

Since the evidence used to support screening decisions is often indirect or incomplete, it is hardly surprising that screening recommendations made by different experts and organizations vary widely. Underlying biases or beliefs may result in different conclusions being drawn from the same data.

As a rule, guidelines developed by groups of experts from different fields are less likely to be biased than those issued by an organization representing doctors whose members perform the tests and procedures. Perhaps the most influential of these multidisciplinary committees has been the US Preventive Services Task Force, a government-sponsored group of 20 experts who reviewed evidence on the usefulness of 100 measures, including screening, aimed at preventing 60 different illnesses and conditions. The goal of the US Task Force, which issued its first report in 1989 and an updated version in 1996, was to prevent disease while avoiding unnecessary tests and procedures.

Recommendations of the US Task Force are sometimes at odds with those of other health or medical groups. For example, the US Task Force recommends mammography screening for breast cancer in women over 50 but not for younger women. In contrast, the American College of Radiology, the American Cancer Society, and others support routine mammography screening starting at age 40.

Screening recommendations made by the US Task Force in its 1996 report and other groups are given in tables 2.1 and 2.2. For a list of screening tests for infants and children, see chapter 27.

SCREENING IN SPECIAL SITUATIONS

Depending on the illness, certain groups are often targeted for testing. The risk of certain diseases increases as a result of certain predisposing conditions. For example, people who have colon polyps have an increased risk of colon cancer and should be regularly screened. Other common factors or conditions that may justify screening are described below.

Family history of a disease. The predisposition to a disorder may be inherited. For example, women with a mother or sister who developed breast cancer in both breasts before menopause may be predisposed to developing breast cancer. These women are usually advised to begin mammograms earlier than women with no family history of breast cancer. Similarly, experts advise people with a family history of very high cholesterol levels (familial hypercholesterolemia) to have their cholesterol level tested in childhood and monitored regularly. These examples point up the importance of knowing your family medical history and reporting it accurately to your doctor.

Occupational exposure. Workers exposed to a disease-causing substance should be screened for early signs of the disease. For example, dyestuff and rubber workers have an increased risk of bladder cancer. Screening them for this is essential because early removal of bladder tumors may cure the cancer. Likewise, miners and factory workers exposed to asbestos, cadmium, coal tar pitch, and hematite have a high risk of lung cancer.

TABLE 2.1 Screening Guidelines for Healthy Adults (Aged 18–50)

Screening Test[1]	Age																										
	18	19	20	22	23	24	25	26	28	29	30	32	34	35	36	38	40	41	42	43	44	45	46	47	48	49	50
For both sexes																											
Blood pressure[2]	•		•	•		•		•	•		•	•	•		•	•	•		•		•		•		•		
Cholesterol[3]			•				•				•			•			•					•					•
Fecal occult blood																											•
Sigmoido-scopy[4]																											•
For women																											
Clinical breast exam[5]			•		•			•		•		•		•		•	•	•	•	•	•	•	•	•	•	•	•
Mammog-raphy[6]																	•		•		•		•		•		•
Pap smear[7]	•	•	•		•			•		•		•		•		•		•			•			•			•

[1]Each of these screening tests is recommended by at least two organizations, the US Preventive Services Task Force (USPSTF) and the American College of Physicians (ACP), unless otherwise noted. This schedule is appropriate for apparently healthy adults who have no symptoms. Anyone who is at increased risk of a particular disease because of personal or family history should consult with his or her doctor about the advisability of additional or more frequent tests.

[2]Also recommended by the American Heart Association and the Joint National Committee on Detection, Evaluation, and Treatment of High Blood Pressure.

[3]Also recommended by the American Heart Association and the National Cholesterol Education Program Panel on Detection, Evaluation, and Treatment of High Blood Cholesterol in Adults. The USPSTF recommends this test in middle-aged men and suggests that testing in young men, women, and the elderly may be clinically prudent.

[4]The American Cancer Society recommends this test. The ACP recommends it every 3 to 5 years after age 50, or an air contrast barium enema every 5 years after age 50. The USPSTF recommends either fecal occult blood test or sigmoidoscopy.

[5]The ACP and the USPSTF recommend this exam annually after age 40. The American Cancer Society recommends it every 3 years from ages 20 to 39 and annually thereafter.

[6]The ACP and the USPSTF recommend this exam annually after age 50. The American Cancer Society recommends it every 2 years from ages 40 to 49 and annually thereafter.

[7]The ACP and the USPSTF recommend that women can discontinue this test after age 65 if they have had consistently normal tests in the past decade. The American Cancer Society recommends continuing this test throughout life.

TABLE 2.2 Screening Guidelines for Healthy Adults (Aged 51–76)

Screening Test[1]	Age																									
	51	52	53	54	55	56	57	58	59	60	61	62	63	64	65	66	67	68	69	70	71	72	73	74	75	76
For both sexes																										
Blood pressure[2]		•		•		•		•		•		•		•		•		•		•		•		•		•
Cholesterol[3]					•					•					•					•						
Fecal occult blood	•	•	•	•	•	•	•	•	•	•	•	•	•	•	•	•	•	•	•	•	•	•	•	•	•	•
Sigmoidoscopy[4]			•			•			•			•			•			•			•			•		
For women																										
Clinical breast exam[5]	•	•	•	•	•	•	•	•	•	•	•	•	•	•	•	•	•	•	•	•	•	•	•	•	•	•
Mammography[6]	•	•	•	•	•	•	•	•	•	•	•	•	•	•	•	•	•	•	•	•	•	•	•	•	•	•
Pap smear[7]			•			•			•			•			•			•			•			•		

[1] Each of these screening tests is recommended by at least two organizations, the US Preventive Services Task Force (USPSTF) and the American College of Physicians (ACP), unless otherwise noted. This schedule is appropriate for apparently healthy adults who have no symptoms. Anyone who is at increased risk of a particular disease because of personal or family history should consult with his or her doctor about the advisability of additional or more frequent tests.

[2] Also recommended by the American Heart Association and the Joint National Committee on Detection, Evaluation, and Treatment of High Blood Pressure.

[3] Also recommended by the American Heart Association and the National Cholesterol Education Program Panel on Detection, Evaluation, and Treatment of High Blood Cholesterol in Adults. The USPSTF recommends this test in middle-aged men and suggests that testing in young men, women, and the elderly may be clinically prudent.

[4] The American Cancer Society recommends this test. The ACP recommends it every 3 to 5 years after age 50, or an air contrast barium enema every 5 years after age 50. The USPSTF recommends either fecal occult blood test or sigmoidoscopy.

[5] The ACP and the USPSTF recommend this exam annually after age 40. The American Cancer Society recommends it every 3 years from ages 20 to 39 and annually thereafter.

[6] The ACP and the USPSTF recommend this exam annually after age 50. The American Cancer Society recommends it every 2 years from ages 40 to 49 and annually thereafter.

[7] The ACP and the USPSTF recommend that women can discontinue this test after age 65 if they have had consistently normal tests in the past decade. The American Cancer Society recommends continuing this test throughout life.

Pregnant women. Pregnant women are routinely screened with blood and urine tests and blood pressure readings for conditions that may put them or their babies at risk (see chapter 25). Detecting the abnormalities early can sometimes avert complications. Screening tests are also used to detect a malformation or an incurable disease in the fetus. The early warning can give parents time to prepare emotionally for this situation or offer them the opportunity to consider ending the pregnancy. However, the benefits of diagnostic tests performed in pregnant women must be weighed against the risks. For example, with amniocentesis, there is a 0.5% to 1% risk of losing the baby. Although this risk is relatively low, the defects that amniocentesis can detect are also relatively uncommon. The test is offered routinely only to pregnant women aged 35 and older because the risk of having a child with Down syndrome, which can be detected by amniocentesis, increases sharply after that age.

Workers responsible for the lives of others. Railroad engineers, bus drivers, and others whose jobs can affect the well-being of others, are sometimes required to take drug or alcohol tests. School and health care workers may be tested for tuberculosis. Although these requirements sometimes generate controversy, the compelling need to protect the public's health is usually found to outweigh the individual's right to privacy.

MOST COMMON AND BENEFICIAL SCREENING TESTS

Together, coronary heart disease and cancers of the colon, breast, and cervix are responsible for almost 600,000 deaths in the United States each year. Many of these deaths could be prevented by early detection. The rest of this chapter summarizes our current knowledge about tests for these diseases. (If you have concerns about a test that is not recommended, see the accompanying box on evaluating screening tests.)

Coronary Heart Disease

Coronary heart disease is the leading cause of death in the United States, and accounts for about 1.5 million heart attacks every year. Two of the leading risk factors for coronary heart disease, high blood pressure and high blood cholesterol, can go undetected for years because they rarely produce symptoms until it is too late. But screening for these conditions is relatively simple.

Blood Pressure Measurement. High blood pressure affects almost one in five Americans. It is a risk factor not only for coronary heart disease but also for congestive heart failure, stroke, kidney disease, and visual problems (retinopathy). Measurements taken with a blood pressure cuff, or sphygmomanometer, are highly accurate if performed correctly, although the results may be distorted by such factors as

Evaluating Screening Tests

Occasionally, your doctor may suggest a screening test that is not recommended in this chapter. You may also wonder about tests that have been suggested by a friend or reported in the media. When in doubt about having a particular screening test, ask your doctor the following questions:

1. Is the disease for which screening is suggested sufficiently common or serious to justify taking the test?
2. Am I in a high-risk category for this disease?
3. Is the test accurate? What are the false-positive and false-negative rates?
4. Is the test safe? What are the risks?
5. Is the test painful?
6. If the disease is detected, how effective is available treatment?
7. What are the consequences of not having the test?
8. Is there a less invasive test that is just as reliable (eg, an exercise perfusion test instead of coronary angiography)?

malfunctioning equipment, patient anxiety, and misreading of values by the examiner.

Most authorities agree that blood pressure levels in adults should be less than 140/90 mm Hg. Lowering high blood pressure significantly reduces the risk of death from heart disease and stroke. The US Task Force recommends that everyone aged 3 years and older have regular blood pressure checks. The typical guidelines are at least every two years if you have normal blood pressure and annually if you have elevated blood pressure, although your doctor may recommend a different schedule.

Cholesterol Measurement. Cholesterol plays an important role in clogging the coronary arteries that supply oxygen to the heart muscle. People with very high blood cholesterol levels have more coronary heart disease than those whose cholesterol levels are low. Studies also show that middle-aged men with exceptionally high cholesterol levels can reduce their risk of heart disease by lowering their cholesterol. But what about everyone else?

Advisors to the National Cholesterol Education Program believe that all people should have their levels measured and should try to lower them if they are too high. Others point out that only a relatively small number of people with coronary heart disease have extremely high cholesterol, and that most people who die from this disease have normal or only slightly elevated cholesterol. People with only slightly raised cholesterol may not benefit from lowering it. Further, the evidence that women, young men, and the elderly can lower their heart disease risk by lowering their cholesterol is not as strong as it is for middle-aged men, who have been the subject of many more studies.

Finally, some experts note that lowering cholesterol with drugs rather than through dietary and exercise changes may be risky because some of these medications can have serious side effects.

The US Task Force advises that periodic measurement of cholesterol is most important for middle-aged men. The group says, however, that it may also be prudent in young men, women, and the elderly. Experts generally recommend that you have your cholesterol checked every five years, or more often if it is elevated or if your doctor deems it necessary.

Defining High Cholesterol. The risk of coronary heart disease begins to rise when cholesterol levels exceed 200 milligrams per deciliter of blood (mg/dL). Levels between 200 and 240 mg/dL are considered borderline high, and those over 240, high. Levels between 200 and 239 can sometimes be reduced through changes in diet and exercise habits. Although some experts recommend drug therapy when levels exceed 240 mg/dL, others reserve medications for higher levels (eg, 280 mg/dL).

Recent research suggests that apart from the absolute cholesterol level, the risk of heart disease is also determined by the ratio between the two major types of cholesterol in the blood: high-density lipoprotein (HDL, the "good" cholesterol) and low-density lipoprotein (LDL, the "bad" cholesterol). For that reason the National Cholesterol Education Program recommends getting a blood test that provides this breakdown.

Colorectal Cancer

Colorectal cancer is the second biggest cancer killer in the United States (behind lung cancer). Of the people whose cancer is detected before it spreads beyond the colon or rectum, 74% survive at least ten years. Of those with widespread disease, only 5% survive as long. The two main screening tests for colorectal cancer are fecal occult blood test and sigmoidoscopy. The digital rectal (finger) exam is considered far less accurate.

Fecal Occult Blood Test. In this test, stool samples are collected on three consecutive days and examined microscopically for the presence of blood, which may indicate a premalignant or cancerous growth (however, blood in the stool is frequently caused by certain drugs, foods, or benign disorders like hemorrhoids). The American College of Physicians and the American Cancer Society recommend annual tests for everyone over age 50, but the US Task Force recommends this for people aged 50 or older only if they have close relatives with colorectal cancer or if other factors place them at an increased risk. The test can be performed by a doctor or at home with an easy-to-use test kit. (See additional US Task Force recommendations under sigmoidoscopy.)

Sigmoidoscopy. In this test, a viewing instrument is inserted into the rectum and colon. Neither patients nor doctors are generally enthusiastic about this test, which is uncomfortable, embarrassing, and expensive. There is also a risk of a perforated colon in about one in every 5,000 to 7,000 people screened.

A study published in the *New England Journal of Medicine* has found that screening by sigmoidoscopy reduces the risk of dying from cancer of the rectum or lower colon by nearly 60%, and many physicians recommend screening for all of their patients aged 50 or older. The American College of Physicians and the American Cancer Society recommend that all adults have sigmoidoscopy every three to five years beginning at age 50. The US Task Force also recommends screening for colorectal cancer with fecal occult blood testing or sigmoidoscopy. The Task Force concludes that there is insufficient evidence to determine which of these screening methods is preferable.

It's important to point out that these procedures do not prevent cancer, but they can detect it at its most curable stage. Colon cancer, for example, is 95% treatable if it is diagnosed while it's still confined to the top lining of the colon or rectum.

Breast Cancer

Breast cancer is the most common malignancy in women and kills more women in the United States than any other cancer except lung cancer. Until about 1987, the incidence of this cancer in the United States was on the increase, but it has since leveled off and may even be decreasing slightly. A surge in the number of new breast cancers from the late 1970s to mid-1980s is attributed to improved diagnosis because many women started mammography screening at that time, and many small cancers were discovered several years earlier than usual.

Women with a mother or sister who had breast cancer before reaching menopause are thought to have a higher risk of developing it also, but they account for only a small proportion of all women who develop the malignancy. The predominant risk factor is advancing age: between the ages of 30 and 50, the risk increases almost tenfold, and continues to rise as women get older.

The three screening tests usually considered for breast cancer are breast self-examination, a clinical breast exam, and mammography.

Breast Self-Examination (BSE). This screening method is cheap and easy to perform, as illustrated in figures 2.1a–c. Studies of its effectiveness show conflicting results. This may be because women do not always examine their breasts thoroughly enough, perhaps because they are not confident about their ability to do so. In addition to being able to detect cancer, a woman who examines her breasts regularly may spare herself unnecessary diagnostic procedures by being able to tell her doctor which lumps have been in her breasts for years and require no new examination. On the downside, breast self-examination may lead to anxiety and unnecessary surgery when benign lumps are discovered.

The US Task Force concludes that since the evidence on the usefulness of breast self-examination is inconclusive, there is no reason to urge all women to start examining their breasts; on the other hand, there is no reason for women who already practice BSE to stop. In contrast, the American Cancer Society recommends that women examine their breasts every month starting at age 20.

Breast self-examination is a simple, 5-minute routine that the American Cancer Society urges all women over the age of 20 to perform monthly. This should be done during the week following menstruation, when breasts are less likely to be swollen and tender. After menopause, simply pick a date that is easy to remember, such as the first of the month. Any unusual swellings, lumps, sores, nipple discharge, or other changes should be brought to your doctor's attention as soon as possible. The basic steps in breast self-examination are illustrated in figures 2.1a–c.

Clinical Breast Exam. Virtually all experts agree that women aged 40 and over should have their breasts examined annually by a physician. The US Task Force also suggests that women with a family history of breast cancer start having the examinations earlier, for example, at age 35; and the American Cancer Society recommends that women aged 20 to 40 have their breasts checked by a physician every three years.

Mammography. Breast X-rays, or mammograms, can detect small growths and abnormalities that are difficult or impossible to feel. Experts agree that in women aged 50 or older, regular mammograms help reduce breast cancer deaths. The US Task Force recommends that all women between the ages of 50 and 75 have mammograms every one to two years, while the American Cancer Society and the American College of Radiology recommend them annually for this age group.

Screening of younger women is much more controversial. There is no conclusive evidence that mammography improves survival in this population group. Most studies have failed to show any benefits, while those that have were either too limited or designed in a way that made their results unreliable. Proponents of mammography in younger women rely largely on the assumption that such screening *should* be beneficial. Yet younger women's breasts are more dense than older women's, and some doctors note that this may be one reason mammography is proving less effective in younger women.

The American College of Physicians does not recommend mammography screening for women under 50. The US Task Force concurs, unless a woman has a family history of breast cancer; in this case, she should start earlier, for example, at age 35. The American

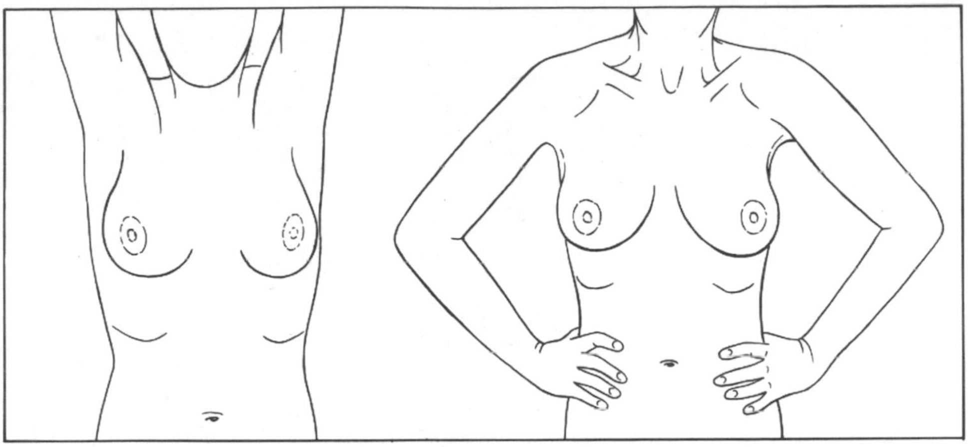

FIGURE 2.1a Begin with a careful visual examination of your breasts while standing in front of a mirror. With your arms in different positions (at your sides, raised over your head, hands on your hips, and chest muscles tensed), note whether the breasts are symmetrical and look for any changes in shape, depressions or bulges, dimples, sores, color of the skin and area surrounding the nipples, and direction in which the nipples point.

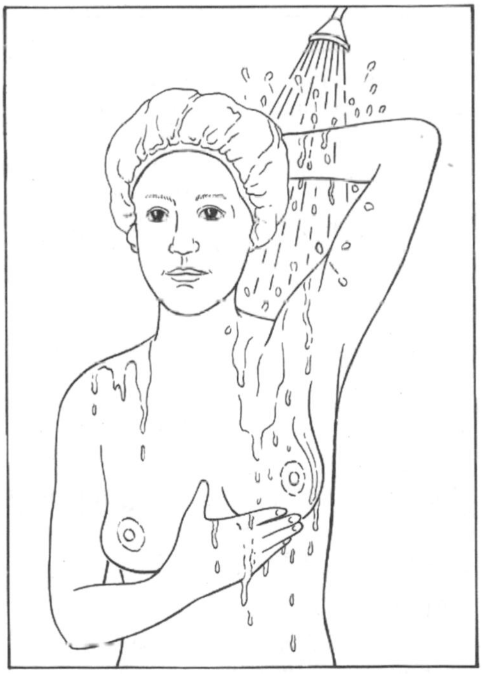

FIGURE 2.1b Start the physical examination while taking a shower or bath. (Wet soapy breasts are easier to examine because there is less skin resistance, and any lumps or thickening are easier to detect than when the breasts are dry.) Place one hand behind your head, and with the other, carefully examine the breast, feeling for any unusual lumps, thickening, or other changes. Repeat on the other side.

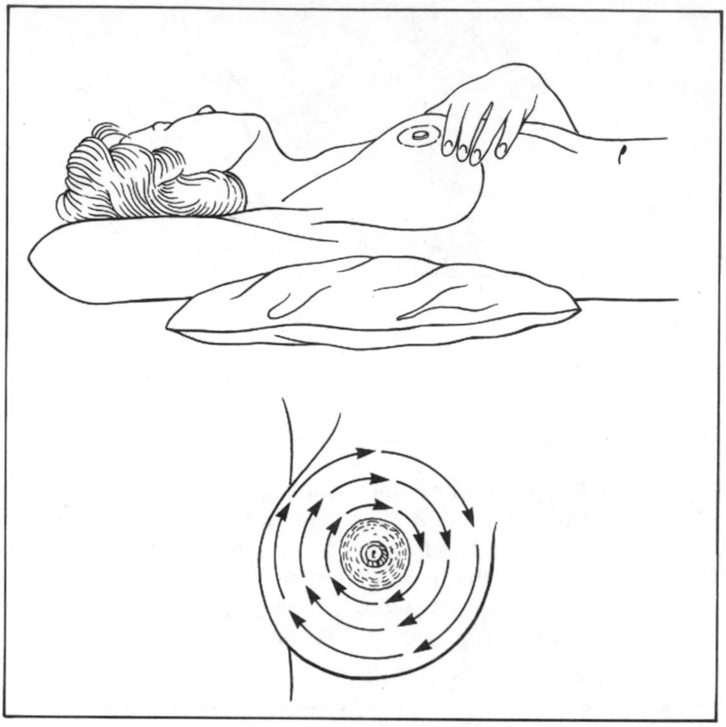

FIGURE 2.1c Next lie down on your back with one arm tucked behind your head and a pillow placed under your back; use your fingers to carefully examine all areas of the breast. One method is to move in circles from the outer portion toward the nipple. (Some women find it easier to go from top to bottom rather than in circles; what's important is to make sure you feel all portions of each breast.) Again, you're feeling for any changes or unusual lumps, thickening, or swelling.

Cancer Society, the American College of Radiology, and other medical professional groups recommend mammography every one to two years for women aged 40 to 49. The National Cancer Institute believes that a woman under 50 should make this decision together with her doctor. In light of these differing opinions, this seems the best course.

Cervical Cancer

In the past 30 to 40 years, mortality from cervical cancer has plunged by almost 70%, and screening programs are believed by some to be responsible. The major screening test for cervical cancer is the Papanicolaou (Pap) smear or test, in which a sample of cells from the cervix is scraped with a cotton swab or spatula and examined under a microscope.

Pap Smear. All the guidelines agree that women should start having Pap smears for cervical cancer when they become sexually active. Screening can stop at age 65, when the risk of cervical cancer drops, but only if previous smears have been consistently normal. Experts disagree on the frequency of testing. The US Task Force recommends that women have the Pap test every one to three years, and that the timing be determined by their doctors, depending on the presence of risk factors such as having multiple sexual partners. A 1980 consensus conference convened by the National Institutes of Health recommended that women have two consecutive annual tests and, if these are normal, continue having the test at intervals of one to three years. The American Cancer Society and the American College of Obstetricians and Gynecologists believe women should start having annual Pap smears at 18, whether they are sexually active or not; after three consecutive normal tests, smears may be performed less frequently at the discretion of the woman's physician.

Prostate and Testicular Cancers

With more than 317,000 new cases diagnosed each year, cancer of the prostate gland is by far the most common malignancy in men. About 41,000 men die of prostate cancer each year, making it second only to lung tumors in cancer mortality among males. According to American Cancer Society statistics, the incidence of prostate cancer rose by 65% between 1980 and 1990. However, it is likely that this apparent rise is due largely to improved methods of detection and increased screening rather than an actual increase in the incidence of the cancer itself.

In contrast to prostate cancer, testicular cancer is relatively rare, with about 7,400 new cases and about 400 deaths a year. This type of cancer tends to occur in young men, generally between the ages of 15 and 34. Early detection and treatment usually produces a cure.

The major screening tests for these cancers of the male reproductive tract are testicular self-examination, a clinical examination of the prostate, and a blood test to measure prostate specific antigen (PSA).

Testicular Self-Examination. This simple self-examination should be done monthly by all males, beginning during adolescence (see figure 2.2).

Clinical Prostate Exam. This is done during a digital rectal exam in which a physcian inserts a gloved finger into the rectum and then palpates, or feels, the prostate gland for enlargement, nodules, and other abnormalities. The American Cancer Society recommends that all men over the age of 40 undergo this examiniation yearly.

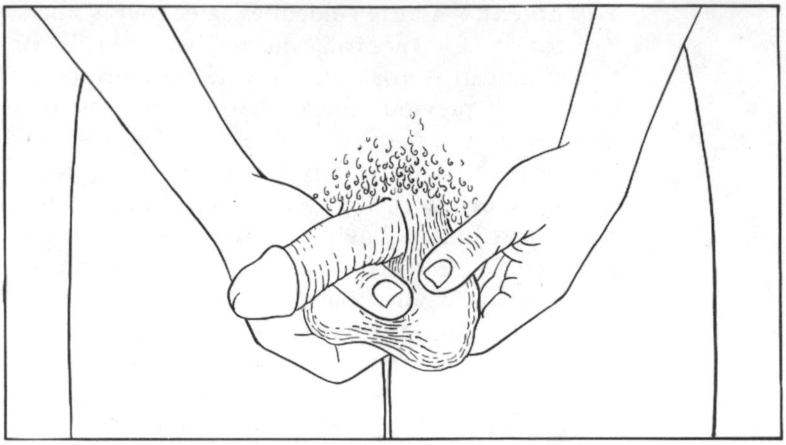

FIGURE 2.2 Testicular self-examination should be done after taking a warm bath or shower to relax the scrotum and make any lumps easier to feel. While standing, roll each testicle between your thumb and fingers. A normal testicle is egg-shaped and feels firm and smooth; any lumps or changes in texture should be checked by a doctor.

PSA Test. High blood levels of PSA indicate an enlarged prostate, possibly due to cancer. The American Cancer Society recommends an annual PSA test for all men over the age of 50.

3

Lee D. Katz, MD

Diagnostic Imaging

Tests Covered in This Chapter:

HISTORICAL OVERVIEW

As we approach the twenty-first century, we can safely say that diagnostic medicine has witnessed more revolutionary changes in the last 50 years than occurred in the previous 2,000 years. From the time of Hippocrates (about 400 BC) until the 1800s, physicians had little in the way of diagnostic aids: About all they could do was listen to a patient's description of symptoms, feel the pulse and perhaps make a superficial examination, and then rely on their experience and rather sketchy knowledge of diseases to make a diagnosis. Because the available treatments were equally lacking, it didn't make much difference whether or not the diagnosis was correct—the patient would either recover pretty much on his or her own or succumb to the disease.

A major breakthrough came in 1819 when Rene T. H. Laennec, a French physician, was trying the hear the heartbeat of a young woman with suspected heart disease. To amplify the sound, he rolled up a sheaf of paper into a cylinder and placed one end to the woman's chest and the other to his ear. Pleased with the results, he went on to fashion a crude stethoscope that was little more than a tube. It would still be several decades before doctors accepted the idea of listening to a patient's chest through a long tube, but by the 1860s there were dozens of different stethoscopes, including a model (Golding Bird's) that had a flexible tube, an earpiece, and a dome-shaped cup to be applied to the patient's chest. By the turn of the century, variations of this stethoscope had become a symbol of modern medicine and remain an essential diagnostic tool used by all physicians. More important, this device paved the way for the many other kinds of scopes that advanced diagnostic medicine into the twentieth century. Starting in the late 1950s, doctors began performing complete physical examinations, which might include using an ophthalmoscope to examine the eyes, an otoscope to peer into the ears, and a proctoscope to look inside the rectum and lower colon. (Still to come were dozens of today's high-tech scopes equipped with fiber optics, magnifying devices, and miniature cameras.)

By the 1970s, the physical exam began to take second billing to chemical or laboratory studies. The concept of taking a single vial of blood, spinning off the serum in a machine, and obtaining a score or more of tests results was mind-boggling. Indeed, this era soon became known as the Age of the Chemical Exam.

Diagnostic medicine is again undergoing tremendous change, and this time, various imaging techniques—X-rays, computed tomography, ultrasound, and magnetic resonance, among others—are leading the way into the Age of Imaging.

Like the invention of the stethoscope, the field of radiology also had a somewhat serendipitous beginning. In 1895, Wilhelm Conrad Roentgen, a German physicist, discovered X-rays while experimenting with metallic salts, electrical current, and a vacuum tube. He noticed that when electrical current passed through the salts in his tube, it could produce a strange phosphorescent image that lingered even after the current was shut off. He deduced that the image was created by invisible radioactive rays generated in his tube, and he quickly determined that these rays could pass through wood and other solid materials. He was also an avid photographer, so the next step was to capture these images on film. The first X-ray was of his wife's hand, clearly showing her bones and wedding ring. For his discovery of X-rays, Roentgen was awarded the first Nobel Prize in physics in 1901, and his invention of X-rays forever changed the practice of medicine. Within a few years, doctors discovered that soft tissues could be made visible on X-rays by introducing various opaque substances such as barium, iodine dyes, and other contrast materials.

Now, just one hundred years following Roentgen's discovery, computers can combine hundreds of X-ray images to provide two- and three-dimensional cross-sectional views of any part of the body. But X-rays are not the only invisible substances that can penetrate the body to produce images of internal organs. The use of sound waves (sonar) has given rise to a relatively new and rapidly expanding field of ultrasonography; and the use of radio waves generated by magnets has led to the development of magnetic resonance imaging (MRI).

OVERVIEW OF NONINVASIVE IMAGING TECHNIQUES

General Radiology

Virtually everyone is familiar with diagnostic X-rays—the basic radiologic technique—but many do not realize that the underlying principle is quite simple. To make an X-ray image, the area to be examined is placed between a metal cassette holding the film and the X-ray tube. The heat generated by electrical current passing through this tube produces a beam of radioactive particles. The X-ray can penetrate body tissue, but it is stopped by lead and other metals; this is why a lead shield is used to protect parts of the body that are not being X-rayed. Metal plates in the X-ray tube housing help collimate the radioactive beam (make the rays parallel) and focus it on the body part under examination.

X-rays pass most easily through air and soft tissue, but are stopped when they encounter bone, which is made up of calcium, phosphate, and other minerals. When the film, which is covered with millions of microscopic particles of silver, is developed, the particles that have interacted with the X-rays will be embedded on the film. If no interaction took place, the silver will wash away. Thus, if you look at a chest X-ray, the lungs appear black because the X-rays easily pass through their air spaces and interact with the silver on the film. In contrast, the ribs appear white because they are bone and do not let the X-rays pass through them as easily to react with the silver on the film, which is washed away during processing.

X-rays pass through soft body tissues—muscles, tendons, nerves, blood vessels, intestines, and other organs—but with a more or less uniform density. To obtain X-ray images in which an internal organ stands out, a contrast material is introduced into the body. Depending on what is being examined, this may be swallowed or inserted (for example, the barium drink or enema that is given before X-raying the intestinal tract), or injected into a vein or artery.

The major drawback to X-ray examinations is that they expose the body to ionizing radiation, which carries certain health risks. Although the amount of radiation exposure from a routine X-ray examination is not enough to be dangerous for most people, there are important exceptions. Even a low dose of X-rays can cause birth defects when a fetus is exposed to them during critical stages of development. Radiation exposure can also damage the male sperm and female eggs and result in genetic defects. X-rays and other radiation exposure have a cumulative effect, so receiving frequent examinations over a period of time increases the risk of cancer. For these reasons, X-rays are contraindicated during pregnancy unless they are absolutely necessary, in which case the mother and fetus should be protected with a lead shield; and routine X-ray screening tests, such as an annual chest X-ray, are no longer recommended.

Fluoroscopy

Fluoroscopy is a special X-ray technique in which a real-time image is projected onto a television monitor as it is being created. Its use is limited by the fact that it delivers a continuous X-ray beam, although at a reduced dose compared to a single conventional radiograph. However, it does have important uses. For example, fluoroscopy aids in the accurate movement of a catheter through the circulatory system during such procedures as cardiac catheterization (see chapter 5) and is then used to track the flow of contrast material through the coronary arteries and other vessels or structures of the heart. It is also very important in following oral or rectal contrast agents when studying the gastrointestinal tract.

Computed Tomography (CT) Scans

Computed tomography expands on the basic principles of radiology. Instead of having a fixed X-ray beam directed through one part of the body and onto film, during a CT scan, an X-ray tube rotates around the patient and generates hundreds of images as it makes its 360-degree circle. These images are received on a series of special plates affixed to the rotating gantry. Data received by these detectors are transmitted to a computer, which reconstructs them to create two-dimensional cross-sectional views of the body. In some examinations, only a single organ may be examined—for example, the brain or spine. In others, the patient may be placed on a moving table, which results in multiple imaging "slices" (similar to slicing through a loaf of bread).

Depending on the part of the body under examination and the nature of the suspected disorder, either an oral or an intravenous contrast medium (or both) may be administered. If the abdominal organs are being examined, for example, two sets of scans may be taken: one without a contrast medium, and the second after injection of an opaque dye into a vein. The contrast agent commonly contains an iodine substance, which may cause flushing and perhaps nausea. People allergic to seafood, which is high in iodine, may experience such adverse reactions to an iodine dye.

Despite the large number of images taken during a CT scan, the total amount of radiation delivered is sometimes less than in a conventional X-ray study. It still poses a risk to a developing fetus and, therefore, should be avoided during pregnancy. Some people who are claustrophobic or are intimidated by medical equipment may find undergoing a CT scan stressful; in such cases, a mild sedative taken beforehand can help alleviate their anxiety.

It is essential to remain as motionless as possible throughout the examination. Children or people who are unable to remain still for any length of time may be sedated for the examination.

Nuclear Scans

Nuclear scans are imaging studies or scans performed after a small amount of a radioactive isotope, such as technetium or thallium, is injected into a vein. After a varying amount of time has elapsed (depending on the organ that is being examined), a radionuclide detector, or gamma scintillation camera, is placed over the area to measure how much of the isotope has been absorbed by the organ or tissue. Cross-sectional images may be taken with a tomographic scanner.

Nuclear scans have many uses, including the following: to detect tumors and other abnormalities of the bones, brain, gallbladder, kidneys, thyroid gland, and many other organs; to assess blood flow to areas of the heart, brain, and other organs; to pinpoint areas of gastrointestinal bleeding; to observe how long it takes for the stomach to empty, or to confirm reflux of stomach contents into the esophagus; and to determine the life span of red blood cells and detect various metabolic abnormalities.

Nuclear scans are based on the principle that specific radionuclides will be absorbed by healthy tissue at a certain rate over a specific period of time. Marked deviations from what is normal indicate possible disease. In a nuclear bone scan, for example, an unusually high absorption of technetium MDP may indicate a tumor, inflammation, or a fracture.

Positron-Emission Tomography (PET) Scans

Positron-emission tomography combines nuclear scanning with biochemical analysis. It is designed to monitor body processes (eg, blood flow) as well as metabolism. A chemical compound is attached to a radioactive isotope, which decays into a positive electron, or positron.

Special gamma detectors record the process, and tomographic scans provide cross-sectional views of the organ being studied.

Recent advances in PET scanning now make it possible to visualize many body processes for the first time. For example, doctors can now study how specific areas of the brain work by injecting a compound of radioactive glucose (the main fuel used by the brain) and then mapping its pattern of distribution. The technique can also be used to accurately measure the extent of muscle damage after a heart attack (see chapter 5) and to monitor the effects of various drugs on body tissue, which is especially important in assessing the effectiveness of cancer chemotherapy.

Unfortunately, the use of PET scanning is limited by the high cost of the necessary equipment, which includes a cyclotron, sophisticated laboratory facilities, computer equipment, and a team of highly trained specialists.

Ultrasound Studies

Ultrasonography, a noninvasive imaging technique that uses high-frequency sound waves instead of ionizing radiation, is an outgrowth of sonar technology developed to detect submarines and other underwater objects. Sound waves travel through different densities at varying speeds, and when they encounter solid material, they are reflected back. Thus, an ultrasound transducer not only generates the sound waves but also receives their echoes. Besides not exposing patients or technicians to radiation, the technique has a number of other distinct advantages: The ultrasound machine is a portable, self-contained unit that doesn't require special installation other than an electrical outlet; ultrasound is ideal for examining a developing fetus; it is also useful during surgery and other diagnostic procedures because it gives doctors a precise location of internal structures.

The recent addition of Doppler technology has greatly expanded the usefulness of conventional ultrasound. The Doppler principle is based on the fact that as a noise-producing object, such as a police siren, approaches, its sound gets louder and louder until the object passes, after which its sound becomes fainter and fainter. Similarly, the sound of blood coursing through an artery becomes louder as the blood approaches the ultrasound transducer, and fainter as it flows away from it. Thus, Doppler ultrasound is helpful in detecting occluded blood vessels, such as the carotid artery in the neck.

In a typical ultrasound examination, a conducting gel is applied to the skin overlying the body part to be examined. The patient then lies on an examination table or bed while the doctor or technician passes the transducer over the area. The reflected sound waves are converted into images, which are viewed on a monitor. When a desired image appears, the operator can store the image and print it on traditional film.

Ultrasound is commonly used to examine abdominal organs, such as the liver, spleen, gallbladder, and pancreas; the kidney, bladder, and uterus; the heart; and the thyroid gland. A recent innovation in which ultrasound is combined with various endoscopic techniques allows a more precise examination of internal organs. For example, the back of the heart can be examined via a transducer incorporated into the end of an endoscope inserted in the esophagus. Similarly, the prostate can be examined by a transducer inserted into the rectum, and the uterus and other female reproductive organs can be visualized using a transducer inserted into the vagina.

Magnetic Resonance Imaging (MRI)

A powerful new diagnostic tool, magnetic resonance imaging uses a magnetic field to create two-dimensional images showing a cross section of an internal organ or structure. The images are similar to those generated by CT scanning, but do not require ionizing radiation to produce. In some instances, MRI provides more detailed images than CT scans; for example, it provides a better contrast between normal and diseased tissue, especially for the soft tissues of the body.

The technique is based on the principle that the most abundant atom in the body is hydrogen, which is present in every water molecule. When placed in a powerful magnetic field like that of an MRI machine, the nuclei of these hydrogen atoms line up in one direction, just as compass needles point to the poles of the earth's magnetic field. When energy from radio waves is directed into the field of the body part that is being examined, the nuclei are temporarily moved out of alignment. When the radio waves stop, the nuclei return to their alignment, giving off their own energy in the process. The machine's computers record the duration and intensity of these signal changes and convert the data into information that produces an image showing the internal structure of the part being examined.

MRI is especially powerful in examining the brain and spinal cord, the joints, and soft tissues of the body. It also provides a painless, noninvasive method to evaluate inflammatory conditions and infections, assess blood vessels and blood flow, and assess cartilage and ligament injury to the knee and shoulder joints.

During MRI, the patient is placed on a narrow platform that slides into the long tube that houses the round, donut-shaped magnet. The patient may be fitted with earphones to help block out some of the loud noise of the magnet in operation and to be able to hear instructions from the technician or doctor conducting the examination. People who are claustrophobic, agitated, or disturbed by the loud noise may be given an antianxiety medication before the examination. There are also open MRI machines that are less noisy and not as confining as the closed models but have other limitations. In some brain examinations, a contrast substance (gadolinium) may be injected into a vein. This relatively harmless substance can enter the brain and help distinguish tumors from surrounding structure.

Although MRI is safe for most people, anyone with internal metal fragments or implanted objects such as a pacemaker or aneurysm clips should *not* undergo MRI because the magnet may move the object and cause serious injury. (Metal dental fillings are safe, however, although some people experience a tingling sensation in their teeth.) If you have any type of implanted prosthesis or have worked as a metal grinder, be sure to tell the doctor or technician, who can determine whether or not the examination is safe for you.

The high cost of MRI (about $1,000 or more per examination) is another limiting factor. The machines, which are very expensive, are not widely available in small hospitals or rural areas. However, MRI has been shown to be cost-effective in many cases by preventing unnecessary surgery costing many thousands more in doctor, hospital, and operating room expense.

INVASIVE IMAGING PROCEDURES

Arteriography

Although X-rays, ultrasound, MRI, and other imaging studies are basically noninvasive, a growing number of these techniques are being used in combination with procedures that *do* require inserting various tubes or instruments inside the body. The arteriography (X-rays of the blood vessels) during cardiac catheterization is a familiar example. In this procedure, fluoroscopy is used to visualize the coronary arteries and other structures after a catheter has been threaded through blood vessels to reach the heart. A contrast medium is injected into the blood vessels or other structures being examined to make them more visible on the fluoroscopy monitor and when eventually recorded on film. This technique may be used to visualize the blood vessels of the legs, brain, liver and spleen, kidneys, and intestines. In cases of bleeding or vascular malformations, occlusion devices can be used, which may prevent dangerous surgery.

Because these invasive procedures require the insertion of catheters or other instruments into the body, they entail a certain amount of discomfort and also carry more risk than noninvasive studies. Possible complications include bleeding at the site where the instrument is inserted, an allergic reaction to the contrast medium, occlusion or perforation of a blood vessel, and in rare instances, a stroke or heart attack. For this reason, invasive procedures are usually carried out in a hospital or other clinical setting where nursing and other emergency medical services are readily available. They also should be performed by a physician and staff who have had special training in the procedures. Invasive procedures tend to be more costly than other imaging studies. Because of this and their increased risk of complications, doctors generally order them only after other tests have failed to provide the necessary information. And there are instances in which the information they yield cannot be obtained any other way. For example, cardiac catheterization and arteriography are essential preliminary tests performed before coronary bypass surgery. In a growing number of invasive procedures, a radiologist may double as a therapist. For example, in cases in which a patient may require long-term intravenous therapy, a radiologist may be asked to insert an infusion catheter that can be used to administer antibiotics or cancer chemotherapy.

X-RAYS

General information

Where It's Done	Who Does It	How Long It Takes	Discomfort/Pain
Doctor's office, radiology unit, outpatient clinic, or diagnostic clinic.	Technician, radiologist, or other doctor.	5–10 minutes.	None, but some people find it uncomfortable to remain still during the procedure.
Results Ready When	**Special Equipment**	**Risks/Complications**	**Average Cost**
Often in a few minutes; may take longer in some cases.	X-ray unit, which varies for special studies such as mammography.	Small risk from radiation exposure; use of contrast agent can cause allergic reaction.	Depends on the study and the number of X-rays taken.

Other names Radiography.

Purpose

- To detect pneumonia, congestive heart failure, broken bones, tumors, and other abnormalities.
- To screen for breast cancer (mammography).

How it works

- Electrical current passing through an X-ray tube produces a beam of ionizing radiation that can pass through the body part being examined to produce an image on film.
- A contrast medium, such as barium or another iodine-based compound, may be injected or inserted into the body to better define intestines, blood vessels, or other soft internal structures.

Preparation

- You will be asked to remove clothing, jewelry, and other metal objects from the area being X-rayed and to position the body part being examined over a film cassette.
- If appropriate, a lead shield will be placed over other parts of the body to minimize unnecessary exposure to the X-rays.

Test procedure

- The technician or other person taking the X-ray will check your position and bring the X-ray unit into proper alignment over the part of the body under examination.

- The technician will then step out of the area and press a button to take the picture.
- During the actual X-ray, it is essential that you remain motionless.

Variations

There are many different types of X-rays; the following are among the most common:

- *Abdominal studies*, in which a plain film of the the abdomen, flat and upright, is used to detect stones, abnormalities, and bowel dilation. These studies also provide an indirect look at the liver, spleen, gallbladder, and kidneys.
- *GI studies*, which may cover the upper gastrointestinal (GI) tract (esophagus, stomach, and duodenum, the upper part of the small intestine) and the lower GI tract (lower small intestine, colon, and rectum), or both. These are usually done after swallowing barium, a chalky contrast medium, or having it infused through the rectum (a barium enema). Also called upper and lower GI series, these studies are done to detect polyps and other tumors, abnormal narrowing or obstructions, ulcers, and diverticula, pouches that bulge out from the intestinal walls (see chapter 8).
- *Mammography*, in which special X-ray equipment is used to produce detailed images of the breast. Mammography is especially useful in detecting early breast cancer (see chapter 26).
- *Renal studies*, which entail X-raying the kidneys, are usually done after injecting a contrast medium into a vein. A series of X-rays is then taken to show the renal outline and collecting system and structures of the kidneys, as well as the ureters (the tubes that carry urine from the kidneys to the bladder) and the bladder itself (see chapter 12 for more detailed descriptions). Sometimes this study is combined with a CT scan.
- *Extremity exams*, which are X-rays of the joints, usually after injection of a contrast medium. These X-rays are especially useful in assessing arthritis, sports injuries, and other common joint problems. During the procedure, the doctor may manipulate the joints to take X-rays from different angles. Fluoroscopy is sometimes used to observe the joints in motion. Companion studies, including CT scans, MRI, or arthroscopy, may be carried out at the same time (see chapter 13 for more details).
- *Chest X-rays*, which are done to study the lungs, heart, rib cage, and other bones of the chest, are probably the most common imaging study. Typically, the X-rays are taken from both the front and side views, and can detect such problems as pneumonia, congestive heart failure, tumors, or fluid in the lungs; an enlarged heart; and broken or abnormal bones. At one time, a routine chest X-ray was included in the annual physical exam; this is no longer done, but routine chest X-rays are still taken upon hospitalization and before any surgical procedure.

- *Dental studies*, which are usually done every two years to detect cavities and other dental problems.
- *Hysterosalpingography (HSG)* is one of several X-ray studies of the female reproductive tract. It entails taking X-rays of the uterus and fallopian tubes after injection of a contrast medium (see chapter 11).

After the test

- You can get dressed and resume your usual activities.
- If a contrast medium was used, you should drink extra fluids to speed its excretion by the kidneys.

Factors affecting results

- Any movement as the X-rays are being taken will result in blurred images.
- Metal objects will show up on the films; application of talcum powder before some studies, such as mammography, can produce misleading images.

Interpretation A radiologist or other medical specialist will interpret the films.

Advantages

- X-rays are relatively inexpensive compared to CT scans and other imaging studies; the equipment is readily available in most hospitals and many doctors' offices.
- The examinations are painless and quick.

Disadvantages

- X-rays involve exposure to radiation, which has a cumulative damaging effect. Those done during pregnancy can result in birth defects.
- Plain X-rays often do not provide adequate details about internal organs, blood vessels, and other soft-tissue structures.
- Intravenous contrast agents may make patients sick, although this reaction passes quickly.

FLUOROSCOPY

General information

Where It's Done	Who Does It	How Long It Takes	Discomfort/Pain
Doctor's office, radiology unit, or outpatient diagnostic clinic.	Technician, radiologist, or other doctor.	Varies according to nature of test.	None, but there may be discomfort from companion tests such as arteriography.
Results Ready When	**Special Equipment**	**Risks/Complications**	**Average Cost**
Usually immediately, although time may be needed to interpret other studies done at the same time.	X-ray unit, fluorescent screen, and perhaps video camera and monitor.	Same as for X-rays.	Varies depending on the companion study.

Other names Moving X-rays.

Purpose

- To guide placement of a catheter during arteriography and other procedures.
- To assess lung movement and function.
- To detect obstructions of the airways or blood vessels.

How it works

- This is a variation of X-ray technology in which a continuous X-ray beam is used to assess an organ or object in real time. Although the beam is on continuously, the dose is low compared with the amount of radiation from a traditional X-ray.
- The images are projected onto a fluorescent screen; a video camera and monitor may also be used.

Preparation Same as for X-rays; additional preparation is needed if a contrast medium is to be used or if the test is a companion to another examination, such as cardiac catheterization.

Test procedure Depending on the nature of the examination, you may be asked to assume different positions, cough, breathe in and out, and perform other maneuvers while being exposed to the X-ray unit.

Variations Fluoroscopy is usually done in conjunction with other studies, including extremity exams, chest X-rays, dental studies, and hysterosalpinography (see above).

After the test You will be free to return to your regular activities, unless these are restricted due to the companion procedures.

Factors affecting results Movement other than that requested by the examiner may alter results.

Interpretation A radiologist or other medical specialist interprets the results.

Advantages The test is noninvasive and allows X-ray examination of an organ in real time. This may be done in conjunction with the administration of a contrast agent that is given orally (upper GI), rectally (barium enema), intra-articularly (arthrography), or intra-uterinely (HSG).

Disadvantages It is contraindicated during pregnancy.

COMPUTED TOMOGRAPHY (CT) SCANS

General information

Where It's Done	Who Does It	How Long It Takes	Discomfort/Pain
Hospital radiology unit or outpatient diagnostic clinic.	Radiologist or technician.	30–45 minutes.	None unless contrast medium is used; some people find it uncomfortable to remain still during the test.

Results Ready When	Special Equipment	Risks/Complications	Average Cost
Often in a few hours; may take longer in some cases and other places.	Revolving CT scanner (camera), X-ray and computer equipment, and monitor.	Slight risk from radiation exposure; use of contrast agent (dye) can cause allergic reaction.	$$$

Other names Computed axial tomograph (CAT) scans.

Purpose

- To obtain a two-dimensional view of a cross section of the brain or other internal organ.
- To detect tumors, bleeding, and other abnormalities that may not show up on an ordinary X-ray.

How it works

- Multiple X-rays are taken as the CT X-ray tube revolves around the patient.
- A computer calculates the amount of X-ray penetration through the specific plane(s) of the body part(s) examined, and gives each a numeric value (density coefficient).
- This information is fed into a computer, which translates the values into different shades of gray.
- These images are displayed on a television monitor and photographed as a series of two-dimensional images depicting a cross section of the part under examination.

Preparation

- You will be shown the CT machine and asked to express any concerns.
- If you experience claustrophobia in small, enclosed spaces, you may be given a mild sedative to quell your anxiety.
- If an intravenous contrast agent is to be used, you will be asked to abstain from ingesting food and water for at least four hours beforehand.
- Before entering the unit, you will be asked to remove any jewelry or other objects that may interfere with clear X-ray images.

- If CT scans of the abdomen and/or pelvis are being done, you may be asked to drink a flavored barium drink.

Test procedure

- You will be asked to lie on a narrow examination table, which slides into the scanner (see figure 3.1).
- As you lie as motionless as possible, the CT tube revolves slowly, taking multiple X-ray images, which are reconstructed into two-dimensional views of a cross section of the body.
- The table is then moved slightly to take another set of images through another plane of the body; typically, three to seven planes are imaged, but this varies according to the part of the body under examination.
- In some instances, the entire length of the body may be scanned; in others, only a relatively narrow section.

Variations

- CT scanning may be performed in conjunction with other imaging studies and diagnostic procedures, such as X-rays of the joint or spinal column (eg, arthrography or myelography). This allows more detailed images of the entire joint structure than can be obtained from X-rays alone.
- A relatively new innovation is *spiral CT imaging,* which allows for continuous scanning as the gantry table slides through the unit. This technique cuts the amount of time needed for whole-body scanning.

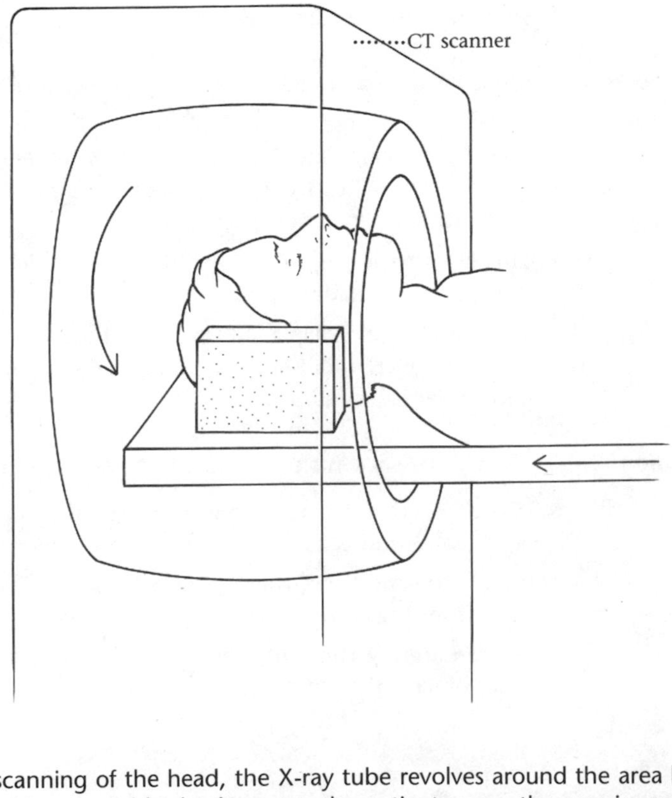

FIGURE 3.1 In CT scanning of the head, the X-ray tube revolves around the area being examined as the table slowly moves the patient across the area in question.

After the test

- You may be asked to wait while a radiologist quickly reviews the images to make sure that the part of the body under study has been adequately photographed.
- If necessary, you may be asked to return to the scanner for additional images. Otherwise, you will be able to resume normal activities.
- If an intravenous contrast medium was used, you will be instructed to drink extra fluids to speed its removal from the body.
- You should also watch for delayed allergic reactions, such as hives, a rash, itching, or perhaps a rapid heartbeat. Such symptoms usually appear within two to six hours; in severe cases, an antihistamine or steroid medication may be prescribed to ease discomfort.

Factors affecting results

- Obesity, movement during the examination, and the presence of metallic objects can interfere with obtaining clear images.
- In some cases, excessive gas or fecal material in the intestines can give misleading results in an abdominal CT scan

Interpretation A radiologist will interpret the scans.

Advantages

- CT scanning provides a painless, noninvasive method of obtaining a detailed view of internal organs.
- In many instances, CT scanning eliminates the need for more invasive procedures, such as arteriography (see chapter 16).

Disadvantages

- The test is costly and may not be available in small hospitals and rural areas.
- It is contraindicated during pregnancy, and may not be suitable for those who are very obese.

NUCLEAR SCANS

General information

Where It's Done	Who Does It	How Long It Takes	Discomfort/Pain
Diagnostic clinic, radiology lab, or hospital.	Radiologist or qualified technician.	20–30 minutes per scan over up to 72 hours.	Some discomfort as radioactive material is injected; lying still during screening may be uncomfortable.

Results Ready When	Special Equipment	Risks/Complications	Average Cost
A few days, but some sooner.	Radionuclide scanner and camera; video unit and monitor.	Radioactive substance is hazardous to fetus.	$$$

Other names Bone, renal, thyroid, lung scans, gallium scans, myocardial perfusion scans, MUGA scan, white blood cell scan, bleeding scan, among others.

Purpose

- To detect tumors and other abnormalities.
- To assess blood flow to specific parts of the body.
- To detect abnormal functioning of the stomach, liver, gallbladder, spleen, and other organs (eg, to determine whether stomach contents are backing up into the esophagus or if the stomach is emptying too fast or too slowly).
- To locate obstructed blood vessels or ducts.
- To study certain metabolic processes.

How it works Nuclear scans detect certain abnormalities by determining how long it takes for an organ or body tissue to absorb a small amount of injected radioactive material. Any deviation from what is normal warns of possible disease—for example, failure of the gallbladder to concentrate the radioactive material may point to a blocked duct.

Preparation

- This varies according to the type of test.
- Many do not require any special preparation.
- For some, such as a gallbladder scan or determination of stomach emptying time, a meal may be given; for others, such as a cardiac scan done in conjunction with an exercise stress test, fasting may be required.

Test procedure

- You will be taken to a nuclear medicine unit where a radioactive substance will be injected into a vein.
- After waiting a certain amount of time (this varies according to the part of the body being examined), you will be instructed to lie on a table under a gamma scintillation camera or other radionuclide detector.
- A computer translates signals from the scanner into images, which are recorded on X-ray or Polaroid film. They may also be projected onto a video monitor.
- In many instances, the scans are repeated at different intervals, for example, every few hours (see figure 3.2).

Variations

- *Bone scans,* which are done to detect tumors, infection, and to assess arthritis and other joint conditions, fracture healing, and various bone diseases (see chapter 13).
- *Cardiac scans (perfusion study, MUGA, and PET scans),* which are done to assess the amount of blood reaching the heart muscle, evaluate the amount of damage after a heart attack, study the heart's pumping function, or study the metabolism of the heart muscle (see chapter 5).
- *Fibrinogen uptake scans,* which help locate clots (thrombosis) in the deep veins (see chapter 6).

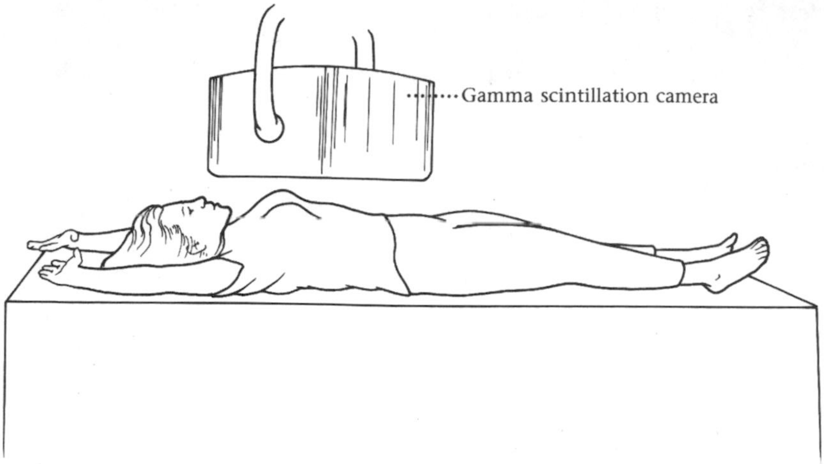

FIGURE 3.2 Nuclear Scan

After a radioactive substance such as thallium is injected into a vein, the patient lies on a table under a gamma scintillation camera, which measures how much of the substance has been absorbed by the organ or tissue under examination.

- *Gallium scans,* which are used to locate certain tumors, areas of inflammation, and abscesses. Typically, the entire body is scanned six, 24, 48, and 72 hours after an injection of radioactive gallium. Areas of unusual concentration of gallium indicate abnormalities that may require further workup.
- *Gastrointestinal scans,* which are done to pinpoint areas of bleeding, assess emptying of the stomach, and detect reflux of stomach acids into the esophagus. The gallbladder and liver are other digestive organs that are scanned for abnormalities such as blocked ducts and inflammation (see chapter 8).
- *Lung scans* (ventilation/perfusion scanning), which are done to detect a possible pulmonary embolism and some other abnormalities (see chapter 7).
- *Red blood cell studies,* which are done over a two- to three-week period in patients with hemolytic anemia to determine how long their red blood cells are surviving. The liver, spleen, and heart are also scanned during this procedure (see chapter 16).
- *Renal scans,* which are done to assess various kidney disorders, including tumors, abscesses, cysts, and abnormal blood flow (see chapter 12).
- *Thyroid scans,* which are used to assess the functioning of this gland, and also to determine whether or not thyroid nodules are producing hormones (see chapter 9).

After the test The amount of time it takes for the body to rid itself of the radioactive material varies according to the type of isotope used, but in most instances it is gone in 14 to 48 hours. This can be hastened by drinking extra fluids.

Factors affecting results

- Some scans, such as those of the gallbladder, can be affected by fasting.
- A residue of radioactive materials from other studies can also alter test results.

Interpretation A radiologist and other medical specialists interpret the results, comparing them with the normal uptake of radioactive material by the organ being studied.

Advantages

- These scans can provide highly detailed information.
- Because only a trace amount of radioactive material is used, there is no risk of radiation exposure except to a developing fetus.

Disadvantages

- Sometimes the results are difficult to interpret.
- The tests are also costly.
- Nuclear scans are contraindicated during pregnancy.

POSITRON-EMISSION TOMOGRAPHY

General information

Where It's Done	Who Does It	How Long It Takes	Discomfort/Pain
Diagnostic clinic, radiology lab, or hospital.	Radiologist or qualified technician.	60–90 minutes.	Some discomfort as radioactive material is injected; IV line may also cause minor discomfort.

Results Ready When	Special Equipment	Risks/Complications	Average Cost
A few days, but some sooner.	Cyclotron, CT scanners, computer; video unit and monitor; and perhaps other lab equipment.	Radiation exposure is hazardous to fetus.	$$$

Other names PET scanning.

Purpose

- To assess various metabolic processes, including brain activity.
- To measure the size and effect of a heart attack.
- To assess the effectiveness of drugs on specific tissue.

How it works

By combining nuclear scanning techniques and chemical analysis, PET scanning enables researchers and doctors to observe how certain body organs work.

Preparation

- Two IV lines may be used—one to inject the radioactive substance and the other to obtain blood samples.
- It is not necessary to fast beforehand, but you should abstain from alcohol, caffeine, tobacco, and mood-altering drugs (both stimulants and tranquilizers) for 24 hours before the test.

Test procedure

- The radioactive substance is injected, after which the person may be asked to perform specific activities, depending on the purpose of the test.
- Someone undergoing a PET brain scan, for example, may be asked to perform certain cognitive functions, such as doing a mathematical calculation or remembering a sequence of words. To block out other stimuli, the person may be asked to wear a blindfold and earplugs.
- Tomographic scans taken during the procedure show how the organ is metabolizing the injected substance.

Variations

PET scanning is an evolving technology with numerous diagnostic and research applications.

After the test

You can resume your normal activities, although you may be warned to stand up slowly to avoid feeling faint or dizzy.

Factors affecting results

Stimulants or drugs that alter metabolism can result in misleading or inaccurate results.

Interpretation

A radiologist or other specialist reviews and interprets the scans.

Advantages

It provides information that cannot be obtained by any other means.

Disadvantages

The technology is still new, very costly, and available for the most part only in major medical and research centers.

ULTRASOUND TESTS

General information

Where It's Done	Who Does It	How Long It Takes	Discomfort/Pain
Doctor's office, clinic, or hospital bedside.	Technician or doctor.	15–60 minutes.	None.

Results Ready When	Special Equipment	Risks/Complications	Average Cost
Immediately if a doctor is there to view sonograms; otherwise, up to a few days.	Ultrasound transducer, monitor with oscilloscope screen, and video and/or strip recorders; other equipment varies according to the purpose of the test.	None, although concomitant tests may entail some risk.	$$ (Cost varies depending on the part of the body being examined and other concomitant tests, eg, exercise stress test.)

Other names Doppler ultrasound, echography, sonography, and ultrasonography.

Purpose

- To examine internal organs for any abnormalities in structure or function.
- To observe the heart, liver, spleen, and other organs in real time (see chapter 5).
- During pregnancy, to evaluate the fetus for normal development and gestational age.
- To evaluate blood flow through specific vessels, usually with the aid of a Doppler transducer (see chapter 6).

How it works

- The ultrasound transducer emits harmless, high-frequency sound waves, which bounce off the internal structure(s) under examination and are echoed back to the transducer. These echoes are amplified and displayed on a monitor; they can also be displayed as tracings on videotape or graph paper.
- The study may also include M-mode recordings, in which the tracings show the organ in motion over a period of time (see echocardiography, chapter 5); two-dimensional views of an organ's spatial anatomy; and Doppler studies (see the variations described below).

Preparation

- The patient lies on an examining table with the part of the body to be examined exposed.
- A conductive gel is applied to the skin over the area under examination.

Test procedure

- You lie quietly as the person performing the examination moves the transducer over the skin surface while watching the monitor.

- You may be asked to shift positions to obtain other views of the organ(s) under study.

Variations

- *Breast sonography*, in which a woman lies face down on an examination table that includes a special water tank containing an ultrasound transducer. The transducer beams sound waves into each breast as it is immersed in the water. (Alternatively, each breast may be examined with a handheld transducer.) The resulting sonograms may be used as an alternative or in addition to information obtained from regular X-ray mammograms (see chapter 26).
- *Doppler studies*, in which a special transducer is used to direct sound waves into a blood vessel, which are reflected back by moving red blood cells (see figure 3.3). The transducer then transforms these echoes into wave forms that can be recorded. There is also an audio

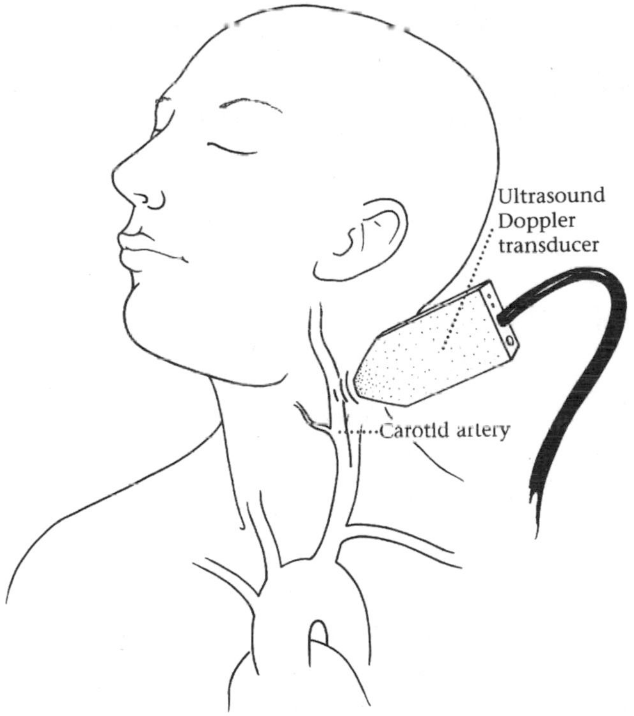

FIGURE 3.3 Carotid Artery Doppler Sonography

A special transducer directs sound waves into a blood vessel. An audio receiver amplifies the sound of blood moving through the vessel, allowing an examiner to detect areas of obstructed blood flow, not only by the visual image but also by sound.

receiver that amplifies the sound of flowing blood, which is then transmitted by an audio speaker. Faintness or absence of such sounds indicates an obstruction to blood flow. Color may be added to the blood to provide better information about changes in the pattern or velocity of blood flow. The results are based on wave-form analysis.

- *Internal ultrasound studies*, in which special transducers are inserted into various body organs, to achieve a more accurate picture of nearby structures, such as the back of the heart from inside the esophagus (see chapter 5), the uterus from inside the vagina (see chapter 11), or the prostate gland from inside the rectum (see chapter 10).
- *Ultrasound in conjunction with other procedures*. Increasingly, ultrasound is used to guide or augment other tests, for example, to safely guide withdrawal of amniotic fluid during amniocentesis (see chapter 25), or to observe the heart in action during and after an exercise stress test (see chapter 5).

After the test The gel is removed, and you can resume your usual activities unless a doctor gives other instructions, as may be the case when ultrasound is performed in conjunction with other tests.

Factors affecting results

- Obesity may distort sound waves and make some organs difficult to examine.
- The presence of barium, gas, and other materials used in other procedures can distort sound waves; thus, ultrasound tests should be done first.

Interpretation A radiologist or other physician trained to interpret sonograms reviews the tracings and video and audio recordings for abnormalities.

Advantages

- Ultrasound studies, by themselves, are painless, noninvasive, and safe.
- They are ideal for use during pregnancy because they don't require radiation or contrast material, which may be harmful to the fetus.
- They can be used to examine blood flow and an organ in motion; they can also be used to evaluate change over a period of time—for example, the possible expansion of an aneurysm, fetal development, tumor growth, or the progressive narrowing of a blood vessel.

Disadvantages

- Some physical characteristics, such as obesity, may distort the images.
- Some critics charge that ultrasound, which is more costly than X-rays, is overused as a routine screening procedure.
- Accuracy depends on the skill of the operator.

MAGNETIC RESONANCE IMAGING (MRI)

General information

Where It's Done	Who Does It	How Long It Takes	Discomfort/Pain
Diagnostic clinic, radiology lab, or hospital.	Radiologist or qualified technician.	30–90 minutes.	None, but some people find the noise and being in a confined space upsetting.

Results Ready When	Special Equipment	Risks/Complications	Average Cost
Often within a few hours.	MRI scanner, computer, and display screen or monitor; film or magnetic tape recorder.	None, unless the patient has an implanted pacemaker or other implanted metal devices.	$$$

Other names Nuclear magnetic resonance imaging.

Purpose

- To obtain two-dimensional views of an internal organ or structure, especially the brain and spinal cord.
- To assess response to treatment, especially cancer chemotherapy or radiation therapy.
- To assess sports-related injury to bones and joints.

How it works

- MRI uses a powerful magnetic field and radio waves to alter the natural alignment of hydrogen atoms within the body.
- Computers record the activity of the hydrogen atoms and translate that into images.

Preparation

- All jewelry, hair clips, and other metal objects must be removed.
- Some facilities ask patients to disrobe and put on a hospital gown; others allow patients to wear clothing so long as it doesn't have metal parts. (Watches should be removed, and pockets emptied of credit cards and other objects that will be damaged by exposure to the magnetic field or will interfere with the images.)
- A contrast medium may be injected before some studies (eg, gadolinium may be injected before an MRI study of the brain); people who are claustrophobic or have difficulty lying still may be given a sedative. Otherwise, no special preparation is required.

Test procedure

- You will be instructed to lie as still as possible on a narrow table that slides into a tubelike structure that holds the magnet (see figure 3.4).
- A loud thumping or hammering noise will be heard during the test; you may request earplugs or listen to music with earphones to reduce the noise level.

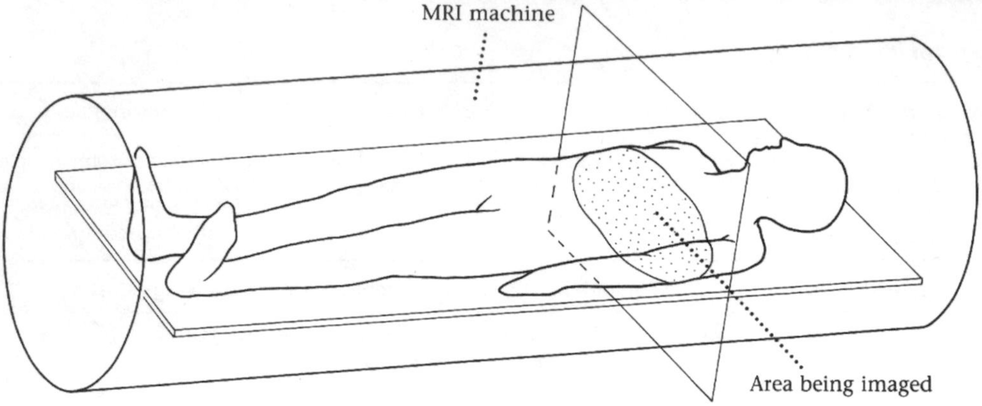

FIGURE 3.4 Magnetic Resonance Imaging

With a patient positioned inside the MRI machine, a two-dimensional image of a cross-section of the body is created by powerful magnets and radio waves.

- At certain points during the test, the noise will stop and you will be able to hear instructions from the doctor or technician administering the test.

Variations Echoplanar MRI is a new technique that allows for rapid accumulation of data such as cardiac motion.

After the test You can resume your pretest activities immediately.

Factors affecting results Movement, extreme obesity, and the presence of metal objects can all affect results.

Interpretation A radiologist or other medical specialist interprets the results.

Advantages

- MRI offers increased-contrast resolution, enabling better visualization of soft tissues. Also, it allows for multiplanar imaging, as opposed to CT, which is usually only axial.
- It provides highly detailed information without exposing the body to radiation. In many instances, it provides more useful images than CT scanning and ultrasound.

Disadvantages

- It is expensive and not available in many small hospitals and rural areas.
- It also cannot be used for patients with implanted pacemakers and certain other metal objects.

ARTERIOGRAPHY

General information

Where It's Done	Who Does It	How Long It Takes	Discomfort/Pain
Outpatient clinic, radiology lab, or hospital.	Radiologist or other doctor.	1–3 hours.	Some pain as anesthetic is injected; prolonged lying on X-ray table may be uncomfortable; dye causes flushing sensation.

Results Ready When	Special Equipment	Risks/Complications	Average Cost
Often within a few hours.	Catheter, X-ray machine, and fluoroscopic equipment; video monitor; other equipment varies according to the purpose of the test.	Bleeding and a bruise where artery is punctured; allergic reaction to dye; slight risk of stroke, kidney failure, or sudden arterial occlusion.	$$$

Other names Angiography.

Purpose To locate and assess narrowing, occlusions, and other abnormalities of various arteries, especially the femoral arteries of the legs; the carotid arteries in the neck; and the arterial systems of the brain, heart, and kidneys. It also displays the vascular anatomy to organs such as the brain, liver, and gastrointestinal tract.

How it works

- X-rays are taken after a contrast agent is injected into the artery under examination.
- The contrast agent, usually an iodine solution, provides the density needed for detailed X-rays of the blood vessels.

Preparation

- Blood tests are done beforehand to make sure that the blood will clot normally.
- You may be instructed to forgo aspirin and other medications that hinder blood clotting for several days before the test, and you will be instructed to fast for at least eight hours before the examination.
- A sedative (eg, a benzodiazepine such as Valium) may be given to help you relax during the examination.
- The area where the catheter will be inserted is thoroughly cleansed and perhaps shaved; you may also be instructed to shower with an antiseptic soap.
- A local anesthetic will be injected into the skin to numb the area prior to the procedure.

- For a lengthy examination, a bladder catheter may be inserted; otherwise, you may simply be instructed to void before going into the angiography suite.
- During the examination, you will wear a hospital gown or sterile drape and lie on an X-ray table. An intravenous line will be inserted in your arm, which can then be used to administer a sedative, pain medication, and other drugs if the need arises.
- ECG electrodes will be affixed to your chest, and a pulse oximeter will be clipped to a finger; these devices allow constant monitoring during the procedure.

Test procedure

- A needle puncture is made, usually in the femoral artery in the groin; a guide wire is threaded through the needle; and the catheter is inserted over this wire and into the artery. (Pressure is applied to the puncture area to minimize bleeding.)
- The catheter is then threaded through the arterial system until it reaches the area to be examined.
- The progression of the catheter is monitored on a fluoroscope monitor to make sure it is positioned properly.
- At this point, the contrast agent will be injected through the catheter, causing a burning or flushing sensation; some patients also experience temporary visual disturbances and a headache, especially if the arteries of the brain are being examined.
- As the contrast agent spreads through the arteries, a rapid series of X-rays is taken by the fluoroscopy unit; these images are intensified, digitized by a computer, and processed almost immediately so that the attending physicians can review them during the examination.

Variations

- *Cerebral angiography*, in which the arteries of the brain are examined for blockages and abnormalities, such as aneurysms or tangles (see chapter 6).
- *Coronary angiography*, in which the blood vessels of the heart are evaluated (see chapter 5).
- *Lower extremity angiography*, in which the arteries of the legs are evaluated (see chapter 6).
- *Renal angiography*, in which the renal artery and other blood vessels in the kidney are examined for narrowing (see chapter 12).

After the test

- As pressure is maintained at the puncture site, the catheter is withdrawn.
- After a few minutes, a sandbag or other weight is placed on the puncture site, and you will be moved to a recovery room where blood pressure, pulse, and other vital signs will be monitored periodically over the next eight hours or so.

- During this time, you will be instructed to drink water, apple juice, or other fluids to prevent dehydration and speed the body's removal of the contrast agent.
- You will also be observed for any delayed allergic reaction or other complications, including possible bleeding, blocked blood flow, abnormal heart rhythms, and stroke (a rare complication).
- If the test is done on an outpatient basis, most patients can go home after two to six hours of observation. However, you may be instructed to remain quiet for the next 12 to 18 hours, to continue applying pressure to the puncture site, and to keep the extremity elevated to prevent swelling.
- If bleeding or other complications arise, you should call your doctor or emergency medical service immediately.
- Depending on the circumstances, most patients can resume normal activities in a couple of days.

Factors affecting results In rare instances, the test may have to be halted if serious complications arise.

Interpretation The angiograms, which may be computer-enhanced, are interpreted by a radiologist or other medical specialist.

Advantages Angiography provides the most accurate information about the state of the arteries.

Disadvantages

- The test is invasive and carries a risk of serious complications, including an allergic reaction to the contrast material, hemorrhaging, stroke, cardiac arrhythmias, arterial occlusion, and infection.
- The test is also expensive and should be performed only by an experienced angiographer.

Peter Jatlow, MD ■ *José C. Costa, MD*

4 An Overview of Diagnostic Laboratory Testing

INTRODUCTION

Although this book is filled with descriptions of elaborate tests, requiring sophisticated equipment, careful patient preparation, and sometimes hours to complete, few of us will ever experience more than one or two of these complicated diagnostic procedures. In contrast, virtually no one reaches adulthood without having a blood or urine test—procedures so routine they create little fanfare and are carried out in laboratories we will never see. Yet these very basic tests provide doctors with a wealth of information about health and disease. This chapter describes how body fluids and tissue samples are collected and what happens once they reach the laboratory.

Testing laboratories, which may be independent or an integral part of a hospital, are generally headed by *pathologists*—experts in identifying the causes of disease and especially the changes produced in the body by disease. These laboratories are generally grouped into two broad and overlapping categories: clinical pathology labs and anatomical, or surgical, pathology labs.

Clinical pathology is concerned with evaluating disease by analyzing blood, urine, and (less frequently) other body fluids. This branch of medical science is predicated on the fact that scores of biochemical processes are constantly going on in the body. As organs do their normal work, they are influenced by hormones, enzymes, minerals, and other chemical substances that come from food or are manufactured by the body. Organs also give off these substances as waste products. At one time or another, these chemicals travel through the bloodstream—and are sometimes found in the urine and other body fluids as well—and thus can be measured.

A level that is higher or lower than the normal range for a person's age and sex may indicate a problem, although these measurements by themselves do not always yield a specific diagnosis. They may reveal or pinpoint disorders in body function that cause a particular health problem or illness, or merely point to the organ or system that needs further study. Sometimes changes up or down, even within the normal range over time, can alert doctors to monitor that organ or system for a potential development, or enable them to monitor treatment or changes in the course of a disorder.

Anatomical pathology is concerned with identifying the causes and consequences of disease in a specific part of the body. This is done by examining samples obtained during surgery or autopsy to identify structural changes in cells, tissues, and organs. This discipline uses tools ranging from the naked eye to powerful microscopes and even molecular analysis of cell genes. Anatomical pathology examinations are among the most reliable ways to establish a diagnosis or, at least, give doctors definitive information on the type of disease suffered by the patient.

HOW TESTS ARE USED

Doctors order laboratory tests to help them establish or confirm a diagnosis, choose and monitor a type of treatment, and determine the prognosis, or outlook, for the patient. Normal laboratory test results can also be helpful in ruling out various diagnoses. Since lab tests are comparatively objective, they can be used to augment the more subjective information the doctor gets from a patient's history and physical examination.

Tests are generally ordered in a branching fashion, going from the general to the more specific, or by choosing a second test that reinforces the conclusion drawn from the first. This strategy can also be cost effective in that more general, broad-based tests are often less expensive than more complex and specific follow-up tests.

Laboratory tests are also ordered periodically to monitor the course of a disease or its response to therapy. Monitoring can help the doctor fine-tune a drug dose, for example, or determine when to stop medication. Lastly, laboratory tests are sometimes ordered as a screening mechanism to detect underlying disease in apparently healthy patients who have no symptoms (see chapter 2).

CLINICAL PATHOLOGY

Types and Sources of Specimens

There are a great many clinical laboratory tests, and they are performed on blood, urine, sputum, and other body fluids, and occasionally feces (see table 4.1). Tests can be performed on *whole blood* (to which an anticoagulant has been added to keep it from clotting), *plasma* (the fluid that remains when whole blood is centrifuged to remove the suspended red and white blood cells), or *serum* (the clear fluid that separates from whole blood that has clotted).

Many of the substances that are measured in blood can also be analyzed in urine or other body fluids, although the results will have different reference (normal) ranges. For example, glucose, a form of sugar, is not normally found in urine, but it is in blood, where it is about twice as concentrated as it is in cerebrospinal fluid (the fluid that surrounds the brain and spinal cord).

Besides blood, urine, sputum, and cerebrospinal fluid, other body fluids commonly examined in clinical laboratories are bronchial or pleural washings (fluids from the lungs and bronchial tubes), gastric or stomach aspirations, serous (or peritoneal) fluids from the abdominal cavity, and joint fluids. The various methods for obtaining these various body fluids are described below.

Blood. Blood is most commonly drawn via venipuncture or finger sticks.

Venipuncture. Blood is usually drawn from a vein on the inside of the elbow. If your doctor orders this venipuncture procedure, the nurse or technician will first wrap a tourniquet (usually a rubber hose) around your arm above your elbow to compress the blood vessels and limit the flow of blood in the veins that would normally return to the heart. You will then be asked to make a fist, which will make your vein stand out more prominently. The skin on the inside of your elbow will be cleaned with a swab or piece of cotton dampened with alcohol, and a sterile needle inserted into your vein. A coupling device attached to the needle allows blood to be drawn automatically by vacuum pressure into rubber-stoppered tubes. When a tube is filled, it can be removed and additional ones attached, depending on the amount of blood needed.

The needle is then withdrawn from the vein, and the tourniquet removed if it hasn't been removed earlier. (Needles are always disposed of after one use so that there is no chance of spreading infection.) The entire procedure generally takes less than five minutes. You will be told to apply pressure to the puncture site with a piece of cotton for a few minutes. A small bandage may be placed over the site; this bandage can be removed in less than an hour. You should refrain from using your arm to carry heavy loads or do strenuous chores for about half an hour.

If for any reason blood cannot be drawn from an arm vein, the one inside your wrist or on the back of your hand can be used

DID YOU KNOW?

Blood-drawing tubes are color-coded by stopper, indicating the type of anticoagulant or preservative they contain. For example:

- "Red tops" contain no anticoagulant; thus they allow the blood to clot so that serum can be drawn off.
- "Lavender tops" have an anticoagulant to prevent the blood from clotting.
- "Gray tops" contain a preservative that prevents the breakdown of glucose, a blood sugar.

TABLE 4.1 Common Clinical Laboratory Tests

Clinical laboratories are typically divided into several specialty laboratories, which may include hematology, clinical chemistry, immunology and serology, microbiology, and the blood bank. The tests described in this table are arranged according to the laboratory in which they are usually performed (indicated in boldface).

Hematology: This laboratory examines the formed or cellular elements of blood, which include red blood cells, white blood cells, and platelets (cells necessary for clotting); the amounts of clotting factors; and the types and amounts of hemoglobin, the red pigment in red blood cells. Such disorders as anemias, hemophilia and other blood-clotting disorders, and leukemias are first diagnosed and then monitored in this laboratory. Organizationally, the urinalysis laboratory is often grouped with hematology. Urine is examined both chemically and microscopically.

Test	What It Shows/What It's Used For
Complete blood count (CBC) (includes white blood cell count, red blood cell count, hematocrit, red blood cell morphology and indices) and differential (the proportion of the various types of white blood cells in the blood)	Identifies anemias, some cancers such as leukemias and lymphomas; evaluates blood loss and response to infection. Sometimes only a part of the CBC is performed (eg, white blood cell count or hematocrit). Often used as a general screening test before surgery or as a part of a routine medical checkup.
Platelet count, fibrinogen	Evaluates, diagnoses, and monitors bleeding and coagulation (clotting) disorders.
Prothrombin time (PT), partial thromboplastin time (PTT), and specific clotting factor assays	Monitors anticoagulation therapy (PT, PTT); evaluates bleeding and coagulation disorders such as hemophilia.
Reticulocyte count	Assesses red blood cell production.
Routine urinalysis (includes color; pH; specific gravity; turbidity; chemical analysis for occult blood, protein, ketones, and glucose; and microscopic examination of sediment for red blood cells, white blood cells, bacteria, crystals, and casts)	Indicates kidney and bladder infections and other diseases, certain metabolic and systemic diseases, dehydration, and urinary tract bleeding.

Clinical chemistry: This laboratory is concerned primarily with measuring the amounts or concentrations of various chemical constituents of blood, and less often with simply identifying their presence. The scope of clinical chemistry is very broad, and many different tests can be done to assess various substances found in blood or urine. The major ones are listed below.

Enzymes: Levels of enzyme activity in blood help determine which organs are damaged or diseased and to what extent. When organs or tissues are damaged, enzymes leak out into the blood. The following are examples of enzymes produced by various organs:

Test	What It Shows/What It's Used For
Heart	
Creatine kinase (CK)	Early marker for acute myocardial infarction (heart attack). Also present in skeletal muscle. CK-NB is a form of CK that is mostly found in the heart muscle and provides more specific information about heart damage.

Lactate dehydrogenase (LDH)	Later marker for acute myocardial infarction. Present in all organs and also released into blood in disorders of liver, kidneys, red blood cells, and muscle. Isoenzymes, or forms of the enzyme that are specific for different organs, can help pinpoint the source of LDH elevations.
Liver	
Alanine aminotransferase (AAT, SGOT) and aspartate aminotransferase (AST, SGPT)	Elevated in many types of liver disorders including hepatitis. May also be abnormal with damage to several other organs or tissues.
Alkaline phosphatase	Elevated in obstructive liver disease, in which excretion of bile by the liver is impaired. The causes include gallstones, tumors, and some forms and stages of hepatitis. Also elevated in bone disease, including Paget's disease, vitamin D deficiency (rickets), hyperparathyroidism, and cancer that has metastasized to the bone. Because their bones are growing, healthy children have higher values than adults.
Pancreas	
Amylase and lipase	Elevated in inflammation of the pancreas (pancreatitis), and less often in cancer of the pancreas.

Hormones: Hormone levels in the blood are used to evaluate the function of various endocrine glands and can indicate hyper- (over) and hypo- (under) activity.

Test	What It Shows/What It's Used For
Cortisol	Adrenal gland function.
Catecholamines	Adrenal gland: elevated with uncommon tumor of adrenal gland that can cause hypertension.
Thyroxine (T_4), TSH, T_4 indices	Thyroid gland function.
ACTH, FSH, LH, GH (growth hormone), TSH	Pituitary gland function; directly relates to function of adrenal glands, sex glands, and thyroid gland.
Parathormone	Parathyroid gland function.

Lipids and lipoproteins: These help evaluate risk of coronary heart disease. They are also sometimes used as markers of liver disease and nutritional status.

Test	What It Shows/What It's Used For
Cholesterol	General but not absolute marker of coronary heart disease risk.
High- and low-density lipoprotein cholesterol (HDL and LDL)	Breakdown of cholesterol that provides better estimate of risk than does total cholesterol alone.
Triglycerides	With cholesterol, used to evaluate coronary heart disease risk.

(continued next page)

TABLE 4.1 (continued)

Proteins: These reflect metabolic and nutritional status in a wide variety of disorders, and overproduction in some cancers.

Test	What It Shows/What It's Used For
Albumin	Reduced in some forms of liver and kidney disease, and in malnutrition.
Globulins	Elevated in some chronic infectious and inflammatory illnesses and some blood cancers. This test includes globulins or antibodies produced by the body in response to infections and allergens. Abnormal globulins can be detected in multiple myeloma and related disorders. Protein electrophoresis fractionates serum proteins into various classes, which allows for more specific diagnoses.

Electrolytes: These tests help to identify and evaluate such metabolic disorders as acidosis, alkalosis, malnutrition, dehydration, and various bone, kidney, and endocrine gland disorders. Results of these tests are nonspecific, and can be abnormal in a variety of disorders too numerous to include here (although a few are listed in table 4.2). Electrolytes are also affected by megadoses of vitamins and minerals, and by such drugs as diuretics and antacids.

Marked abnormalities in electrolytes can have important, and sometimes urgent, medical consequences and therefore require rapid intervention and treatment. In seriously ill, hospitalized patients, these tests may need to be monitored frequently, so that any abnormalities can be quickly corrected.

Electrolytes, which may vary individually or in concert with each other, are often measured in a group. The term usually refers to sodium, potassium, chloride, and bicarbonate (some labs report CO_2 instead), but may also include calcium, phosphorus, and magnesium.

Blood glucose (blood sugar): The glucose tolerance test is used to assess the handling of glucose by the body. In one form of diabetes (Type I), it reflects insulin release by the pancreas. In the other (Type 2), it reflects insulin sensitivity of various body tissues, such as liver and muscle. It is also used to assess low blood glucose, although less frequently.

Test	What It Shows/What It's Used For
Glucose, fasting	Diagnoses and monitors diabetes mellitus, evaluates and diagnoses other disorders of carbohydrate metabolism, and diagnoses hypoglycemia (low blood sugar).
Glucose tolerance test	Follow-up test that allows more specific diagnosis of diabetes mellitus after finding elevated fasting blood glucose levels.

Other metabolic products:

Test	What It Shows/What It's Used For
BUN (blood urea nitrogen) and creatinine	Measures these metabolic waste products eliminated by the kidneys. Elevated when kidney filtration function is impaired and in dehydration.

Uric acid	Measures these metabolic waste products derived from proteins. Elevated in gout, in some forms of kidney disease, and with excessive tissue destruction.

Vitamins and trace elements: Vitamin and trace element (mineral) levels can indicate deficiencies that can be responsible for anemias and nervous system and metabolic disorders, as well as excess due to industrial or environmental exposure, which can result in symptoms and signs of toxicity or poisoning. (For testing for substance abuse, see chapter 29.)

Test	What It Shows/What It's Used For
Folic acid	Evaluates anemia.
Vitamin B_{12}	Evaluates anemia and neurological symptoms.
Other vitamins (thiamine, C)	Only very rarely measured to evaluate various unexplained symptoms consistent with vitamin deficiency.
Lead	Unexplained anemia and/or neurological symptoms. Screening of infants and young children for environmental exposure.
Mercury, arsenic	Unexplained neurological symptoms; suspicion of poisoning.

Immunology and serology: This laboratory is involved with identifying antibodies (proteins produced in the body in response to an antigen, which can be an infectious agent, virus, toxin, or other foreign substance) or in the diagnosis of autoimmune diseases (antibodies against the body's own tissues) and immunodeficiency states (indicative of an underactive immune system).

Test	What It Shows/What It's Used For
Antibodies to infectious agents	Exposure to various infectious agents.
Antinuclear antibodies, complement, autoantibodies	Autoimmune diseases, especially systemic lupus erythematosus.
Antistreptolysin O titer	Streptococcal infection, acute rheumatic fever, acute glomerulonephritis, and other streptococcal enzymes.
Heterophil agglutinins and monospot test	Infectious mononucleosis.
Human leukocyte antigen (HLA)	Correlation with disease syndromes, paternity exclusion testing, and transplantation donor and recipient matching (tissue typing).
Immunoglobulins	Immunodeficiency states and certain malignancies, especially multiple myeloma.
Rheumatoid factor	Arthritis classification and diagnosis of rheumatoid arthritis.
VDRL (Venereal Disease Research Laboratory)	Syphilis; if positive, *must be* confirmed with a more specific test.

(continued next page)

TABLE 4.1 (continued)

Microbiology: This laboratory is responsible for the diagnosis of infections by isolating and identifying infectious agents in blood, urine, sputum, feces, cerebrospinal fluid, and other body fluids, and for testing for their sensitivity to various antibiotics used to treat these infections. Bacteria, viruses, parasites, and fungi are identified by using such techniques as staining, microscopic examination, and chemical, immunological, and genetic tests.

Test	What It Shows/What It's Used For
Acid-fast stain	Identifies bacteria that cause tuberculosis and monitors therapy.
Blood culture	Septicemia or "blood poisoning" (bacterial infection of the blood).
Gram stain	Identifies disease-causing microorganisms including fungi in body fluids and wounds.
Microscopic stool examination for ova and parasites	Identifies disease-causing parasites such as amoebae, pinworms, hookworms, etc.
Sputum culture	Identifies disease-causing organisms of the lower respiratory tract; evaluation of pneumonia and bronchitis.
Routine culture and sensitivity (of many body fluids or sites and wounds)	Isolates and identifies disease-causing organisms; tests for effective antibiotic therapy .
Cell culture	Identifies disease-causing viruses.

Blood bank: This area is responsible for the selection and preparation of appropriate, compatible blood components (red blood cells, platelets, and plasma) that are safe for transfusion into patients. Blood products are also tested to be sure they are free from infectious diseases such as HIV and hepatitis viruses B and C. This laboratory also evaluates transfusion reactions by diagnosing their cause, determining whether or not it is safe to proceed with a transfusion, and selecting further components that are safe for transfusing. The blood bank may have a donor service to draw units of blood for general use and for autologous transfusions (for elective-surgery patients who wish to donate their own blood before surgery so that it will be available to them if they need it).

Test	What It Shows/What It's Used For
ABO group and Rh type, or type and cross match	Establishes blood group (A, B, AB, or O) and Rh type (positive or negative) to ensure compatibility of transfused blood between donor and recipient.
Antibody screening	Ensures that blood is safe for transfusion.
Direct Coombs'	Tests for antibodies on surface of red blood cells in autoimmune hemolytic anemias, transfusion reactions, and erythroblastosis fetalis (newborn hemolytic disease).

instead. For hospitalized patients, blood at times is obtained from the intravenous tubing used to deliver fluids directly into a patient's vein. Some tests are done on blood drawn from an artery instead of a vein, but these are rare. Because of the increased risk of bleeding, however, arterial blood is drawn by a doctor.

Preparation for blood drawing is minimal. You may be instructed to refrain from eating or drinking anything except water for about eight hours before blood is drawn. These so-called fasting specimens guard against interference from the elements in food or liquids that may cause inaccurate test results. Blood glucose and triglycerides (a constituent of fats) are examples of tests that should ordinarily be done on fasting specimens. For many, if not most, tests, however, non-fasting (random) specimens are fine.

The amount of blood that will be drawn depends on the total amount needed for a particular test, as well as the amount needed in each tube to mix with an anticoagulant or preservative to achieve the desired effect. While one or more tubes of whole blood may be drawn, usually only a fraction of it is needed, but that fraction may come from the whole blood, plasma, or serum. To put this in perspective, your body contains about 100 ounces, or 3 quarts, of circulating blood. A typical tube contains only about ⅓ of an ounce. A drop of blood, serum, or plasma is often enough to do one test, and sometimes many, on an automated instrument. This drop is equal to about $2/1000$ of an ounce—a trivial amount compared to the total amount available in your body.

> **PATIENT TIP**
>
> Medications can interfere with some tests. Always advise your doctor of any drugs you are taking. Sometimes a medication must be stopped before a test is performed, but usually notification is all that is necessary.

Finger sticks. If an even smaller amount of blood is needed (to check for anemia if you are planning to donate blood, for example) or if your veins are too small or too fragile for a venipuncture, blood can be obtained by sticking a finger with a small, sharp blade. This is frequently done in children. An earlobe or a heel (especially in newborns or infants) can also be used.

For a finger stick, the nurse or technician will wash your skin with alcohol and then make a quick prick with the blade designed to obtain blood from capillaries—hair-sized vessels that connect the smallest of veins to the smallest of arteries. He or she will then gently squeeze your finger to produce drops of blood that are gathered into micropipettes (tiny glass or plastic straws) or very tiny tubes. Because capillaries are so small, they usually produce only enough blood for a few tests, and the blood flow quickly ceases. There are no precautions to take after the test; you may not even need a bandage.

Urine. Urine for analysis can be obtained in several different ways. The most common method is a *random* (also called a *"spot" specimen* that is used for the standard chemical and microscopic urinalysis. It simply requires you to urinate into a cup, jar, bottle, or tube. The container must be thoroughly clean and dry, but it needn't be sterile. If the specimen is not directly examined, or sent within a few hours to a laboratory, it should be refrigerated.

A *clean catch specimen* requires that you thoroughly clean your external genital area with a mild soap and water and then dry off the area before urinating into a clean, dry container. This is because skin naturally contains bacteria that could obscure bacteria from your urinary tract or falsely indicate an infection. Your doctor will commonly ask for a clean catch specimen if a kidney or bladder infection is suspected.

If a *sterile urine specimen* is needed to identify a specific bacterium, a doctor or nurse will obtain it by catheterization. While you are lying down, a catheter—a thin, flexible tube—is inserted into the outer opening of your urethra, the tube through which urine from your bladder leaves your body. Urine is then drained into a sterile specimen container. This technique is often used for patients who cannot urinate voluntarily. If that is the case, the catheter may be left in place.

Sometimes your doctor may request a *timed test*, which measures the quantity of a substance excreted in the urine over a period of time—typically 24 hours, but occasionally two, six, or 12 hours. For a *24-hour urine tes*t, you begin by voiding and discarding the first specimen. This is because the substance being measured has to be estimated over an exact period of time. Including the first specimen, which has been building up in your bladder over an unspecified amount of time, will throw off the measurement of the substance (such as a hormone) being tested. After discarding the first specimen, you collect the rest of the urine you void over the specified time period in a clean plastic jug, which may contain a preservative (for specific instructions, see chapter 12). In the laboratory, the total volume of urine is measured and an aliquot, or sample of the total volume, is used for the analysis.

Sputum and Other Specimens. Sputum (phlegm) is the product of a deep cough and can be collected directly into a clean, widemouthed plastic or glass specimen container. Sometimes you may be asked to cough directly into a Petri dish. This round, shallow glass or plastic dish with a cover contains a gel-like substance, or medium, in which bacteria will grow.

Other body fluids (cerebrospinal, pleural, abdominal, or joint) are obtained by aspiration. After a local anesthetic is injected or applied to your skin, a fine needle is injected into the appropriate body cavity or joint, and a small amount of fluid is aspirated (withdrawn). The fluid can then be examined for its microscopic cells or chemical constituents, or cultured for infectious agents.

Feces specimens need to be collected directly into a clean, dry cardboard or plastic container.

Laboratory Profiles

When you go for a routine checkup or for evaluation of a specific symptom, your doctor will often order a set list of tests called a laboratory, chemical, or biochemical profile. This standard series of tests is done on a single blood or urine specimen. The reasoning behind this is that screening tests occasionally lead to an unsuspected finding, and with modern automated instruments, as many as 30 common tests can often be done for the same cost as four or five tests ordered separately. Although laboratories differ, the most common component tests are among those described in the laboratory sections of this chapter (for a typical group of tests, see table 4.2).

The value of laboratory profiles is somewhat controversial, however, since such broad screening tests rarely lead to the diagnosis of unsuspected illnesses. Moreover, they can result in abnormal findings in the absence of disease, possibly leading to unnecessary workups. The trend among doctors now is to be very selective and to order tests based only on specific patient complaints. In fact, since March 1996, Medicare policy has been to cover only specific blood tests considered medically necessary based on symptoms, family history, or risk profiles for a specific disease. Although many private health insurers continue to pay for laboratory profiles, such organizations as the American College of Physicians (ACP) recommend that they not be done on healthy patients without specific risk factors.

A more effective variation of the general profile concept is an organ profile. This is ordered when a patient has symptoms that suggest a disease of a specific organ or organ system. Common examples would be a liver profile, a lipid profile, or a thyroid profile. In these instances, the tests comprising the profile, when considered in the context of one another, provide a much more complete picture of the condition of an organ or organ system than any single test by itself. In a sense, a complete blood count (CBC), which includes a hematocrit, red and white blood cell counts, a hemoglobin measurement, and a white blood cell differential, can be considered a hematology profile. Similarly, profiles can be customized according to a clinical problem.

Testing Technology

Automation and computerization have increased dramatically in clinical pathology laboratories, allowing lab staff to keep up with the high volume and array of tests now available. Conversion from manual to automated procedures means that tests can be done rapidly, in large batches, with very small or "micro" amounts of specimens, and by fewer staff. The computer-calculated results are highly accurate because the potential for human error that can occur with each step of multiple-step processes has been eliminated.

Many clinical chemistry tests are routinely processed on large instruments called multichannel analyzers, by only one or two techni-

TABLE 4.2 Common Blood Profile Tests and What They *Most Often* Mean

Test	Increase May Mean	Decrease May Mean
Albumin	N/A.	Malnutrition; liver or kidney failure; gastrointestinal malabsorption.
Alkaline phosphatase	Liver disease; biliary tract disease; some bone diseases.	Rare congenital disease.
Bilirubin	Liver disease; hemolytic anemia.	N/A.
BUN (blood urea nitrogen)	Kidney failure; dehydration, blood in gastrointestinal tract.	Liver failure.
Calcium	Parathyroid gland hyperfunction; thyroid gland hyperfunction, certain cancers; various bone diseases, Vitamin D intoxication.	Kidney failure, parathyroid gland hypofunction; malnutrition; GI malabsorption; Vitamin D deficiency.
Chloride	Acid-base imbalance resulting from gastrointestinal, adrenal, and renal disease.	Gastrointestinal loss; some kidney disease; adrenal gland hyperfunction, acid-base imbalance.
CO_2	Acid-base imbalance from a variety of causes including respiratory failure and vomiting.	Acid-base imbalance from a variety of causes including kidney disease, diabetic acidosis, and diarrhea.
Creatinine	Kidney failure; dehydration.	N/A.
Glucose	Diabetes mellitus; adrenal gland hyperfunction; intravenous glucose fluids.	Excess insulin, liver failure, adrenal gland hypofunction, starvation.
Phosphorus	Kidney failure; parathyroid gland hypofunction.	Parathyroid hyperfunction; malnutrition; GI malabsorption; vitamin D deficiency.
Potassium	Kidney failure; adrenal gland hypofunction; acid-base imbalance.	Diuretic therapy; diarrhea; vomiting; adrenal gland hyperfunction; acid-base imbalance.
SGOT (AST)	Liver disease or damage; heart injury; muscle injury.	N/A.
SGPT (ALT)	Liver disease.	N/A.
Sodium	Dehydration; adrenal gland hyperfunction; some kidney disease; diabetes insipidus.	Kidney failure; adrenal gland hypofunction; gastrointestinal loss; diuretics; overhydration; kidney, liver, and heart failure.
Total protein	Multiple myeloma; chronic infection or inflamation.	Malnutrition; liver or kidney failure; gastrointestinal malabsorption.
Uric acid	Gout; kidney failure; some blood malignancies; tissue destruction.	Some uncommon congenital diseases.

cians, generating up to 20 different test results per minute on a single patient's blood specimen. Various instruments allow for about 80% of tests in clinical chemistry to be highly automated. The remaining 20% of technically complex and highly specialized tests that are less automated or performed manually can consume more than half of laboratory staff time.

Automation has not only enhanced speed and accuracy, but has also allowed computerized reporting of test data. Often different analyzers from different laboratories can be linked, enabling laboratories to produce a single report of a patient's tests from all laboratories. For hospital patients these reports can be generated daily, or even more frequently, and can show data from previous days for purposes of comparison or creating comprehensive records. Results from the laboratory can even be displayed directly on terminals in patient care units.

Clinical laboratories use all of the technologies described below in analyzing test data.

Immunoassays. This group of laboratory techniques is used to identify such diverse substances as infectious diseases, hormones, vitamins, drugs, cardiac enzymes, and antigens (proteins) associated with cancer. These techniques are exquisitely sensitive and, in some instances, capable of measuring less than a billionth of a gram of a biological substance.

Immunoassay technology is based on the antigen-antibody response, that is, the ability of the body to develop antibodies (proteins made by the immune system) to protect against antigens (proteins on the surface of invaders such as bacteria, viruses, or allergens). Since there is a specific antibody for each specific antigen, it is possible to test for one using the other. That is, if one is placed in close proximity to the other, such as happens when a small amount of a known antigen is placed in a test tube that is then filled with blood that contains an antibody for it, they will bind together and can be identified by using a special marker.

Immunoassay testing relies on tagging antibodies or antigens with different markers such as radioisotopes, enzymes, or fluorescent chemicals, in order to make the substance tested for visible. For example, in radioimmunoassay (RIA), the antigens are tagged with a radioisotope; in some nonisotopic immunoassay, with a special dye that shows up as glowing particles under a fluorescent microscope. In enzyme-linked immunosorbent assay (ELISA)—an increasingly popular technique used in such diverse circumstances as testing for allergies and antibodies to the HIV virus—the antibodies are tagged with enzymes.

There are many types of immunoassays. In addition to RIA and ELISA, the most common ones include enzyme-multiplied immunoassay technique (EMIT), fluorescence polarization immunoassay, and enzyme immunoassay.

DID YOU KNOW?

The development of immunoassay technology was considered so significant that its inventors were awarded a Nobel Prize. This technology has become so ubiquitous that it is done manually in specialized laboratories, on automated instruments, in doctors' offices, and in some instances, even at home, as is the case with over-the-counter pregnancy tests.

Spectrophotometry. This technique measures the intensity of color formed when the substance being tested for reacts with added chemical reagents. It is the basis for most automated tests performed on multichannel analyzers. Applications vary from highly automated tests to simple procedures for blood sugar testing that can be performed at home.

Electrophoresis. This technique is based on the differences in movement of electrically charged particles under the influence of an electrical current. The size, shape, and electrical charge of the particles will affect the direction, distance, and rate of movement and can be used to distinguish between two substances, such as different proteins. There are several variations on this technique, including the following:

Serum protein electrophoresis. Separates serum proteins, which is useful in diagnosing and monitoring multiple myeloma and related disorders, evaluating and monitoring chronic inflammatory conditions, and evaluating and managing kidney disease, liver disease, and nutritional status.

Immunoelectrophoresis. Proteins are separated in an electrical field and further identified by reaction with specific antibodies. This is most often used for diagnosing and classifying multiple myeloma, and also for diagnosing some immunodeficiency states.

Hemoglobin electrophoresis. Separates the various types of hemoglobin (red pigment in red blood cells). Used in diagnosing sickle-cell anemia, thalassemia, and related congenital blood disorders.

Chromatography. A technique for separating substances on the basis of their molecular size, or physical or chemical properties, which is used to measure drugs, some proteins, and hormones, among other substances. Variations of this technique are based on the medium in which the chromatography is performed. These include high-performance liquid chromatography (HPLC), thin-layer chromatography (TLC), and gas-liquid chromatography (GLC).

Mass Spectrometry. In combination with chromatographic techniques described above, this technology makes possible very specific identification and measurement of substances on the basis of their physical structure. It is widely used in screening for illicit drug use, to provide definitive confirmation when an initial immunoassay screen is positive.

Atomic Absorption and Flame Emission Spectrometry. When a solution is converted to the gaseous state in a hot flame, dissolved metals, depending on the conditions, will either emit or absorb light at a wavelength that is characteristic of that element. A type of spectrophotometer measures the amount of light emitted or absorbed. Many trace metals can be measured by these techniques, including the amount of lead in the blood, a measurement of great importance in pediatrics.

Specific Ion Electrode. The potential, or voltage, of specially designed electrodes is altered when exposed to certain elements (ions) in the blood that are critical for normal metabolic functioning. The current generated by the electrode is a measure of the amount of the substance present. This technology is used in many multichannel automated analyzers, as well as smaller instruments that are devoted to urgent laboratory services. Critically important tests that employ specific ion electrodes include those used to measure levels of the electrolytes sodium, potassium, bicarbonate, and calcium.

Automatic Blood Cell Counters. Used in the hematology laboratory for automated counting and typing of blood cells (CBC). These are commonly used for evaluating and monitoring anemia, infection, bleeding, leukemias, and cancer chemotherapy, for screening before surgery, and for general health screening.

Flow Cytometry and Molecular Diagnostics. Two relatively new techniques that are used in both anatomical pathology and clinical pathology laboratories. (For more information, see the discussion of new diagnostic technologies below.)

Test Results and Interpretation

Test results from clinical pathology laboratories are usually represented as numbers, or occasionally, as positive or negative, meaning that the substance or disorder being tested for is or is not present. The numerical values are usually expressed as the amount of a substance present in a given quantity of body fluid. For example, the amount of phosphorus is given in milligrams per deciliter (100 mL) of blood (mg/dL).

For most numerical values, there is a range of what is considered normal. These so-called reference ranges can vary with such factors as sex and age. For example, the normal concentration of serum alkaline phosphatase, a bone enzyme, may be up to three times greater in growing children than in adults. Reference ranges can also vary according to the population being considered. For example, hospitalized patients may have a range of results that differs from that of healthy outpatients.

Although reference ranges are often relatively wide, any given individual may have a narrower range of what is normal. Thus, you may have a test result that falls within the normal range for the general population and still have a disorder. There is no way to perfectly estimate ranges because, in general, only 95% of a population is statistically described by a reference range. Thus, it is also possible for the remaining 5% to fall outside a reference range and still be healthy.

Finally, reference ranges can vary from laboratory to laboratory, depending on the technology used to analyze test results. For these reasons, reference ranges are not given in this book.

Specificity and Sensitivity. The most reliable tests are those that are both sensitive and specific, and thereby minimize the incidence of false-positive and false-negative results. "Sensitivity" refers to the ability of a test to correctly identify individuals who *have* a given disease or disorder. "Specificity" refers to the ability of a test to correctly exclude individuals who *do not have* a given disease or disorder.

A false-positive result indicates a disease in a patient who in fact does not have the disease, and these must be minimized to achieve high specificity. A false-negative result indicates that there is no disease in a patient who does have the disease, and these must be minimized to achieve high sensitivity.

An ideal test that is 100% sensitive and specific would detect everyone with a given disease but no one without it. Few, if any, tests achieve this, although many come close. Yet even with the most specific and sensitive tests, misapplication can cause difficulties. For example, even a highly specific test used in a segment of the population that is known to have very few cases of a disease (defined as a low prevalence) can have a high likelihood of yielding a false-positive result in healthy individuals. An illustration of this would be the PSA test for prostate cancer performed on males less than 40 years old: many of the positive results will be false.

Tests are only a piece of the diagnostic process; your doctor's judgment is critical. Presented with clinical laboratory results, your doctor must interpret the information in the context of your history and physical examination, as well as other diagnostic tests. If your test results are negative but your doctor suspects (based on your symptoms and complaints and the physical exam) that you have a specific disease, he or she may elect not to rule it out but to repeat the test or order a different test for the same disorder. The results of several tests taken together can provide a better evaluation of a disorder than a single test alone.

Alternatively, if you have an abnormal test result but no signs or symptoms of a particular condition, your doctor may suspect a false-positive result, which might be caused by elements in your diet or a medication you're taking, or simply because you're one of a small percentage of the population that falls outside the reference range. Finally, if your tests were ordered for monitoring purposes, your doctor may consider changes in results to be more important than any absolute value.

PATIENT TIPS

- Abnormal test results do not always indicate disease.
- Findings can be affected by factors ranging from medications to diet to athletic conditioning.
- Some tests are more likely than others to produce false-positive results. There is also the possibility of laboratory error.
- Diagnosis or treatment should not be finalized on the basis of a single test, especially if you have no symptoms.

ANATOMICAL PATHOLOGY

Types and Sources of Specimens

There are now very few areas in the body that cannot be sampled for analysis, and virtually no organs from which tissue or fluid cannot be obtained, thanks to great advances in surgical techniques and the development of flexible endoscopes and miniaturized instruments for diagnostic sampling. It is now possible, for example, to sample the heart muscle of cardiac transplant patients to test for potential rejection reactions. Biopsies of the intestine and stomach are easily obtained through flexible endoscopes. Common biopsy sites include the bone marrow, breast, gastrointestinal tract, kidney, liver, lung, lymph nodes, skin, thyroid, and even the brain. Fluids in the chest, abdomen, joints, or spinal column can also be sampled and examined for abnormal cells.

Tissue specimens are generally obtained by biopsy, a procedure in which a sample of a patient's tissue is taken in order to establish a diagnosis, or sometimes to monitor the progress of treatment. The sample is usually small in size or quantity and comes from a site known as a *lesion*—any tissue that is changed in structure due to injury or disease. (Ulcers and tumors are examples of lesions.)

Cells lining tissues can be sampled by scraping and examined as cytological preparations. Cells in fluids can be prepared by depositing them on a slide. Large volumes of body fluids are obtained by tapping or puncturing a body cavity and suctioning off the liquid through a needle or catheter. The fluid is then spun in a centrifuge to separate out cells so they can be examined under a microscope.

Depending on the patient's condition, the nature of the suspected illness, and the biopsy site, tissue and fluid can be obtained in a doctor's office or in various settings in a hospital. These include operating rooms and special procedure rooms in, for example, the gastroenterology or radiology department. Unlike clinical pathology samples, biopsies are usually obtained by a doctor rather than a laboratory technician. The tissue samples are then sent for analysis to one of the following three divisions of the typical anatomical pathology laboratory:

1. *Surgical pathology*. Surgical pathologists examine all the biopsies and tissues removed in the operating room and similar settings. Tissues are examined with the naked eye (grossly) and, in most cases, processed so that they can be examined under a microscope. Surgical pathologists work very closely with surgeons and provide consultation during an operation by microscopically examining tissues by frozen section. This method (see below) helps determine the best surgical procedure for a particular case. For example, during surgery for breast cancer, the decision about how much of the breast to remove or whether to also remove the lymph nodes under the arm will be made in consultation with a surgical pathologist.

2. *Cytology*. The cytopathologist examines cells obtained from scraping the surface of tissues, from body fluids (such as stomach aspirations or bronchial washings), or from fine-needle aspirations. The objective is to identify abnormal cells that suggest

cancerous or precancerous conditions or, less often, infectious organisms.

3. *Autopsy service.* Autopsies, or postmortem examinations, entail a visual (gross or macroscopic) examination and description of the whole body as well as the internal organs and structures, followed by microscopic and sometimes chemical and microbiological examinations of organs and tissues. The objective is to verify and correlate clinical and pathological findings, all diagnostic tests, and diagnoses (as well as to uncover missed diagnoses) and to establish the effectiveness of therapy. This investigation establishes the cause of death in the majority of cases. Autopsies can benefit living relatives by uncovering genetic and environmental diseases, and the general population by providing reliable data about the prevalence of certain diseases.

Types of Biopsies and Cytology Examinations

Many types of biopsies are done to obtain tissue or cells for examination to establish a diagnosis. The most common ones are the following:

- *Excisional biopsy.* Removal of an entire, usually small, lesion with a scalpel. Less often, an entire organ is removed as a means of treatment.
- *Incisional biopsy.* Removal of a selected part of a large lesion with a scalpel.
- *Fine-needle aspiration (FNA).* Removal of a column of cells by drawing them through a fine needle. Microscopic examination of the cells can help diagnose tumors or lumps near the surface of the skin or on deep-seated organs, or can help determine the next step in diagnostic testing.
- *Needle biopsy.* Removal of a core of tissue from a lesion or organ located deep within the body.
- *Endoscopic biopsy.* Removal of tissue from the interior of an organ or body cavity using an endoscope for visual guidance. Tiny surgical tools are sometimes passed through the flexible tube of the endoscope and used to obtain the biopsy.
- *Frozen section.* Removal of selected tissue from a patient in the operating room and then rapid preparation of the tissue for microscopic examination by freezing it with liquid nitrogen. This facilitates a very quick diagnosis, which enables the surgeon to carry out the appropriate surgical procedure.
- *Pap smear.* Removal of cells from the cervix (tip of the uterus) using a tiny brush and small spatula.

Testing Technology

There are several ways in which biopsied tissue is prepared for examination. The three main techniques are usually employed in specialized laboratories within the department of pathology. These techniques (and their respective labs) are as follows:

1. *Histology.* After the pathologist examines a gross tissue specimen and selects certain parts of it for further microscopic evaluation, these selected tissues are processed and then cut into extremely thin slices measuring about 0.0000236 of an inch thick, the equivalent thickness of one cell. After being affixed to glass slides, they are stained with various types of chemical dyes that will reveal certain structures of tissues based on their chemical properties. The slides are examined under a light microscope for structural and cytological alterations that indicate disease. Tissue is usually kept in reserve once the slides are made. The pathologist can then order additional "deeper cuts," called recuts or levels, of the tissue to complete the examination.
2. *Immunohistochemistry.* In this laboratory, tissue specimens are prepared in a similar manner; however, the slides are stained using specific antibodies that can be targeted to recognize specific components of the cell. This technique, which has replaced many of the special tissue stains previously used, enables the pathologist to identify a type of tumor by the substances it contains. These same substances can be used as tumor markers to identify cancer cells that may have spread to the bone marrow or lymph nodes.
3. *Electron microscopy.* In this laboratory, selected tissue samples are examined under very high magnification—many thousands of times that achieved with the light microscope. Before examination, the tissue must be cut into sections even thinner than those used for histologic evaluation—about 0.0000036 of an inch. With the electron microscope, the pathologist can see viruses and minute components of the cell. This level of detail can be especially important in the diagnosis of kidney diseases and in the classification of some types of tumors.

New Diagnostic Technologies with Multiple Applications

The following two technologies have had a rapidly growing impact on surgical pathology and virtually all other aspects of diagnostic laboratory testing as well. It is likely that over the next decade they will revolutionize the diagnostic laboratory.

1. *Flow cytometry.* With this technology, white blood cells are mixed with fluorescent antibodies that bind to specific components on the surface of cells, or with dye that binds to genetic material (DNA) within the cell. Using the amount and type of light emitted by the cells containing the antibody or dye, the flow cytometer determines the quantity and type of white blood cells. In other instances, flow cytometry analyzes the amount of DNA in

tumor cells. The first technique is used to diagnose certain leukemias and lymphomas, and the second (known as ploidy) to evaluate the probable behavior of certain tumors, including breast cancer. This allows the doctor to better determine the patient's prognosis and to select the most appropriate therapy.

2. *Molecular diagnostics (DNA/RNA analysis).* These new techniques enable the specific identification of minute amounts of genetic material in fetal and adult tissues, tumor cells, and infectious agents. Oligonucleotides (chemicals closely related to genetic material), each of which will attach or bind to a specific gene or part of a gene, can be used for prenatal diagnosis by identifying genetic abnormalities in fetal cells that indicate inherited or congenital disorders. Oligonucleotides can be used to classify white blood cells (lymphocytes) as benign or malignant, and can detect early genetic changes in tissue cells that indicate potential for malignant transformation. This technique also enables exquisitely sensitive identification of genetic material from infectious agents in tissues and body fluids, allowing much more rapid and specific diagnosis than traditional microbiological methods. These techniques have social implications and ramifications for forensic medicine as well: They can be used to establish paternity and to identify criminal suspects by the nearly unique DNA pattern in a drop of their blood or other body fluids.

Test Results and Interpretation

Anatomical pathologists present their results in a written report that represents a personal consultation to the physician requesting the test. Typically, the report reflects the thought process involved in rendering a diagnosis. First, the gross specimen is described in detail. This is done because the tissue is usually disposed of after the sections for microscopic examination are made. There may be a written description of the microscopic slides, but since they are kept indefinitely and can be retrieved for further review at any time, this is not always done. Finally, a diagnosis is recorded.

Occasionally a definitive diagnosis cannot be made. In some instances the diagnosis may contain qualifiers such as "suspicious of" or "compatible with," or a probability may be stated. At times, the diagnosis may be deferred because the pathologist is unable to immediately determine one. For example, the slides may show an abnormality, but the precise nature of it cannot be established. Or a tumor may be identified, but the pathologist cannot be absolutely certain whether it is benign or malignant. Or a malignant tumor may be identified, but its cell type is not known, making it difficult to choose the best therapy. Sometimes a note or comment following the diagnosis and, occasionally, a new biopsy are needed to do further tests.

The practice of anatomical pathology is usually a group practice. Difficult as well as enigmatic diagnoses are made after a great deal of professional consultation among colleagues. Even after a consensus is reached, second opinions may be sought from subspecialty experts. This very personal process makes test interpretation labor-intensive work, but the consequences of a diagnosis and the sometimes grave events it can set in motion mandate this.

II SPECIFIC TESTS

Barry L. Zaret, MD

5 The Heart

Tests Covered In This Chapter

The case of Gerald S., a 67-year-old professor and electrical engineer:

My symptoms started with a vague feeling of tightness and shortness of breath during any strenuous activity. Although I tried to ignore the feelings, I knew it was my heart. Ten years earlier, I had suffered a mild heart attack, and then underwent coronary bypass surgery. Two years later, I had a couple of ministrokes, and had to have surgery to clean out the carotid artery in my neck. Ever since that operation, I had been free of symptoms and in good health, even though my doctor and wife kept nagging me about my high cholesterol and excess weight. With some trepidation, I went to see my cardiologist. My blood pressure, electrocardiogram, and chest X-ray were all normal, but my cholesterol was too high. I was put on a stronger cholesterol-lowering drug, and my doctor also prescribed a nitroglycerin patch for my angina. It helped but still did not completely eliminate the problem.

The Tests Gerald was then referred for additional tests, which included an echocardiogram, an exercise stress test, a thallium scan, and finally, cardiac catheterization and angiography. These tests confirmed that Gerald's previous bypass grafts were no longer functioning and that several other coronary arteries were badly diseased. On a more positive note, a Doppler study of the carotid arteries in Gerald's neck confirmed that these arteries were not seriously blocked, lessening the risk of a stroke during a second coronary bypass operation.

The Outcome During an eight-hour operation, a cardiovascular surgeon moved both the left and right mammary arteries in Gerald's chest wall to his heart. He also made a graft from a vein in Gerald's leg to bypass another clogged vessel. Gerald soon left the hospital to recuperate at home, returning to work four weeks later and feeling strong and optimistic that he could again lead an active, productive life.

INTRODUCTION

The case of Gerald S. illustrates a common sequence of tests performed in patients with coronary artery disease. The process starts with questions, a physical examination, and simple, relatively inexpensive tests like an electrocardiogram and a chest X-ray. Gerald's case also illustrates a common dilemma that doctors face daily: no test is perfect, and when looking at results, we must weigh them against our experience and what you, the patient, tell us. Gerald's initial screening tests did not point to a serious problem—his blood pressure and ECG were normal, but his cholesterol (268 mg/dL; see chapters 2 and 14) was definitely higher than desirable. However, Gerald's medical history, age, uneasiness, and persistent angina told his doctor that more tests were needed. His abnormal exercise stress test and thallium scan set the stage for more invasive testing, which ultimately confirmed the need for bypass surgery.

WHAT YOUR DOCTOR LOOKS FOR WHEN EXAMINING YOUR HEART

Your doctor begins a cardiovascular workup by examining the heart and measuring your blood pressure while sitting quietly. A high reading may mean that your heart is having to work too hard to pump blood because the small arteries are constricted and putting up too much resistance (see figure 5.1 for an overview of the structure and function of the heart). Or it may simply mean that you're nervous or are still feeling the effects of a recent cup of coffee. This is but one example of how your doctor looks at various clues and sorts out information to arrive at a diagnosis.

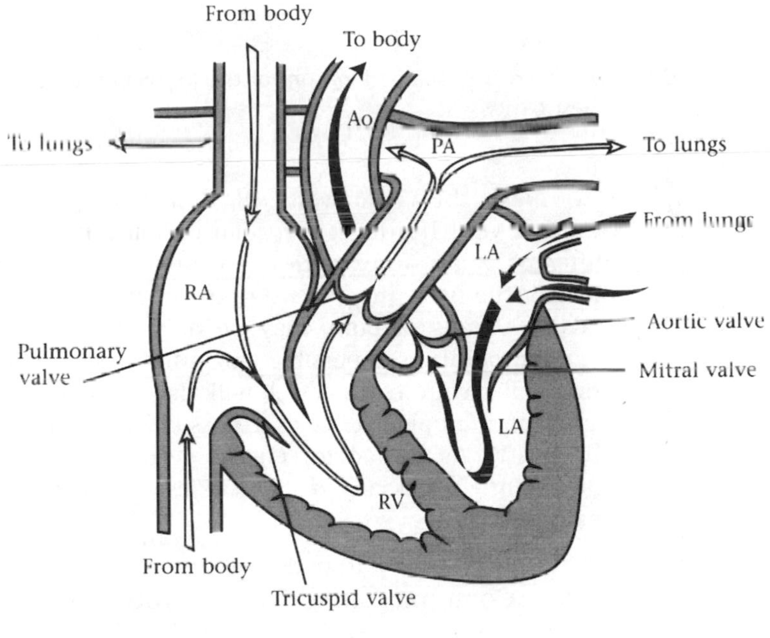

FIGURE 5.1 Overview of the Heart

The heart is made up of four chambers: the right (RA) and left (LA) atria, which are the two upper chambers that receive blood, and the right (RV) and left (LV) ventricles, which are the pumping chambers. After oxygenated blood has circulated through the body, it is returned to the heart through a network of veins that culminate in the superior vena cava and inferior vena cava, which empty into the right atrium. This blood passes through the tricuspid valve into the right ventricle, which pumps it through the pulmonary valve and into the pulmonary arterios (PA), which transport it to the lungs. Here, carbon dioxide and other wastes are exchanged for a fresh supply of oxygen; the newly oxygenated blood is returned to the heart through the pulmonary veins into the left atrium. It passes through the mitral valve into the left ventricle, the heart's major pumping chamber, which forces it through the aortic valve into the aorta (Ao), the body's largest artery, which feeds it into smaller arteries to again circulate through the body.

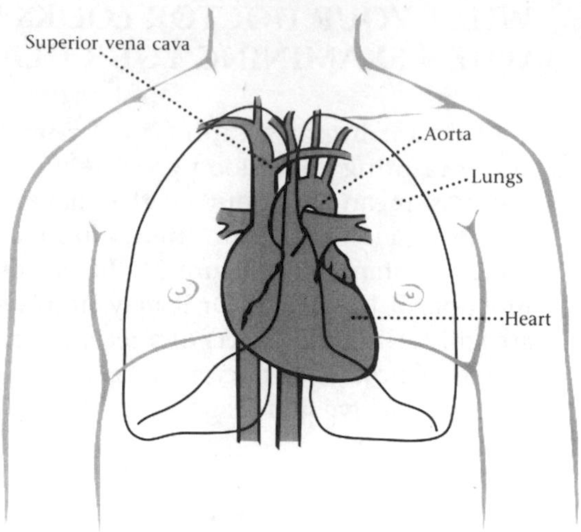

FIGURE 5.2 The heart is positioned in front of the lungs in the central part of the upper chest cavity.

Next, the doctor will feel, or palpate, different pulses to learn whether your heartbeat is regular and strong. It's important to check different pulses—the arteries in your wrist, above the elbow, on both sides of the neck, in your groin, in the back of the knees, and in your ankles—because a pulse may be normal in one place and weak in another, pointing to possible clogging of certain arteries. The pulse in the jugular vein in your neck will also be checked. (A swollen jugular vein, for example, indicates a possible backup of blood returning to the heart.) As the doctor checks your pulses, he or she also looks for swelling, especially of the ankles, which may be a sign of heart malfunction.

Common Cardiovascular Problems

Coronary artery disease, also called arteriosclerotic heart disease or coronary heart disease, in which fatty deposits clog the blood vessels that nourish the heart muscle.

High blood pressure, also referred to as hypertension, in which the heart must pump harder to force blood through the arteries.

Heart valve disease, either due to stiffness or narrowing (stenosis) of the valve, or a failure of the valve to close properly, which leads to leakage (insufficiency or regurgitation).

Heart failure, in which the heart is unable to pump enough blood to meet the body's needs.

Cardiac arrhythmias, which refer to any abnormality in the heart's normal rhythmic beating.

Cardiomyopathies, in which the heart becomes enlarged and the heart muscle weakens.

Congenital heart defects, which are structural abnormalities that develop before birth.

Infections and inflammation of heart tissue, such as *endocarditis* (an infection of the heart lining and valves), *pericarditis,* an inflammation of the membrane surrounding the heart (the pericardium), and *myocarditis,* inflammation of the heart muscle itself.

Signs and Symptoms Arising from the Heart

In some instances, a heart attack is the first obvious sign of heart disease and may result in sudden death. In many cases, however, there are warning signs and symptoms, although they may not be recognized as such. If you develop any of the following symptoms, see a doctor as soon as possible:

- Shortness of breath (dyspnea).
- Chest pain (angina pectoris).
- Palpitations and other irregular heartbeats (cardiac arrhythmias).
- Swelling (edema), especially of the ankles and feet.
- Unexplained fatigue.
- Dizziness and fainting (syncope).
- Blue coloration (cyanosis), especially of the lips, under the nails, and of the mucous membranes.

Listening through a stethoscope is another important aspect of the heart exam. By placing the stethoscope on different parts of your body, a doctor can listen to the sounds of your heart, lungs, and blood vessels; and each sound provides important clues about how well your heart and blood vessels are functioning. For example, a crackling sound as you take a deep breath may mean that there is too much fluid in your lungs because your heart cannot pump hard enough to prevent the lungs from becoming waterlogged.

Symptoms of a Heart Attack

A heart attack always demands immediate emergency treatment. Still, persons having a heart attack wait an average of six hours before seeking help, often thinking the symptoms are due to indigestion, stress, or some other cause. It is always best to err on the safe side and call your local emergency medical service if you have any of the following symptoms:

- Chest pain or discomfort lasting more than two minutes. The pain of a heart attack is often intense or crushing; in other instances, it is a dull, aching sensation.
- Spread of the pain to the shoulders, neck, arms, back, or jaw.
- Shortness of breath.
- Light-headedness, dizziness, or fainting.
- Pulse that is rapid, shallow, or irregular.
- Sweats, which may be drenching.
- Nausea and vomiting.
- Feelings of weakness.
- Pallor or bluish tinge of the lips and fingertips.
- Feelings of extreme anxiety.

The heart produces different sounds during each beat; your doctor listens for abnormal clicks, rubs, murmurs, snaps, and other sounds as you breathe and move about. Also, by placing a stethoscope over different arteries, a doctor can tell whether blood is flowing normally. For example, a turbulent sound, called a *bruit*, points to a buildup of fatty deposits in the artery.

During another important part of the physical examination, your doctor looks into your eyes with a lighted magnifying instrument. This is to inspect the tiny blood vessels that are visible inside the eyes—the only place in the body where arteries can be seen directly. Abnormalities such as tiny ruptures, tangles, or narrowing or swelling of blood vessels indicate damage from high blood pressure, diabetes, or other disorders.

ELECTROCARDIOGRAM

General information

Where It's Done	Who Does It	How Long It Takes	Discomfort/Pain
Doctor's office or clinic, or at hospital bedside.	Technician, nurse, or doctor.	5 minutes.	None.

Results Ready When	Special Equipment	Risks/Complications	Average Cost
Immediately.	ECG machine and electrodes.	None.	$

Other names Resting electrocardiogram, ECG, or EKG.

Purpose

- To detect heart problems or blockages in the coronary arteries.
- To draw a graph of the electrical impulses moving through the heart.
- To record heart rate and the regularity of heartbeats.
- To diagnose a possible heart attack or other heart disorders.

How it works Electrodes, or leads, attached to the chest, neck, arms, and legs record the pathway of electrical impulses through the heart muscle (see figure 5.3).

Preparation

- The chest, arms, and legs are exposed.
- Gel may be applied to the chest, neck, arms, and legs for better electrical conduction to the leads. (In some instances, chest hair may also be shaved for better conduction.)

Test procedure You lie quietly on your back while the heart's electrical impulses are recorded on the graph paper.

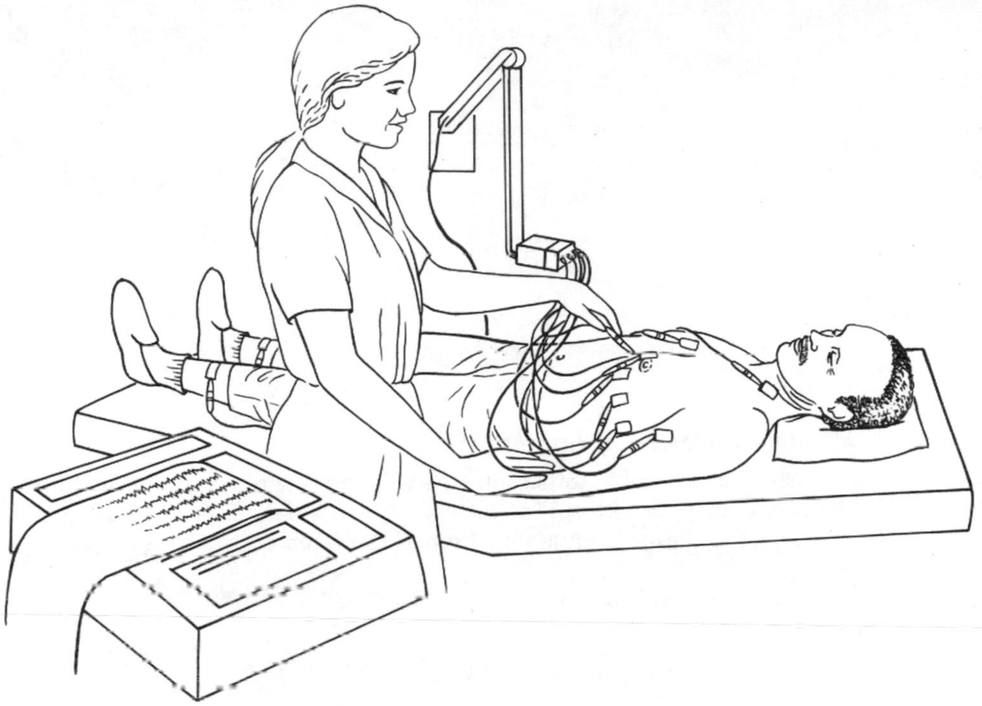

FIGURE 5.3 **A Resting Electrocardiogram**

To make an ECG, electrodes are attached to specific points over the heart, on the neck, and on the arm and legs.

After the test Leads are removed and gel (if used) is wiped off. Unless the test detects heart problems, you can immediately resume your normal activities.

Factors affecting results

- Movement or faulty placement of the leads.
- Imbalance of electrolytes in your blood (eg, too much or too little calcium, potassium, magnesium, or sodium).
- Thickening of the heart muscle.
- Low body temperature.

Interpretation

- A doctor examines the ECG tracings for abnormalities, sometimes with the help of a computer.
- An ECG can be transmitted over phone lines for evaluation at a diagnostic center or clinic.

Advantages

- It's painless, noninvasive, safe, inexpensive, and easy to perform.
- The necessary equipment is widely available.

Disadvantages

- It doesn't always permit an accurate diagnosis.

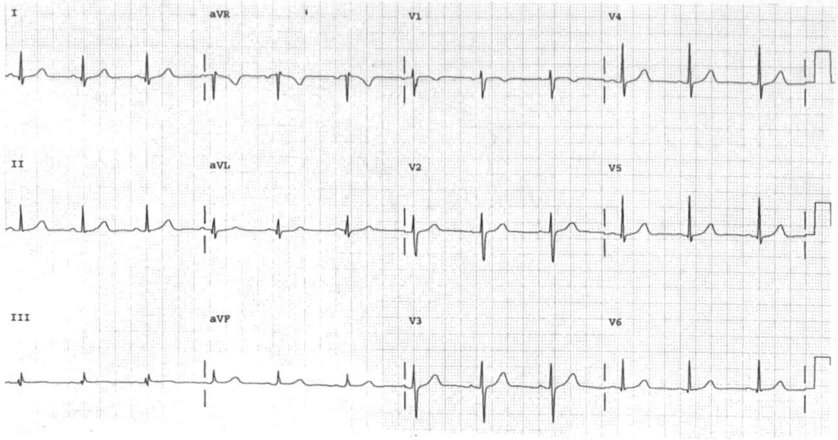

FIGURE 5.4a **Normal Electrocardiogram (ECG)**

The letters along the top of this ECG strip indicate readings obtained from specific leads, or sensors. For example, V-1 to V-6 are from the leads placed across the chest; the others are from leads placed on the arms and legs.

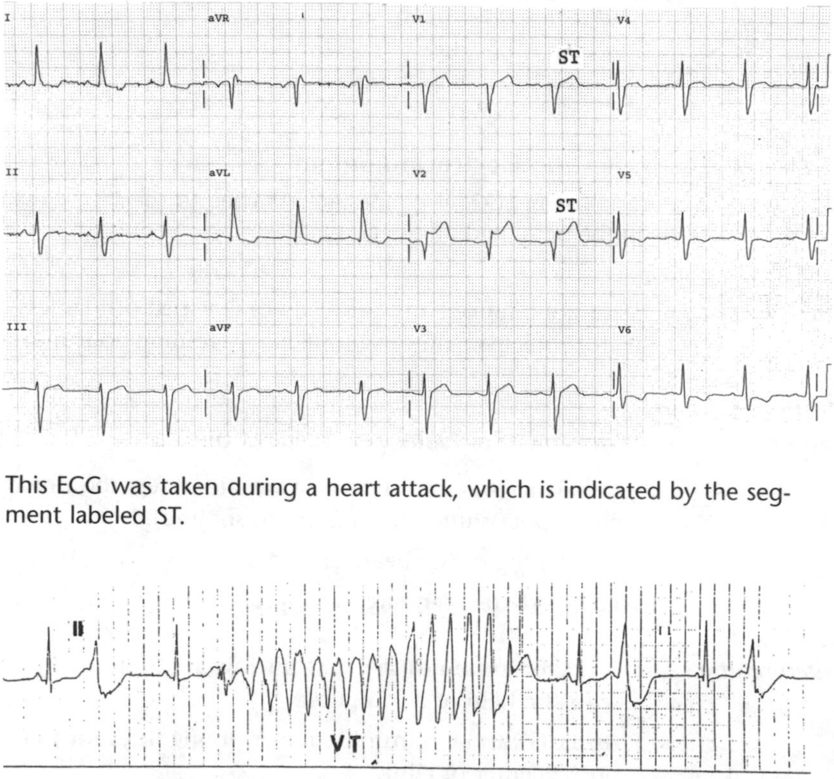

FIGURE 5.4b This ECG was taken during a heart attack, which is indicated by the segment labeled ST.

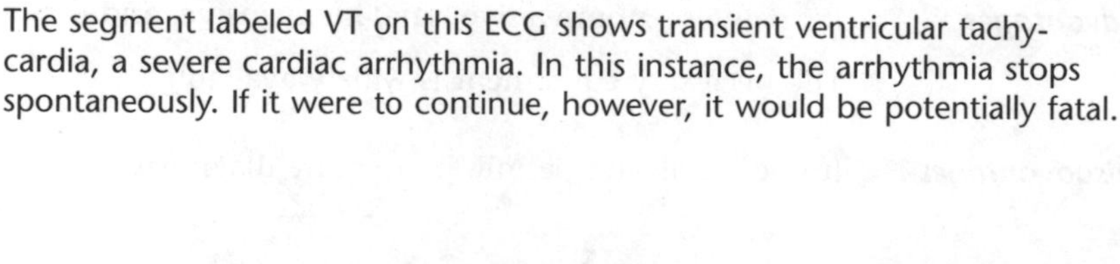

FIGURE 5.4c The segment labeled VT on this ECG shows transient ventricular tachycardia, a severe cardiac arrhythmia. In this instance, the arrhythmia stops spontaneously. If it were to continue, however, it would be potentially fatal.

- It can be normal despite a serious heart problem (a false-negative result).

The next step

- If the electrocardiogram is normal and you are not experiencing symptoms of a heart disorder, no further testing is needed.
- If the ECG or symptoms point to a disturbance in the heart's normal rhythm, Holter monitoring—a 24-hour ECG—may be ordered (see below).
- If the ECG shows increased electrical activity in the heart, which can indicate thickening of the heart wall, a follow-up echocardiogram may be ordered.
- If the ECG indicates a heart attack, intensive treatment is started immediately to minimize its damage and stabilize the patient.

HOLTER MONITORING

General information

Where It's Done	Who Does It	How Long It Takes	Discomfort/Pain
Monitor is hooked up in doctor's office or diagnostic lab.	Technician, nurse, or doctor.	Monitor is left on for 24 hours or more.	None, although the monitor may be cumbersome and interfere with bathing or showering.

Results Ready When	Special Equipment	Risks/Complications	Average Cost
Within a few days after removing the monitor.	Portable ECG monitor, chest ECG leads, tape or digital recorder, and a computer to analyze the ECG.	None.	$$

Other names 24-hour ECG or long-term continuous electrocardiographic recording.

Purpose To record heartbeats over an extended period, during normal activities—which may identify problems undetected by an electrocardiogram.

How it works A portable ECG monitor is connected to ECG leads attached to your chest to measure and record the pathway of electrical impulses through the heart muscle.

Preparation

- ECG leads are attached and taped in place to prevent displacement. Chest hair may be shaved.
- The monitor is usually worn in a shoulder harness or can be carried in a pocket or attached to your belt.

Test procedure

- A continuous ECG is made as you go about your daily activities.
- You may carry out normal, everyday activities, but be alert to irregular heartbeats, chest pains, and other symptoms.
- Keep a careful diary recording your various activities (exercise, eating, etc.), and record the time and circumstances of any symptoms. Some monitors allow this to be done electronically, highlighting specific portions of the ECG recording during the symptoms.
- Don't let the leads get wet. If a lead comes loose, don't try to reattach it yourself. Go to the lab or doctor's office to have it reattached.

After the test You return to the doctor's office or lab to have the monitor and leads removed.

Factors affecting results

- Mechanical failure such as battery malfunction, a faulty monitor, scratching, or moving a lead.
- Use of certain drugs—legal or illicit—that can alter heart rhythms.
- Stress, hyperventilation (overbreathing), exercise, and straining (these activities should be recorded in your diary).

Interpretation The ECG recording is scanned by a computer for abnormalities; abnormal recordings, along with your diary of activities, are reviewed by a doctor.

Advantages

- It allows ECG monitoring over an extended period and is used to detect heart rhythm disturbances.
- It can be used by people who cannot undergo exercise stress tests to detect intermittent serious heart problems such as intermittent arrhythmias and silent ischemia (periods of insufficient oxygen supplied to the heart muscle) occurring during normal activities and not necessarily detected in the laboratory.

Disadvantages It may not detect serious arrhythmias or other problems if they do not happen to occur during the test period. If this happens and symptoms continue, another type of monitor may be employed ("event-triggered").

The next step Holter monitoring allows an ECG to be recorded over an extended period—usually at least 24 hours. During this time, arrhythmias or signs of silent ischemia may be uncovered that are not evident during a brief ECG performed in a doctor's office. Further testing depends on what shows up on the extended ECG.

SIGNAL-AVERAGED ELECTROCARDIOGRAM (SAECG)

General information

Where It's Done	Who Does It	How Long It Takes	Discomfort/Pain
Doctor's office or clinic, or at hospital bedside.	Technician, nurse, or doctor.	30 minutes.	None.
Results Ready When	**Special Equipment**	**Risks/Complications**	**Average Cost**
Immediately.	ECG machine and computer.	None.	$$

Other names Late potential study.

Purpose To detect late electrical potential currents that may be present after the heart muscle has been activated. This electrical activity usually occurs in damaged parts of the heart muscle and indicates risk for development of an abnormal heart rhythm.

How it works

- A regular ECG is taken, for a prolonged period of time, usually 30 minutes.
- A computer superimposes the ECG signals over an average ECG signal to check for abnormalities.

Preparation Same as for an ECG.

Test procedure You lie quietly while the heart's electrical impulses are recorded on the graph paper.

After the test Same as for an ECG.

Factors affecting results Same as for a resting ECG.

Interpretation Same as for an ECG.

Advantages It can provide information on arrhythmic potential that is missed by a resting ECG and Holter monitoring.

Disadvantages Same as for an ECG.

The next step Because this test provides clues to potentially serious cardiac arrhythmias, a positive result calls for further tests that may include electrophysiology studies.

EXERCISE STRESS TEST

General information

Where It's Done	Who Does It	How Long It Takes	Discomfort/Pain
Doctor's office, clinic, or hospital.	Doctor with nurse or technician.	5–20 minutes.	May provoke angina, leg fatigue, muscle aches, and shortness of breath.

Results Ready When	Special Equipment	Risks/Complications	Average Cost
Preliminary results immediately. Final analysis takes several days.	ECG machine, leads, blood pressure cuff, and exercise treadmill or cycle.	Slight chance of heart attack during exercise (1 in 100,000), cardiac arrhythmia, cardiac insufficiency, and cardiac arrest.	$$

Other names Stress test, exercise tolerance test, and electrocardiographic exercise test.

Purpose

- To help in the evaluation of possible coronary artery disease.
- To determine safe levels of exercise and exercise guidelines, especially if you have angina or other symptoms of coronary disease or heart failure.
- To help in the evaluation of heart health following a heart attack, coronary angioplasty, and bypass surgery, and to help detect ischemia (episodes of insufficient oxygen supply to the heart muscle).

How it works

- After being connected to leads for an electrocardiogram, you exercise on a treadmill or stationary bicycle until your heart rate reaches a certain level, or until you are exhausted or develop symptoms such as chest pain or dizziness.
- Your blood pressure is monitored periodically throughout the test.
- To get more data about the state of your heart and coronary arteries, radioactive isotopes may be injected through an intravenous (IV) line, and a gamma scintillation camera may be used to follow their uptake into the heart muscle; or an electrocardiogram may be obtained.

Preparation

- In general, you shouldn't eat or smoke for at least two hours before the test, but follow your doctor's specific instructions.

- Wear comfortable walking or running shoes or sneakers, and shorts or loose-fitting exercise pants. Women may wear a loose-fitting top that opens in the front.
- A physician or other health care provider should be present with a defibrillator and other emergency equipment.

Test procedure

- ECG leads are attached to your chest.
- Your blood pressure is measured, and the blood pressure cuff is left in place to allow regular blood pressure measurements during the test.
- Your heart rate, ECG pattern, and blood pressure will be monitored as you exercise at increasing levels of intensity.

Special precautions

The test should be stopped immediately if you develop any of the following symptoms:

- An unsteady gait, mental confusion, glazed expression, grayish or cold, clammy skin—all signs of cardiac insufficiency.
- Dizziness or fainting.
- A drop in blood pressure.
- Severe angina.
- Cardiac arrhythmias.

Variations

Patients with orthopedic problems, arthritis, or other conditions that make it impossible to exercise on a treadmill or cycle may be given a drug to increase their heart rate. (For other variations, see the descriptions of exercise echocardiography and myocardial perfusion scan below.)

After the test

- Depending on the test results, you should rest until your blood pressure, heart rate, and other vital signs return to normal.
- If there are no complications, the ECG leads are removed, and you can resume normal activities.

Factors affecting results

- Certain medications such as antianginal drugs may alter the results by increasing your exercise tolerance. These drugs may be discontinued for a day or so beforehand, unless the test is meant to assess their effectiveness.
- Medications such as digitalis can produce a false-positive, or abnormal, result.

Interpretation

A doctor studies the ECG tracings, and also assesses your performance and symptoms during the test.

Advantages

- This test offers a simple, noninvasive method of assessing heart function during vigorous activity, and is generally safe when performed in the proper setting.
- It can disclose or confirm abnormalities, such as silent ischemia, that do not produce symptoms, providing a safe and relatively inexpensive (albeit less accurate than an exercise radioisotope scan or electrocardiogram) method of diagnosis and assessment. It is often the first approach to diagnosis after a routine office evaluation and ECG.

Disadvantages

- Results are often unreliable: 15% to 40% of exercise stress tests produce false-positive results. Women are more likely than men to have a false-positive exercise stress test.
- Patients with an abnormal resting ECG usually shouldn't undergo an exercise stress test.

The next step Test results may be used to develop an exercise prescription as part of a cardiovascular conditioning or rehabilitation program. Abnormal results may point to a need for further tests, including an exercise stress test or myocardial perfusion scan, or cardiac catheterization and angiography.

EXERCISE ECHOCARDIOGRAPHY

General information

Where It's Done	Who Does It	How Long It Takes	Discomfort/Pain
Same as for exercise stress test.	Doctor with nurse or technician.	20–90 minutes.	Same as for exercise stress test.
Results Ready When	**Special Equipment**	**Risks/Complications**	**Average Cost**
Same as for exercise stress test.	Same as for exercise stress test, plus ultrasound equipment.	Same as for exercise stress test.	$$$

Other names Stress test with echocardiography.

Purpose Same as for exercise stress test, and also to evaluate the heart muscle and valves in action.

How it works The heart is evaluated with ultrasound before and after an exercise stress test. This test may also be performed using a drug (dobutamine) that mimics the effects of exercise.

Preparation Same as for an exercise stress test and echocardiography.

Test procedure Same as for an exercise stress test, plus the following:

- An echocardiogram (see page 103) is taken before and after exercise.
- The test may also be performed with a medication, given through an intravenous tube, that mimics the effects of exercise and can therefore substitute for the exercise portion of the test (dobutamine). This is valuable in patients who cannot exercise.

After the test Same as for an exercise stress test.

Factors affecting results Same as for echocardiography and an exercise stress test.

Interpretation The test is evaluated for the development of abnormal contractions (heartbeats) during exercise. This suggests an inadequate blood supply to the heart muscle.

Advantages Same as for an exercise stress test, and also it's a noninvasive way to evaluate function of the heart muscle and valves and detect coronary disease.

Disadvantages Same as for an exercise stress test, and also the equipment is expensive and not available at all testing centers.

MYOCARDIAL PERFUSION SCAN

General Information

Where It's Done	Who Does It	How Long It Takes	Discomfort/Pain
Diagnostic clinic, doctor's office, or hospital outpatient department.	Doctor and a nurse or technician.	2–4 hours.	IV needle may be bothersome. Test may provoke angina, leg fatigue, and muscle aches. Remaining in position for imaging may be uncomfortable.
Results Ready When	**Special Equipment**	**Risks/Complications**	**Average Cost**
A few hours to several days.	ECG machine and leads, blood pressure cuff, IV line, treadmill or exercise bicycle, gamma scintillation camera.	Radioactive isotopes should not be administered during pregnancy.	$$$

Other names Myocardial perfusion scintigraphy, MIBI stress test, exercise radioisotope scan, thallium imaging, thallium scan, thallium, MIBI or tetrofosmin scintigraphy, and perfusion imaging.

Purpose

- To assess the amount of blood reaching the heart muscle.
- To identify areas of heart muscle lacking an adequate blood supply as a result of a heart attack.
- To identify blocked coronary arteries and evaluate the effectiveness of coronary bypass grafts or angioplasty.

How it works

- Following an exercise stress test, you are injected with radioisotopes, such as thallium, MIBI (Cardiolite), or tetrofosmin (Myoview), that concentrate in heart muscle and can be tracked by a gamma scintillation (or detection) camera.
- The radioisotope circulates through the body and collects in the heart, revealing heart areas receiving insufficient amounts of blood.
- The gamma scintillation camera photographs your heart shortly after the injection and again several hours later, allowing doctors to compare thallium uptake immediately after exercise and again after rest.
- If MIBI or tetrofosmin is used, a second injection at rest is necessary.
- Because the test has two sections (four hours apart), evaluation may be performed on the same day or on consecutive days.

Preparation

- You should not consume or use alcohol, caffeine, or tobacco (or any other source of nicotine) for 24 hours before the test.
- Do not eat anything for at least three hours before the test.
- You may be instructed to stop certain medications before the test.
- At the test site, blood pressure is measured, and ECG leads are attached to your chest, arm, and leg.
- An IV line is started in your arm.

Test procedure

- You exercise at increasing levels (as for an exercise stress test).
- Near the end of the test's exercise portion, the radioisotope is injected into the IV line, and you resume exercising for another minute. This allows the substance to travel through your body and concentrate in the heart muscle.
- If you are unable to exercise, a drug such as dipyridamole (Persantine), adenosine (Adenoscan), or dobutamine can be used to increase blood flow before the radioisotope is injected.
- After you stop exercising, you are positioned on a narrow examination table directly under the gamma scintillation camera. One or both arms are placed on a rest over your head, and the camera takes multiple pictures. In many instances, it rotates slowly around you, thereby producing three-dimensional images (SPECT or single-photon emission computed tomography).

After the test

- After the initial pictures are taken, you return for a second set of scans. Between sessions, you should remain relatively quiet, even though you may be permitted to leave the testing center. You can drink water or other plain, noncaloric beverages, but you should not eat.

- In some instances, another set of scans is made 24 hours later. In these cases, your doctor will give specific instructions regarding food consumption and other activities.

Factors affecting results

- The consumption or use of caffeine, alcohol, nicotine, and certain other drugs.
- Inadequate exercise before or after injection of the radioisotope.

Interpretation The ECG taken during the exercise test and the scans are examined for abnormalities by a physician trained in nuclear cardiology. "Cold" spots on the scan (areas of decreased radioisotope uptake) indicate heart muscle areas receiving inadequate oxygen due to blocked or narrowed coronary arteries or a previous heart attack.

Advantages

- It provides more information about the heart muscle and its blood supply than a conventional exercise stress test.
- It's more accurate than exercise testing.

Disadvantages

- Some people are disturbed by the closeness of the camera; lying still for 30 to 45 minutes may also be uncomfortable.
- It's more expensive than routine exercise testing and requires an intravenous injection of a radioactive isotope.

The next step Results indicating diseased coronary arteries may be confirmed by cardiac catheterization and angiography.

MUGA SCAN

General information

Where It's Done	Who Does It	How Long It Takes	Discomfort/Pain
Diagnostic clinic, hospital outpatient department, doctor's office, or hospital bedside.	Doctor and technician.	10–15 minutes for preparation, plus 20–30 minutes under the scintillation camera.	Minor discomfort from IV line insertion.
Results Ready When	**Special Equipment**	**Risks/Complications**	**Average Cost**
A few hours to several days.	ECG machine and leads, IV injection, scintillation camera, and computer.	Slight risk from use of technetium, a radioactive substance that should not be used during pregnancy.	$$

Other names Multigated graft acquisition, cardiac blood-pool imaging, and equilibrium radionuclide angiocardiography.

Purpose

- To provide information about the heart's pumping (left ventricular) function by measuring the ejection fraction (the amount of blood that is pumped with each heartbeat) as well as measuring ventricular filling, the flow of blood into the pumping chamber.
- Also used to evaluate the function of the right ventricle (the chamber that pumps blood to the lungs) and to diagnose heart wall abnormalities.

How it works An injection of a radioactive isotope (technetium) temporarily "labels" the patient's red blood cells, and a gamma scintillation camera linked to a computer follows the blood moving through the heart. An ECG triggers the computer system, and data from several hundred heartbeats are collected and analyzed.

Preparation There is no special preparation.

Test procedure

- After ECG leads are attached, the technetium is injected, usually into an arm vein.
- You lie on an examination table under the gamma scintillation camera, and hold still without speaking during the scanning process.
- Images are viewed on a video screen and recorded on a computer for later viewing and interpretation.

After the test You may return to normal activities.

Factors affecting results

- Movement during the test.
- Abnormalities in the ECG.
- Irregular heartbeat.

Interpretation A computer is used to process and analyze the data, which is then interpreted by a doctor trained in nuclear cardiology.

Advantages

- It's noninvasive.
- It assesses the heart's ejection fraction—probably the single most important index of heart performance—and other measures of cardiac function.

Disadvantages The injection of a radioactive isotope is required.

The next step Depending on the results, you may be referred for cardiac catheterization or for treatment of the underlying condition.

ECHOCARDIOGRAPHY

General information

Where It's Done	Who Does It	How Long It Takes	Discomfort/Pain
Doctor's office, testing lab, or outpatient department.	Technician, nurse, or doctor trained in ultrasound.	30–60 minutes.	None.

Results Ready When	Special Equipment	Risks/Complications	Average Cost
Immediately to several days.	Ultrasound transducer, monitor with oscilloscope screen, video and/or strip-chart recorders, and ECG machine.	None.	$$

Other names Cardiac ultrasonography, ultrasound, and Doppler study.

Purpose

- To evaluate various congenital and acquired heart defects.
- To measure the size of the heart and its chambers
- To evaluate the function of the heart muscle and heart valves, and to detect excessive fluid in the pericardium, the membrane that surrounds the heart.

How it works High-frequency sound waves are directed through the body to create an image of the heart and other internal structures (see figure 5.5).

Preparation

- You remove your clothing and jewelry above the waist, and recline on an examination table.
- Gel is applied to your chest to help conduct the sound waves.

Test procedure

- As you lie on the examining table, the tester guides the transducer probe, shaped like a pencil or microphone, over specific areas of your chest. Slight pressure is applied between the skin and transducer.
- From time to time, you may be asked to assume a different position.
- As the transducer passes over the skin, it emits high-frequency, inaudible sound waves used to create images of internal organs and indicate the flow of blood to various parts of the heart.

Variations

- *Doppler ultrasound,* in which a special microphone is used to measure the velocity of blood flow in different parts of the heart.
- *Exercise echocardiogram* (see above), in which the echocardiogram is done during exercise. This provides a better picture of the state of the coronary arteries than an echocardiogram done during rest. If you are unable to exercise, a drug can be used to increase blood flow, mimicking what happens during exercise.

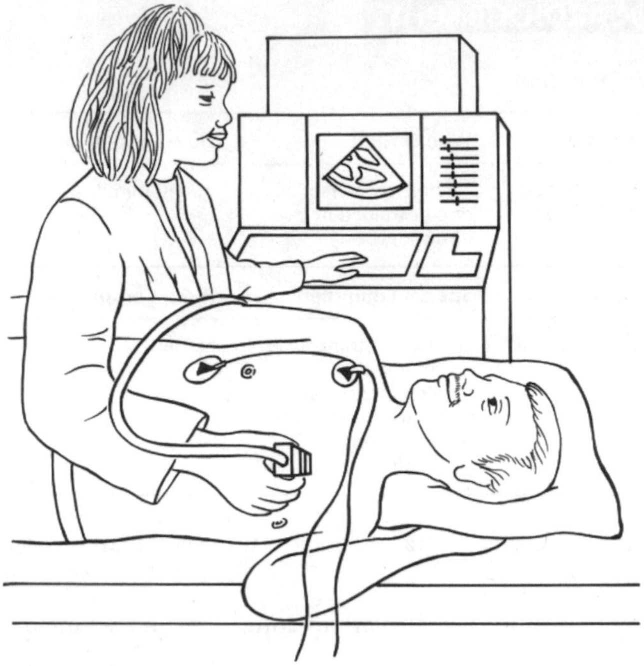

FIGURE 5.5 Echocardiography

As a technician passes an ultrasound transducer over the heart, the echoed sound waves create an image that can be viewed on a monitor and also recorded on paper or tape.

After the test You can return to normal activities.

Factors affecting results

- Other diseases, such as emphysema.
- Chest wall abnormalities, including unusual thickness, which may distort the sound waves.
- Excessive movement.
- Faulty use of the transducer.

Interpretation A doctor trained in interpreting ultrasonography studies the tracings and video images in a number of conditions related to the heart valves, heart muscles, or the outer covering of the heart (pericardium).

Advantages It's painless, noninvasive, and reliable.

Disadvantages

- It doesn't detect narrowed coronary arteries when performed at rest.
- It may not accurately measure the heart's pumping function (ejection fraction) as well as other tests.
- Certain physical characteristics distort the images.

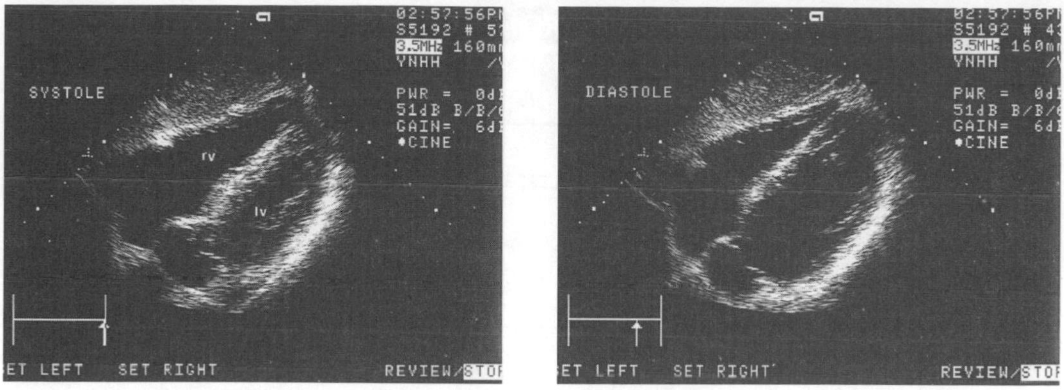

FIGURE 5.6a and 5.6b

These normal echocardiograms are taken during two phases of a heartbeat: (a) shows the heart's two pumping chambers, the left ventricle (lv) and the right ventricle (rv) when they are contracted to their smallest size (systole). During this phase, blood is pumped from the heart. In contrast, (b) shows the same two chambers during diastole, the brief resting period between beats (contractions), when blood flows into them. Note that the chambers appear much larger here than during the systole phase.

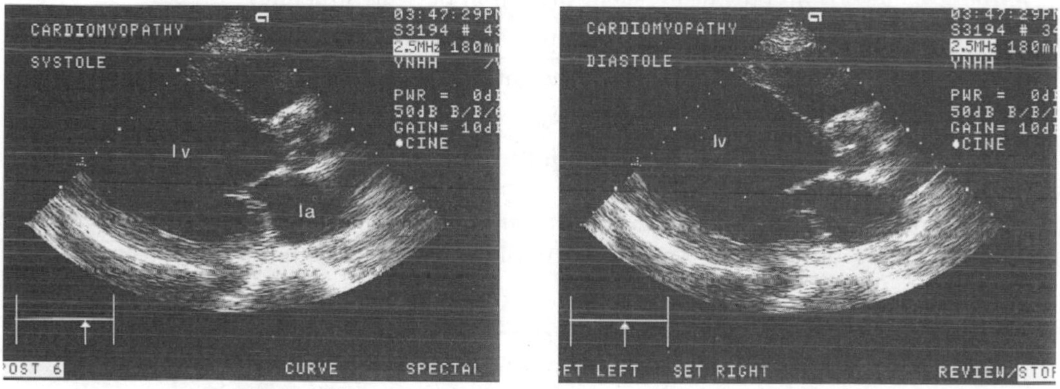

FIGURE 5.6c and 5.6d

These echocardiograms show cardiomyopathy, a serious disorder in which the heart muscle becomes enlarged and weak. Note that unlike figures 5.6a and 5.6b, the two chambers on one side of the heart—the left ventricle (lv) and left atrium (la)—are virtually the same size during both the contraction (systole) and resting (diastole) phases. This indicates that the left ventricle is unable to pump blood adequately from the heart into the circulation.

The next step Cardiac catheterization may be performed if the echocardiogram indicates heart valve disease, a congenital heart defect, or other abnormalities.

TRANSESOPHAGEAL ECHOCARDIOGRAPHY (TEE)

General information

Where It's Done	Who Does It	How Long It Takes	Discomfort/Pain
Diagnostic lab or hospital outpatient department.	Doctor.	30–60 minutes.	Possible gagging and throat discomfort; transducer movement may cause a pressured feeling in the chest.

Results Ready When	Special Equipment	Risks/Complications	Average Cost
A few hours to a few days.	Ultrasound transducer, viewing tube (endoscope), oral suction device to remove saliva, and possibly a mouth guard to protect the teeth.	A possible sore throat for a few days. Possibly, some bleeding in the esophagus; in rare instances, the esophagus may be perforated.	$$$

Other names None.

Purpose

- To provide excellent definition of heart structures.
- To view a heart difficult to examine using conventional echocardiography (for example, if the patient is obese or has a thick chest wall).
- To monitor heart function during cardiac surgery.
- To detect blood clots in the left atrium.

How it works A viewing tube and small transducer are passed down the esophagus, allowing the examiner to transmit sound waves to the heart from inside

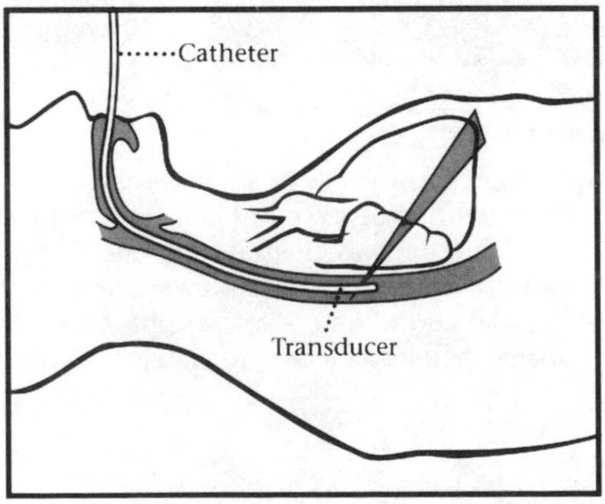

FIGURE 5.7a Transesophageal Ecocardiography

To visualize the back of the heart, a tiny transducer is inserted into a small tube, or catheter, and passed through the mouth into the esophagus until it is positioned immediately behind the heart.

the body (see figures 5.7a–b). (This is similar to a routine endoscopy procedure employed to evaluate the GI tract, described in chapter 8.)

Preparation

- A mild sedative may be given for relaxation.
- The back of the throat is sprayed with a local anesthetic to reduce the gag reflex.

Test procedure

- The endoscope containing the ultrasound transducer is passed through the mouth and throat. You may have to swallow several times to help move it downward.
- The transducer projects sound waves to the heart from the front of the esophagus wall. It may be moved several times to obtain different views of the heart.
- Throughout the test, the sound waves are recorded and analyzed using techniques similar to conventional echocardiography.

After the test

The tube is withdrawn from the throat.

- It takes an hour or longer for the anesthetic to wear off and the gag reflex to return to normal. *Do not* try to eat or drink until the gag reflex is tested, which can be done by touching the back of the throat with a tongue depressor.
- If a sedative was given, you may be drowsy and should not drive for at least ten to 12 hours.
- Abstain from alcohol for a day or so before and after the test, because it increases the sedative effect.

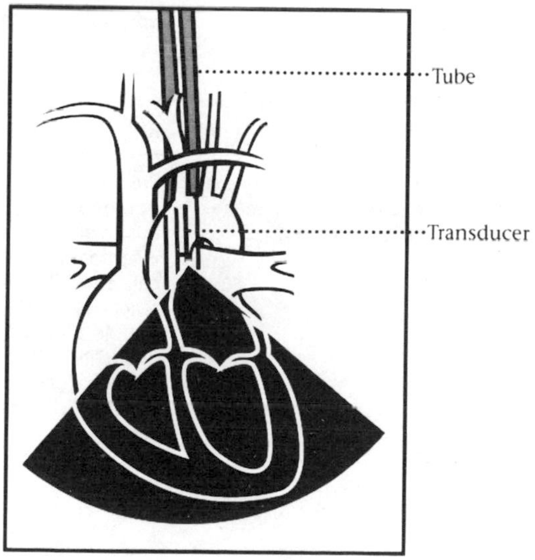

FIGURE 5.7b Images from behind Heart

After the transducer is positioned behind the heart, it can then be manipulated to produce images of the heart chambers and other structures.

Factors affecting results Very few factors affect results. In fact, this test overcomes most of the problems that may be encountered during ordinary echocardiography because the transducer is placed immediately next to the heart.

Interpretation The images and video are analyzed by a doctor trained in interpreting echocardiograms.

Advantages It provides views of the heart that cannot be obtained with conventional echocardiography.

Disadvantages The viewing tube (endoscope) creates some discomfort and risk.

The next step More invasive tests, such as cardiac catheterization, may be ordered if images indicate cardiac abnormalities.

CARDIAC CATHETERIZATION AND ANGIOGRAPHY

General information

Where It's Done	Who Does It	How Long It Takes	Discomfort/Pain
Hospital catheterization lab or special diagnostic center.	Doctor.	2–3 hours plus at least 6–8 hours of rest and observation afterward. In selected cases, the patient may go home the same day; in many instances, you may have to stay in the hospital overnight.	Minor discomfort from IV and anesthetic injection. Dye may cause flushing or burning. Holding position for imaging may be uncomfortable. You may have to remain in bed overnight with your weight on your groin.

Results Ready When	Special Equipment	Risks/Complications	Average Cost
A few hours.	X-ray and fluoroscopic equipment, IV line, catheter, and dye.	Possible clot, bleeding, or blood vessel damage at site of catheter insertion. Dye may cause an allergic reaction, especially in people allergic to iodine or shellfish. Rarely, test may provoke heart attack, stroke, or cardiac arrest.	$$$

Other names Coronary arteriography or cardiac cath.

Purpose

- To evaluate blockage of coronary arteries; to evaluate function of bypass grafts, heart valves, and other heart structures; and to assess coronary circulation and overall heart function.

- To study congenital heart defects.
- To take tissue samples (biopsies) and study heart muscle disorders such as myocarditis, or transplant rejection.

How it works

- A thin catheter is inserted into a blood vessel, usually an artery in the leg or arm, and passed through the blood vessel to the heart.
- Dye is injected to make the coronary arteries and other structures visible on X-rays.
- Fluoroscopy and X-rays provide images of the coronary arteries and other heart structures.

DID YOU KNOW?

- The German scientist who did the first human cardiac catheterization actually did the procedure on himself, with the help of his office nurse.
- Each year, more than one million Americans undergo cardiac catheterization and angiography.
- Of these patients, about 300,000 later undergo balloon angioplasty, while 265,000 later have coronary bypass surgery to improve blood flow to their heart muscle.

Preparation

- Do not eat or drink for 12 hours before the test.
- An IV line will be inserted before the test, and a mild sedative may be administered to ease anxiety.
- If the catheter is introduced from the leg, the groin is shaved to help prevent infection.

Test procedure

- You lie on an examination table under the X-ray monitoring equipment, and remain as still as possible throughout the test unless you are told to shift your position.
- Anesthetic is injected into the leg (or arm).
- A small incision is made in the leg (or arm) to permit insertion of the catheter (see figure 5.8).
- The doctor threads the catheter through the blood vessel to the heart while watching its progress on the video monitor.
- Contrast dye is injected through the catheter, and the doctor views the heart function on the monitor.
- Moving and still X-ray pictures (angiograms) are made for later study and interpretation (see figure 5.9). If a biopsy is needed, a special tweezerlike instrument is inserted through the catheter to collect tissue samples.

PATIENT TIPS

- Be sure to tell the doctor of any allergies, especially to seafood or iodine. Otherwise, you may suffer an adverse reaction to the dye.
- About one in ten patients has an adverse reaction to the dye when it is injected, becoming nauseated and possibly vomiting.

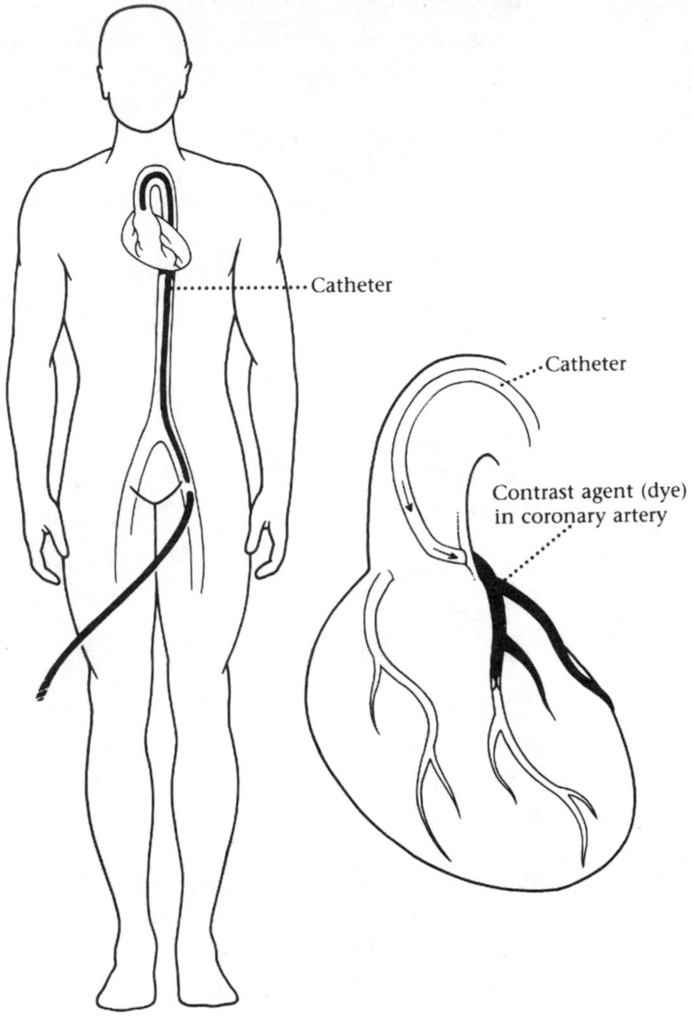

FIGURE 5.8 During cardiac catheterization, the catheter is inserted into a vein in the leg and then threaded upward to the heart. (In some instances, the catheter is inserted into a blood vessel in the arm.) A contrast dye is then injected through the catheter to make the coronary arteries and other heart structures more visible on X-rays.

After the test

- After the catheter is removed, pressure is applied to the incision site until bleeding stops, and a bandage is applied.
- A small sandbag is usually placed over the incision for a few hours to prevent bleeding.
- During the recovery period, your blood pressure and other vital signs are monitored periodically.
- If you have the test as an outpatient, you rest in a recovery room for six to eight hours. Otherwise, you stay in the hospital overnight.

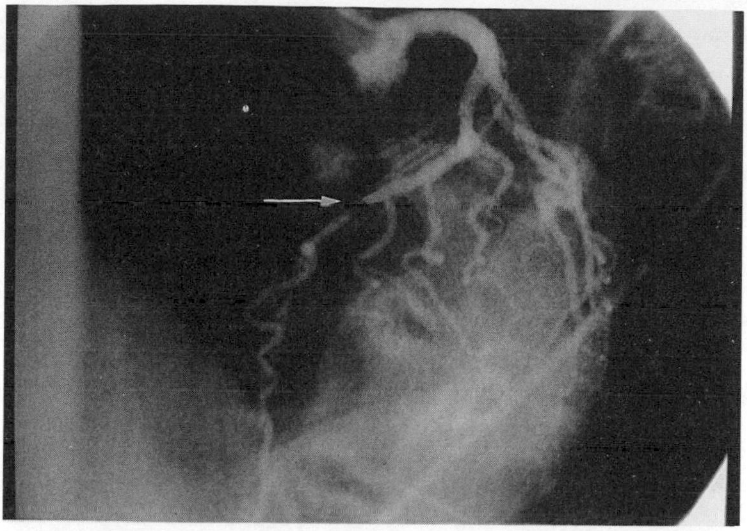

FIGURE 5.9 In this angiogram, the coronary arteries are shown in white. The arrow points to an area of significant narrowing of the left anterior descending coronary artery due to fatty plaque, or atherosclerosis.

- In the first few hours after the test, you will be given apple juice, water, or other clear fluids. Drink as much as you can to speed the kidney's removal of the dye from your body.
- For the first few hours, you are checked every 30 minutes by a doctor or nurse. During this time, you should avoid moving your leg (or arm), and summon help immediately for bleeding or other symptoms.
- If your condition remains stable and there is no bleeding, you can sit up, stand, and walk for a short distance five or six hours after the test. Outpatients can usually leave the testing center seven to eight hours after the test.
- Before you go home, a doctor or nurse should show you how to apply pressure to stop any bleeding at the incision site. If continuous bleeding (not stopping within a few minutes) or other symptoms develop at home, call for an emergency medical crew to take you to the nearest hospital.

Factors affecting results

- Obesity may obscure X-rays.
- Severe arteriosclerosis in the blood vessels of the arms or legs may limit access of the catheter to the heart.

Interpretation The films are studied for narrowed or blocked arteries and other abnormalities.

Advantages The test is reliable, providing the most accurate information about heart structures.

Disadvantages

- It's invasive.
- It carries a risk of a clot (embolism), bleeding, or blood vessel damage at the incision site.

The next step This is usually the definitive diagnostic test that confirms or rules out earlier findings. If the results point to the need for surgical treatment, the next step may be balloon angioplasty, coronary bypass surgery, a heart valve operation, or some other intervention.

POSITRON-EMISSION TOMOGRAPHY

General information

Where It's Done	Who Does It	How Long It Takes	Discomfort/Pain
Hospital lab or special diagnostic center.	Doctor.	2 hours.	Minor discomfort from isotope injection. Holding position for imaging may be uncomfortable.
Results Ready When	**Special Equipment**	**Risks/Complications**	**Average Cost**
A few hours to several days.	Tomographic cameras, positron detectors, and a computer.	Minimal risk of reaction to injected isotopes.	$$$

Other names PET scans.

Purpose

- To assess the viability of and blood flow to the heart muscle.
- To diagnose coronary artery disease, and to study metabolism of the heart muscle.
- At the time of this writing, the tests are often considered experimental in some settings. However, they are likely to be more widely used in the next several years.

How it works

- The test uses special radioactive substances called positron-emitting isotopes that provide more information about the heart muscle than other imaging techniques.
- It can assess the heart muscle's metabolism of glucose as well as the blood flow to the heart, and distinguish viable "stunned" heart muscle from dead (infected) tissue, an important consideration in treatment after a heart attack.

Preparation

- Remove all clothing above the waist.
- Lie on the examination table with arms above the head.

Test procedure

- The heart is localized with fluoroscopy or some other method, and a 10- to 30-minute scan is made with a tomographic camera.
- The positron-emitting isotopes are injected, and after a 30- to 40-minute wait, a second tomographic scan is made.

After the test You can resume normal activities.

Factors affecting results

- Diabetes may alter the result; blood sugar level in most patients must be monitored during testing.
- Extreme obesity may limit imaging.

Interpretation A computer is used to assess the results, which are interpreted by a physician trained in nuclear cardiology.

Advantages The test is noninvasive and provides sensitive and specific information regarding blood flow to the heart muscle and the viability of the muscle itself.

Disadvantages

- It's costly and not widely available.
- You may feel claustrophobic during the scanning procedure.

The next step Same as for myocardial perfusion scan.

ELECTROPHYSIOLOGY STUDIES (EPS)

General information

Where It's Done	Who Does It	How Long It Takes	Discomfort/Pain
Hospital catheterization lab or special diagnostic center.	Doctor specializing in this technique.	2–3 hours plus at least 6–8 hours of rest and observation following the test.	Minor discomfort from IV line insertion and anesthetic injection. Dye may cause flushing or burning. Arms held over the head and legs may become numb. You may have to remain in bed overnight with your weight on your groin.

Results Ready When	Special Equipment	Risks/Complications	Average Cost
A few hours to several days.	Same as for cardiac catheterization.	Same risks as for cardiac catheterization, plus the possibility of serious arrhythmia, which can usually be reversed with electric shock.	$$$

Other names Arrhythmia evaluation.

Purpose

- To evaluate people who either have or may have serious cardiac arrhythmias that are not adequately controlled by drugs. Occasionally performed to evaluate possible arrhythmia as the cause of fainting (syncope).
- Under some circumstances, performed prior to insertion of a pacemaker, defibrillator, or surgery to correct an arrhythmia.
- Used to assess the effectiveness of different drugs and drug dosages.

How it works

- Electrodes, guided into the heart during cardiac catheterization, make detailed recordings of the heart's electrical activity and pathways, and can mimic the patterns of heartbeats that lead to serious arrhythmias.
- Sometimes, a specific abnormal electrical pattern within the heartbeat causing the arrhythmia may be identified. This may be eliminated (ablated) with special radio-frequency catheters during the same procedure.

Preparation Same as for cardiac catheterization.

Test procedure When the electrodes are in place, drugs may be administered to study their effectiveness, or an abnormal electrical pathway may be destroyed.

After the test Same as for cardiac catheterization. Be alert for the recurrence of abnormal heart rhythms.

Factors affecting results

- Medication that can affect heart rhythm may alter the results.
- Other heart problems, such as heart failure or coronary disease, may require treatment before EPS is performed.

Interpretation A physician studies the heart rhythm patterns and decides the best course of treatment.

Advantages The test provides information that cannot be obtained by less invasive methods.

Disadvantages

- It's invasive.
- It carries a risk of serious arrhythmias.

The next step Treatment of the underlying problem may entail drugs, ablation of an electrical pathway, implantation of a pacemaker or automated defibrillator, or surgery.

PACEMAKER OR AICD FOLLOW-UP

General information

Where It's Done	Who Does It	How Long It Takes	Discomfort/Pain
Doctor's office or testing center.	Doctor, technician, or nurse.	A few minutes.	None.
Results Ready When	**Special Equipment**	**Risks/Complications**	**Average Cost**
Immediately or within a few days.	Telephone monitoring equipment.	None.	$

Other names Transtelephonic pacemaker monitoring, or telemetry.

Purpose To check that an implanted pacemaker or AICD (artificial implanted cardiac defibrillator) is functioning properly.

How it works

- A doctor physically examines you about two weeks after a pacemaker is implanted, and again two months later. By that time, the pacing system is usually stable, and regular follow-up tests can be planned.
- After this, you should be examined every three to 13 months, depending on the type of pacemaker or AICD.

PATIENT TIPS

- Avoid strenuous activity during the first eight weeks after a pacemaker is implanted. Use care when moving the arm on the side where the pacemaker is implanted.
- Ask your doctor about checking your pulse regularly. Take it for one full minute at rest and after exercise. If your pulse is 5 beats per minute or more below the recommended range and is accompanied by symptoms, contact your physician or monitoring clinic. A faster rate than the range is okay, but if it is more than 100 recommended beats per minute at rest, call your doctor.
- Avoid exposure to older appliances and microwave ovens that are not well insulated. Avoid frequent switching on and off of electrical equipment. Do not stand right in front of an operating microwave oven. Operating newer appliances is generally safe, but if you suspect electrical interference, move away from the appliance or shut it off.
- Avoid airport metal detectors, which can reset your pacemaker. Ask airport security personnel to physically check your person instead.
- Never have magnetic resonance imaging (MRI) scans, and try to avoid other strong magnetic fields.

Signs of Pacemaker Problems

- Original symptoms recur.
- Muscle twitches near pacemaker.
- Breathing difficulties and shortness of breath.
- Chest pain.
- Dizziness and/or fainting.
- Irritation, redness, or drainage where incision was made.
- Extensive hiccuping.
- Swelling in ankles, lower arms, wrists, or lower legs.

- Depending on the device, testing is also performed in the doctor's office or by using telemetry, a special telephone line that transmits information about the heartbeat and pacemaker function. This is done every two or three months until the pacemaker battery weakens; after that, the pacemaker should be monitored monthly.

Preparation

- You are instructed on how to use the telemetry equipment. Otherwise, the only preparation is making the telephone call.
- Preparation for an in-office follow-up is the same as for an ECG.

Test procedure The pacemaker or AICD signals and battery are checked.

After the test If the battery is failing, it must be replaced.

Factors affecting results None.

Interpretation A physician or nurse will evaluate the electronic signals from the pacemaker battery to make sure it's working properly.

Advantages Telemetry allows checking the pacemaker by phone without going to a doctor's office.

Disadvantages None.

TILT TABLE TEST

General information

Where It's Done	Who Does It	How Long It Takes	Discomfort/Pain
Hospital outpatient department.	Doctor and technician.	20–25 minutes.	Possible dizziness, nausea, and perhaps vomiting.

Results Ready When	Special Equipment	Risks/Complications	Average Cost
Immediately.	An examining table that tilts at various angles.	Test may provoke a heart attack.	$$

Other names None.

Purpose To investigate fainting episodes (syncope), many of which involve an abnormal reflex that causes a fall in blood pressure and a slow heart rate but not an arrhythmia; this condition is called neurocardiogenic syncope.

How it works Abruptly tilting your position so blood drains from your head usually provokes fainting and a fall in blood pressure and heart rate if you have neurocardiographic syncope. Medication may also be used to provoke the response.

Preparation

- An intravenous line is started.
- You are monitored with ECG leads and a blood pressure cuff. A defibrillator and other emergency measures are available.

Test procedure

- After being strapped in place with loosely fitting belts on a tilt table, you lie flat for 15 minutes and are then abruptly tilted to an 80-degree upright position.
- If no symptoms occur, the tilt may be repeated after the administration of a medication.
- An abnormal response involves a fall in blood pressure, slowed heart rate, and other symptoms of fainting or near-fainting.

After the test After a short observation period, you may resume normal activities.

Factors affecting results Other medications may affect results.

Interpretation A physician trained in electrophysiology studies and reports the response.

Advantages The test may provide the best information concerning fainting due to an abnormal reflex.

Disadvantages It should be done only in a hospital or facility where emergency resources are available.

The next step If the test is positive, the abnormal reflex is present, and specific medication will be started.

Richard J. Gusberg, MD

6 The Vascular System

Tests Covered in This Chapter

The case of John P., 80, a retired college dean:

I had been having pain in my calves on and off, so two years ago I had some tests that revealed a circulatory impairment in both my legs. My doctor explained that the pain and weakness, called claudication, is produced during physical activity because the muscles aren't getting enough blood and oxygen. He put me on drug treatment for a while, but even after I stopped it, the pain subsided and everything seemed under control for the next year or so.

Then, while on a vacation during which I'd done some strenuous hiking, my left foot suddenly went numb and cold. Although moving around seemed to get the circulation going again, I decided to see my doctor when I got back. This time the test showed significantly reduced blood flow. I was admitted to the hospital at once and scheduled for surgery. I was told that if the circulation could not be restored, I was facing loss of my leg.

The Tests John had pulse volume recordings (PVRs) and segmental leg pressure measurements (using ultrasound). These noninvasive studies help define the location and extent of the blockage. In John's case, they also confirmed that his leg was in jeopardy. The next step was an arteriogram (see chapter 3), in which a contrast dye is injected into the arteries and followed on an X-ray screen. It showed that while John's abdominal blood vessels were relatively free of atherosclerosis, the arteries in his left leg had a number of blockages causing diminished blood flow. It also confirmed the feasibility of surgery to restore the circulation.

The Outcome John had an arterial bypass, in which a superficial vein taken from the same leg was grafted on one end to an artery in his groin and on the other end to an artery in his lower calf, thus circumventing the blockages. Although he spent the day after surgery in the intensive care unit, John came through the bypass surgery quite well. The first thing he noticed was that his feet were no longer cold and the foot pain was gone. Over the next several months, his condition continued to improve, and he is now walking actively with very little residual pain.

INTRODUCTION

Every day your heart pumps 4,300 gallons of blood through your body via a complex network of blood vessels known as the vascular system. These blood vessels include arteries, which bring blood containing oxygen and nutrients to the various organs and tissues of the body, and veins, which drain the blood from the organs and tissues and carry it back to the heart. Laid end to end, all the blood vessels in your body would stretch some 60,000 miles.

Diseases of the vascular system are common and can cause significant disability and, sometimes, death. Major disorders affecting the arteries fall into several categories.

Aneurysms represent a weakness in an artery wall, commonly the aorta, the major artery exiting the heart. The area fills with blood, balloons out, and in severe cases, eventually ruptures.

Atherosclerosis, also referred to as "hardening of the arteries," results in the buildup of fatty deposits on the inside lining of the arteries, progressing to blockages that can eventually impair blood flow to the organs.

Blood clots can develop in arteries or veins, causing a blockage where they form or traveling in the bloodstream to cause a blockage elsewhere.

Disorders of the veins are much less likely to result in organ-damaging, life-threatening problems. *Inherited structural abnormalities,* which impair the efficiency with which blood drains from the legs back to the heart, are the most common condition. *Venous blood clots* can develop superficially (superficial phlebitis) and in the deep veins of the leg (deep vein thrombophlebitis). In the latter condition, blood clots may travel to the heart and lungs (pulmonary embolization) or result in chronic leg swelling (associated with ankle ulcers).

SIGNS AND SYMPTOMS

Disorders of the vascular system can cause symptoms in various parts of the body, depending on the blood vessels involved and the organs that these blood vessels supply. These signs and symptoms may be chronic and subtle or acute and dramatic, and include the following:

- *Abdominal pain,* which usually occurs after meals and is commonly associated with weight loss. It may reflect insufficient circulation to the intestine.
- *Back or flank pain,* which may indicate impaired kidney function or an acute change (or rupture) of an aortic aneurysm.
- *Bruit,* a noise or murmur heard in a blood vessel when the pulse is checked. In the neck, it often signals a blockage in the carotid artery, which carries blood to the brain. This sound, detected with a stethoscope, reflects turbulent blood flow.
- *Claudication,* pain or weakness that occurs in the calf or thigh muscle during walking or exercising, represents an insufficient supply of blood and oxygen to the exercising muscle. The pain ceases when the exercise stops.
- *Rest pain,* which is pain in the foot (usually across the instep or toes) that occurs at rest, increases when the leg is elevated, and is relieved by standing. It usually reflects markedly impaired circulation and a threatened leg.
- *Ulcers or gangrene,* which may indicate severe impairment in leg circulation, especially when these changes involve the toes.
- *Kidney failure and/or high blood pressure,* which can occur when the arteries supplying blood to the kidneys are blocked.
- *"Ministroke," or transient ischemic attack (TIA),* which may include transient blindness in an eye, speech difficulties, or weakness in an arm or leg, any of which symptoms characterizes impaired circulation to the brain. In TIA, these symptoms disappear within 24 hours. If they persist for more than 24 hours, they indicate a full-blown stroke. These problems may be caused by a correctable blockage in the carotid artery in the neck.
- *Swelling,* especially sudden swelling in the leg, which may indicate a blood clot in the deep veins (thrombophlebitis) or abnormalities in the structure of the veins themselves.

HOW YOUR DOCTOR DIAGNOSES VASCULAR SYSTEM DISORDERS

Blockages

Blockages in the blood vessels may be caused by either the buildup of plaque on the inside lining of the artery walls, a blood clot that is impeding blood flow, or a structural abnormality—or some combination of these factors. How your doctor approaches the physical examination and tests will usually be dictated by the site of your symptom but may go beyond that. For example, atherosclerosis is a diffuse process affecting many blood vessels. Although signs and symptoms might point to one affected organ, thorough evaluation might require assessment of other blood vessels and organs as well. It is also important to assess the presence and extent of risk factors, such as smoking, diabetes, high blood pressure, and high cholesterol levels, that might predispose the patient to this condition. The most common locations of blood vessel blockages are discussed below.

In the legs and surrounding vessels. Leg problems often start with claudication (see above). Although this condition usually remains stable (and only rarely progresses to limb loss), significant blockages or blood vessel problems may require attention. If the symptoms are so severe that they interfere significantly with daily living, intervention may be indicated.

After recording your history, the doctor will feel one or both of your legs, noting the temperature and color and checking pulses, and will then assess blood flow in the legs by performing pulse volume recordings (PVRs), a test that measures blood pressure in the legs and feet (see below).

If the problem has progressed to the point where you experience pain even without exercise, there may not be enough oxygen to keep the tissues and skin alive. You may develop ulcers and gangrene in your feet, particularly your toes. In this case, your doctor may also perform transcutaneous oximetry, which uses a small sensor or probe to measure how much oxygen is reaching the skin (see below). If the results show a low oxygen level and other test results are abnormal, you may be a candidate for blood vessel bypass surgery or angioplasty to restore circulation in your leg. A contrast arteriogram, which lights up the vessels like a road map, highlighting the blockage, is commonly used to verify the need for and feasibility of either treatment. Magnetic resonance angiography (MRA), though still not widely used, provides a way to look at the blood vessels without injecting any dye. It shows great promise as an adjunct to contrast arteriography in certain situations (see chapter 3 for descriptions of these tests).

If the blockage is in the iliac arteries, the two branches of the aorta (at the level of the navel) that supply the legs, you may feel pain in the thighs and hips as well as the calves. This type of blockage can also cause impotence in men.

If the blockage is *in the kidney vessels* and if the kidney doesn't get enough blood, it can produce the chemical renin, which increases blood pressure. If your doctor suspects a blockage in the renal arteries, you may undergo a captopril renal scan (see chapter 12) or a Doppler ultrasound (duplex scan). If the scan suggests a blockage in one or both of the renal arteries, a contrast arteriogram or MRA test will usually be ordered before treating the blockage (see chapter 3).

Even if kidney function is normal, high blood pressure that has developed recently, is poorly controlled with medication, or is suddenly higher may be a sign of a blocked renal artery. Your physician may check for bruits in the abdomen or flank and use ultrasound or other imaging technique to locate and define the blockage.

In the neck. A blockage in the carotid artery, a blood vessel in the neck, can lead to a stroke. Anyone at risk for stroke might display signs and symptoms such as a bruit in the neck or suffer a transient ischemic attack (see above), reflecting impaired circulation to the brain. If your physician hears a bruit in your neck and you are experiencing warning symptoms such as temporary weakness in an arm or leg, he or she would suspect a blockage of the carotid artery and order a Doppler ultrasound of your neck. If the test demonstrated narrowing consistent with the noise and symptoms, you would undergo arteriography or MRA to confirm the blockage. If you have a carotid bruit without symptoms, you might still have an ultrasound to define the severity of the underlying blockage. If the blockage is significant, contrast arteriography might then be used to confirm the diagnosis (see chapter 3 for descriptions of these tests).

In the veins. Your physician may look for a blockage caused by blood clots in the deep veins of the legs (thrombophlebitis) if you are experiencing any unexplained swelling and pain in your leg, though in many cases this type of blockage doesn't produce symptoms. The Doppler ultrasound test would confirm the location. Deep vein clots must be treated more aggressively because there is a risk that the clot will travel and cause an embolism, a blockage of blood flow, especially to the heart or lungs. Blood clots in the superficial veins to do not result in embolism to the heart or lungs.

Aneurysms

Aneurysms, the result of weakness in an arterial wall, rarely cause symptoms until they progress to a usually fatal rupture. Early detection is therefore crucial for preventing rupture. An aneurysm might be detected during a physical examination as a deep pulsation, typically in the abdomen just above the navel, or it might be discovered during an X-ray or imaging test done for some other reason. You are more likely to be monitored for an aneurysm if you have a family history of them.

Aneurysms most often involve the aorta, the major artery carrying blood away from the heart, although the diagnostic process and treatment are the same for those in less common locations. If an aortic aneurysm is suspected, your physician will recommend an abdominal ultrasound. If an aneurysm is identified, it will be treated according to its size, since larger ones are more likely to rupture. Surgery may be recommended to replace the weakened segment of the vessel, in which case you would undergo a cardiac evaluation and a more detailed evaluation of the aneurysm, including a CT scan or contrast arteriography (see chapter 3 for descriptions of these tests). If the aneurysm isn't large enough to warrant surgery, you would have periodic ultrasound evaluations to monitor it—about every three to six months to monitor its growth.

PULSE VOLUME RECORDINGS (PVRS)

General information

Where It's Done	Who Does It	How Long It Takes	Discomfort/Pain
Hospital or clinic.	Specially trained nurse or Registered Vascular Technologist.	30–45 minutes.	Mild pressure in the legs when blood pressure cuffs are inflated.
Results Ready When	**Special Equipment**	**Risks/Complications**	**Average Cost**
Preliminary results, immediately; interpretation by vascular surgeon, in a few days.	Pulse volume recorder with Doppler blood velocity detector, and blood pressure cuffs for legs.	May be inadvisable for people with deep-vein blood clots, bandages or casts that cannot be removed from the legs, trauma, or prior surgery, ulceration or other site that should not be compressed by a blood pressure cuff.	$$

Other names Vascular studies or Doppler segmental pressures.

Purpose To identify locations and extent of arterial blockages and other circulatory disorders.

How it works By noting any differences in blood pressure and flow measurements taken at various locations, it is possible to determine where blockages inhibit circulation.

Preparation

- You must refrain from smoking for at least one hour before the test.
- If you have walked to the testing place, you must rest for at least 20 minutes before the test.
- You remove any clothing covering your legs and recline on an examination table with your extremities at the same level as your heart.

Test procedure

- The technologist examines your legs and checks your pulse at several points.
- Blood pressure cuffs are placed on both arms and several points on each leg: high thigh, above the knee, at the ankle, and at the foot and toe level.
- Each cuff is inflated in turn in order to measure blood volume in the arteries.
- Clear gel is applied to the legs to help conduct sound waves.
- The blood pressure cuffs are tightened slightly, and an ultrasound transducer shaped like a pencil is held against the skin in various locations to measure blood pressure.

- You may be asked to walk on a treadmill for a few minutes wearing the ankle cuff while additional readings are taken.

After the test You are free to resume regular activities.

Factors affecting results In obese people, a standard cuff may not fit the thigh, precluding a reading at that location.

Interpretation Although preliminary test results are available immediately, a vascular surgeon will examine the blood flow and pressure measurements.

Advantages

- This test is noninvasive, painless, and inexpensive.
- It may be used repeatedly to monitor a condition or the results of treatment.

Disadvantages Results may not be definitive enough to begin treatment.

The next step

- If arterial blockages are identified, additional imaging studies (ultrasound, contrast arteriography, or magnetic resonance angiography) may be warranted to determine the best treatment.
- If no further evaluation is required, regular follow-up may be recommended to monitor your condition.
- If your skin is ulcerated, a transcutaneous oxygen measurement may be ordered to check the blood supply to the skin.

TRANSCUTANEOUS OXYGEN MEASUREMENTS

General information

Where It's Done	Who Does It	How Long It Takes	Discomfort/Pain
Hospital or clinic.	Specially trained nurse or Registered Vascular Technologist.	15–20 minutes.	None.
Results Ready When	**Special Equipment**	**Risks/Complications**	**Average Cost**
Immediately.	Transcutaneous oxygen monitor and sensors, contact gel, and adhesive collars.	None.	$

Other names $TCpO_2$ or transcutaneous oximetry.

Purpose

- To assess the severity of arterial blockage.

- To predict the potential for healing of ulcers and amputations.
- To predict the outcome of a revascularization procedure.

DID YOU KNOW?

Transcutaneous oximetry is a technique first developed for use in neonatal intensive care units to obtain data about oxygen levels in ill newborns who cannot withstand repeated blood drawings. It is particularly useful for diabetics, whose blood vessels are sometimes hard to compress, making blood pressure readings unreliable.

How it works A sensor detects oxygen emanating from the skin. As the oxygen flows through the sensor membrane to the cathode, an electrochemical reaction results in electrical current. The amount of current indicates the amount of oxygen reaching the skin.

Preparation

- You disrobe and don a hospital gown.
- The sites where sensors will be applied (chest, calf, foot, or near a wound) are wiped with alcohol, shaved if necessary, and dried. Any surgical dressings are removed.
- Three or more small electrodes are affixed to the skin with contact gel. An adhesive collar around each sensor insures that no oxygen from the surrounding air leaks into the sensor membrane.

Test procedure

- You lie quietly while tiny heaters in each sensor warm the skin to dilate the capillaries (small blood vessels).
- After about 15 minutes, the sensors detect the oxygen. The resulting current flow is measured, and its value, the oxygen level, is displayed and printed on recorder paper.

After the test

- The sensors are removed and the gel is wiped off. Any wound dressings are reapplied.
- You are free to leave and resume normal activities.

Factors affecting results Factors that inhibit the transmission of oxygen, including the following:

- Swelling of extremity.
- Obesity.
- Growths on the skin.
- Cellulitis (inflammation of connective tissue, usually the tissue just beneath the skin surface).

Interpretation Preliminary results are available as soon as the tests are completed. A vascular surgeon studies them further to assess the extent of blockage and to recommend for or against surgery.

Advantages

- It's noninvasive and painless.
- It's especially useful in people on whom pulse volume recordings and systolic pressure readings are not possible because of painful ulcers or very stiff vessels.

Disadvantages It's able to measure oxygen flow only to very small areas.

The next step

- If results indicate a blockage, contrast arteriography or MRA may be ordered to locate it and assess its extent before treatment is initiated.
- If no blockage is indicated, regular follow-up may be recommended to monitor your condition.

Lynn Tanoue, MD ■ *Jack A. Elias, MD*

7 The Respiratory System

Tests Covered in This Chapter

The case of Carole M., a 59-year-old prep school teacher:

I was diagnosed with emphysema at about age 50, but the roots of the disease go back 13 years earlier. My doctor had me take a pulmonary test, and I couldn't handle it. The report on the test said: This patient has signs of lung disease.

By that time I had been smoking at least two packs of unfiltered cigarettes a day for 17 years. I gave up the habit then and there, but the symptoms gradually worsened. The first time I truly noticed the effects was during a ski trip. I was only in my late 40s, but I found I couldn't carry the skis up a small incline. It still took me a few years to finally see my doctor, who sent me to a pulmonary specialist.

Two years after I was diagnosed, my older sister died of emphysema at age 61. She had also been a smoker, and her emphysema was really bad. At the end, she had just 10% lung capacity. Our mother had also died of the disease. The same year that my sister died, I developed acute bronchitis, then asthma.

The Tests The pulmonary specialist ordered a chest X-ray and a pulmonary function test. The latter showed that Carole had obstructive lung disease with a low lung flow rates. Although a lung biopsy is the most definitive diagnostic test for emphysema, Carole's history and symptoms were so classic that the diagnosis could be assumed. Additionally, the doctor said that Carole had asthma and chronic bronchitis.

The Outcome Even though Carole had stopped smoking 13 years before her diagnosis, the damage to her lungs was irreversible. Although she realizes that her disease, like her mother's and sister's, may be fatal, she is doing everything she can to maintain her health. She takes medication to control her asthma and chronic bronchitis. She attended a pulmonary rehabilitation program to learn special breathing exercises and methods of strengthening her diaphragm and abdominal muscles. These help her use her lungs to maximum capacity. She swims almost every day but sometimes finds it hard getting to the classroom.

Although she used to be very active, she has come to accept that there are certain things she just can't do anymore.

INTRODUCTION

The main role of the respiratory system is to bring together air and blood so that oxygen can be taken up by blood and then circulated to every cell in the body. The system also warms and filters the air and removes gases such as carbon dioxide that cannot be used by the body.

In order for oxygen to reach the cells, the air we breathe must first pass through the upper respiratory tract—the nose, throat, and voice box (larynx)—and then the lower respiratory tract—the windpipe (trachea), the airways of the lungs, and the air sacs (alveoli). This chapter focuses on the lower respiratory tract; the upper tract is covered in chapter 18, The Sensory Organs.

The lower respiratory tract begins with the trachea, which divides in the chest into two main bronchial tubes, or airways, one leading to each lung. Each bronchial tube in turn branches off into progressively smaller tubes called bronchi and then again and again into thousands of thin tubes called bronchioles. The bronchioles terminate in some 300 million tiny sacs known as alveoli, whose thin walls contain numerous blood vessels, the capillaries. It is in these interfaces between alveoli and capillaries that the gas exchange takes place: Oxygen from the inhaled air is taken up by the blood, and carbon dioxide, the waste product of metabolism, is removed and exhaled.

The lungs are enclosed by a membrane called the pleura—a two-layered sac. The inner layer is wrapped over the lung; the outer layer is attached to the inside of the chest (thoracic) wall. In a healthy person, the two layers of the pleura are in close contact and slide against each other as the lung shrinks and expands with every breath. The space between the layers, known as the pleural space or cavity, usually contains a small amount of fluid that makes the movements of the lung easy and smooth. If air accumulates in this space, however, the lung may collapse, a condition known as a *pneumothorax*.

COMMON RESPIRATORY DISORDERS

Diseases of the respiratory system are extremely common throughout the world; in the United States, they are responsible for more days missed from school or work than any other type of illness. They encompass a wide variety of disorders due to the multitude of structures that make up the respiratory system and the diversity of their functions. In general, respiratory disorders fall into one of the major categories described below.

Obstructive disorders. As their name suggests, these disorders involve obstruction or narrowing of the airways, which limits air flow through the bronchi and results in shortness of breath, wheezing, or coughing. The most common of these disorders are asthma, chronic bronchitis, and emphysema. While asthma generally is reversible, chronic bronchitis and emphysema are usually persistent. Cigarette smoking is a risk factor for the development of chronic bronchitis and emphysema.

Restrictive disorders. Diseases in this group cause the lungs to be smaller than normal. Some disorders, such as sarcoidosis and pulmonary fibrosis, are characterized by shrinking of the lung as its connective fibers turn into scar tissue. Lung size may be restricted by an abnormal shape of the chest, such as that caused by severe curvature of the spine or deformities of the ribs. Proper expansion of the lungs may be restricted by diseases of the nerves or muscles that control expansion or by diseases of the pleura. Finally, tumors or large amounts of fluids in or around the lung may interfere with its movement and reduce the volume of lung available for breathing.

Infectious disorders. The most common infection of the lower respiratory tract, bronchitis, is a result of inflammation of the airway, and can be caused by bacteria or a virus. Pneumonia, which can be caused by bacteria, viruses, fungi, or parasites, also results in inflammation of the airways and alveoli. Recurrent or chronic respiratory infections may plague people with certain chronic lung diseases, such as cystic fibrosis or bronchiectasis.

Cancer. Lung cancer is the leading cause of cancer death in both men and women. Its symptoms may include a persistent cough, bloody sputum, chest pain, and recurring pneumonia or bronchitis. However, symptoms may be absent until very late in the course of the disease. When it is discovered in advanced stages, the cure rate is generally low. Cigarette smoking is the major risk factor for the development of lung cancer.

Diseases of blood vessels in the lungs. Pulmonary hypertension, or abnormally high blood pressure in the lung, is usually unrelated to high blood pressure in the rest of the body. Its cause may be unknown or it may be due to lung tissue damage or to inflammation of blood vessels in the lung. The pulmonary circulation may also be affected by pulmonary embolism, a serious disorder in which a blood clot travels through the circulation and is trapped in a lung.

Other disorders. The lungs may not function properly because the areas in the brain that control breathing are disrupted or the nerves that supply the muscles of breathing are abnormal. There are also breathing disorders associated with sleep, the most common of which is obstructive sleep apnea, a disease characterized by temporary interruptions of breathing.

SIGNS AND SYMPTOMS OF RESPIRATORY DISEASE

The following signs and symptoms may be caused by disorders of the respiratory system:

- *Cough.* This is a defense mechanism that can help clear the airways of mucus, inhaled toxins, or a foreign body. A cough may be considered productive or nonproductive, depending on whether or not it results in the production of secretions, or sputum. A cough that persists or worsens or is accompanied by high fever, breathlessness, or bloody or copious sputum requires prompt medical attention.
- *Shortness of breath (dyspnea).* Shortness of breath may result from problems in the respiratory system, heart disease, anxiety, and numerous other conditions. When it appears suddenly, particularly if it is persistent or accompanied by other symptoms, it may signal disease and must be evaluated by a doctor.
- *Wheezing.* A high-pitched sound produced while inhaling or exhaling, wheezing occurs when the airways are narrowed or obstructed by abnormal tissue or inflammation, excessive secretions, or even an inhaled foreign body, such as a peanut. It may signal a worsening of obstructive lung disease, particularly asthma.
- *Chest pain.* Chest pain may result from problems in the lungs, pleura, or muscles and bones of the chest as well as from the heart. Chest pain may be caused by serious or relatively minor problems. Since mild chest pain may occasionally signal a life-threatening condition, this symptom must always be taken seriously. The pain may be present all the time or appear only with inhalation (pleuritic chest pain). It may signal infection if it is accompanied by a cough or fever.
- *Coughing up blood (hemoptysis).* Blood coughed up from the airways can be a frightening symptom. It may appear as a pinkish froth, mucus with a bloody streak or clot, or pure blood. It may be a result of persistent coughing or it may signal a serious respiratory disorder. Hemoptysis that does not originate from the digestive tract (in which case it is usually accompanied by nausea and vomiting), a nosebleed, or an injured gum may require immediate medical attention.
- *Cyanosis.* A bluish or purplish coloration of the skin that is most apparent around the lips and under the nails is a sign that the blood is not receiving enough oxygen. It may come on suddenly as a result of acute lung disease or gradually as lung disease progressively worsens. People who have abnormal hemoglobin or who are regularly exposed to certain toxic substances may have chronic purplish or bluish skin. (See also chapter 5.)
- *Swelling.* Swelling (edema) in your arms, legs, and ankles may be a sign of lung disease. Swelling commonly accompanies heart failure, which in turn may be associated with shortness of breath. In fact, the lungs and the heart often produce similar symptoms, and many disorders affect both organs.

- *Respiratory failure.* The most severe sign of lung problems is respiratory failure, which can be acute or chronic. In acute failure, breathing stops suddenly. This may be a result of massive infection, inflammation of the lung, cessation of the heartbeat, or severe lung disease. Chronic respiratory failure is a state in which the lungs cannot oxygenate the blood and/or remove carbon dioxide normally. Symptoms may or may not be present.

HOW YOUR DOCTOR DIAGNOSES LUNG DISEASE

If you have symptoms that suggest a respiratory disorder, your doctor will want to know about your medical history, especially any risk factors for lung disease, such as cigarette smoking, and about any family history of respiratory diseases, such as cystic fibrosis and emphysema. The doctor will ask about workplace or other exposure to materials (such as asbestos and coal) that can damage the lungs, any history of allergies, and any seasonal variation of symptoms. It will be important for you to inform your doctor of anything usual or unusual you believe may be related to your breathing.

During the physical exam, the doctor will check your blood pressure, examine your chest, listen to it with a stethoscope, and look for signs of respiratory disease. The doctor will also percuss your lungs by placing one hand on your chest and thumping it with the fingers of the other hand. The resultant vibration helps in evaluating the size and condition of the lungs.

In many cases, the doctor will also order a chest X-ray. If you have had a previous chest X-ray, the films will be compared to check for new abnormalities. Sometimes a diagnosis can be suggested at this stage or, depending on your symptoms and X-ray findings, more tests may be needed. In general, the more sophisticated and invasive tests are usually performed last.

CHEST X-RAY

General information

Where It's Done	Who Does It	How Long It Takes	Discomfort/Pain
Hospital, commercial lab, or doctor's office.	X-ray technician.	10–15 minutes.	None.
Results Ready When	**Special Equipment**	**Risks/Complications**	**Average Cost**
Several minutes to 1–2 days.	X-ray machine (portable or stationary).	Risks associated with radiation, particularly during pregnancy.	$

Other names Chest radiography, chest roentgenography, and chest films.

Purpose

- To evaluate the lungs, as well as the chest cage, for the presence of abnormalities.
- To evaluate the size of the heart.
- To establish the size and location of an abnormality prior to performing other tests, such as a biopsy.
- To screen for lung disease in people who have occupational exposure to potentially toxic substances such as asbestos.

How it works X-rays (electromagnetic energy emitted by an X-ray tube) are absorbed by the body tissue. When the tissue is exposed to special photographic film, various types of tissue show up as shadows, dark gray areas, or white opaque areas.

Preparation

- You remove clothing and jewelry above the waist and don a hospital gown.
- If your hair is long, you must pin it up on your head so that no locks hang over your chest or shoulders.

Test procedure

- The technician positions you against the X-ray machine.
- You are asked to take a deep breath and hold it without moving while an X-ray picture is taken.
- Pictures are usually taken from the front and the side. Depending on the suspected problem, additional X-rays may be taken at different angles.

After the test

- You dress and are free to leave.
- The film is processed in a developing machine, and X-ray pictures are produced.

Factors affecting results

- If you move during the test, the image may be distorted.
- Images obtained with portable X-ray machines tend to be of poorer quality than those taken with stationary X-ray equipment. Portable X-rays are usually done only if you are hospitalized and physically unable to go to the X-ray department.

Interpretation The doctor studies the X-ray picture and determines whether all chest structures look normal.

Advantages

- It's relatively inexpensive and widely available.
- It's painless and fast.

Disadvantages

- It involves exposure, although minimal, to radiation.

- It may not provide adequate information about lungs and other soft tissues.

The next step

- A normal X-ray usually requires no further testing.
- An abnormal X-ray may require monitoring (observation), confirmation by another test such as a chest CT scan or MRI, or a biopsy of the abnormality.

CHEST COMPUTED TOMOGRAPHY (CT SCAN)

For a full description of this test, see chapter 3.

Other names Computed axial tomography (CAT) scan or computed transaxial tomography

Purpose

- To obtain a better image of the lung and chest structures than with regular chest X-rays.
- To evaluate the potential spread of cancers, including lung tumors.
- To determine the anatomy of chest structures prior to surgery.

Interpretation The doctor studies the images and looks for abnormalities that may signal lung disease.

The next step

- A normal CT scan may require no further evaluation.
- An abnormal CT scan may require monitoring (observation), confirmation by another test such as an MRI or bronchoscopy, or a biopsy.

CHEST MAGNETIC RESONANCE IMAGING (MRI)

For a full description of this test, see chapter 3.

Other names Magnetic resonance scan of the thorax.

Purpose To obtain a better view of chest abnormalities detected by X-rays.

Interpretation The doctor studies the views of your chest on a display screen or on film and evaluates all chest structures.

The next step

- A normal MRI scan may require no further evaluation.
- An abnormal MRI scan may require monitoring (observation), confirmation by another test such as a CT scan or bronchoscopy, or a biopsy.

PULMONARY ANGIOGRAPHY

For a full description of this test, see chapter 3.

Other names Pulmonary arteriography.

Purpose

- To detect abnormalities in the blood vessels of the lung.
- To diagnose a pulmonary embolism.

Interpretation The doctor examines the image obtained with this test, referred to as a pulmonary angiogram, and studies the blood vessels in the lungs for the presence of malformations, narrowing, bulging, or a blood clot.

The next step

- The diagnosis or exclusion of pulmonary embolism by pulmonary angiography is definitive, and treatment is begun or continued.
- The diagnosis of other pulmonary vascular abnormalities may require further interventions.

FLUOROSCOPY

For a full description of this test, see chapter 3.

Other names Image-intensifier fluoroscopy.

Purpose

- To assess the movements of the diaphragm.
- To evaluate the movements of the lungs and other structures in the chest during breathing.

Interpretation The doctor studies the images obtained with this test and looks for abnormalities in the chest or abnormal movements of the lungs, heart, or other structures. This test is usually performed to evaluate the movement of the diaphragm.

The next step

- A normal test indicates that the diaphragm is functioning normally.
- An abnormal test may require that the diaphragm be further evaluated, or that the situation be monitored.

CHEST ULTRASOUND

For a full description of this test, see chapter 3.

Other names Chest wall ultrasonography.

Purpose To check for the presence of excessive fluid in the pleural space.

Interpretation The doctor studies the sonogram for the presence of excess fluid.

The next step

- A negative test indicates no excessive fluid.
- If excessive fluid is detected, medication may be prescribed; monitoring may be done; the fluid may be removed; or your doctor may recommend further evaluation with chest CT, bronchoscopy, or thoracoscopy.

LUNG SCAN

General information

Where It's Done	Who Does It	How Long It Takes	Discomfort/Pain
Hospital or outpatient facility.	Doctor specializing in nuclear medicine and a nuclear medicine technologist.	30–60 minutes.	Minor discomfort when radioactive material is injected intravenously.
Results Ready When	**Special Equipment**	**Risks/Complications**	**Average Cost**
Within days.	Radioactive material, oxygen mask, IV equipment, and gamma scintillation camera.	High blood pressure in the lungs may be temporarily worsened; a very small number of patients (less than 1%) may feel claustrophobic about camera.	$$

Other names Perfusion lung scan, lung perfusion scintigraphy, radionuclide pulmonary scan, and ventilation-perfusion scan.

Purpose

- To assess the ability of the lungs to ventilate (take in air) and the ability of the lungs' tiny arteries (arterioles) to receive blood.
- To detect a blood clot in an artery leading to the lung (pulmonary embolism).
- To assess the function of the lungs in anticipation of lung surgery.

How it works A gamma scintillation camera picks up radiation emitted by the radionuclide particles in your lung tissue or in the arterioles and produces an image showing which portions are receiving air and blood, which is displayed on the screen or printed out on film (for more on radionuclide scanning, see chapter 3).

Preparation

- A regular chest X-ray is usually performed within 12 hours before this test or immediately afterward to identify any abnormalities that would alter the scan.

- Before the scan, you remove clothing and jewelry above the waist.

Test procedure

- For the ventilation part of the test, you are seated and a mask is placed over your nose and mouth.
- You follow specific instructions about inhaling and exhaling, and you breathe in a combination of air and radioactive gas.
- A large scanning camera takes pictures of your chest.
- For the perfusion part of the test, radioactive material is injected intravenously through your hand or arm.
- You sit or lie down and breathe freely as the scanning camera takes pictures of your chest at various angles.
- Sometimes, SPECT (single photon emission computed tomography) technology may be used to produce a three-dimensional lung scan (see chapter 3).

> **PATIENT TIP**
>
> A very small minority of patients feel claustrophobic when the camera is held close to their face. If this bothers you, ask if you can turn your head to the side.

After the test You dress and are free to leave.

Factors affecting results

- Traces of a radioactive substance remaining from a similar test recently performed.
- The presence of pneumonia, obstructive lung disease, or structural abnormalities in the chest.
- Movement during the test will distort the image.

Interpretation If the blood flow through the lungs is normal, the radioactive material will be evenly distributed throughout the lungs. Areas where no radionuclide is seen may signal the presence of an abnormality, such as an obstruction to blood flow or a blood clot. If the airflow to the lungs is normal, radioactive gas will be evenly distributed throughout the lungs. Areas where no radionuclide is seen may signal a mechanical obstruction to airflow. Areas that retain radionuclide for a prolonged period usually indicate areas of trapped gas, such as occurs in obstructive lung disease. Results are expressed in terms of probability of a pulmonary embolism (blood clot), ranging from normal (less than 2% probability), to high (85% to 90%).

Calculation of the percent of blood flow to a given area of the lung may help your doctor predict lung function after lung surgery to remove a piece of lung or a whole lung.

Advantages

- Exposure to radiation from radionuclides is minimal.
- Adverse reactions to radionuclides are extremely rare.

- The test is helpful in the evaluation of pulmonary embolism.
- It is also helpful in preoperative evaluation of lung function.

Disadvantages

- It may detect an abnormality but fail to lead to a definitive diagnosis.
- It involves exposure, although minimal, to radiation.

The next step

- If the patient's symptoms are suggestive of an embolism and the test shows a high probability, the scan is considered a reliable indicator that there *is* an embolism, and no further testing is needed.
- If the patient doesn't have definitive symptoms and the scan is normal, the test is a reliable indicator that there is *no* embolism.
- If the patient's symptoms and the test outcome are not consistent, pulmonary angiography or other diagnostic tests may be recommended to clarify the results.

BRONCHOSCOPY

General information

Where It's Done	Who Does It	How Long It Takes	Discomfort/Pain
Hospital or surgical center.	Doctor (pulmonary specialist or chest surgeon) and radiology technician or respiratory therapist.	30 minutes to 2 hours.	Procedure may cause some irritation in the throat and/or coughing; slight discomfort when IV line is inserted.
Results Ready When	**Special Equipment**	**Risks/Complications**	**Average Cost**
2 days.	Bronchoscope and bronchoscopy instruments.	Bleeding, fever, infection (uncommon), collapse of the lung (in 2–5% of cases), cessation of heartbeat or breathing (very rare).	$$

Other names Flexible fiber-optic bronchoscopy or rigid bronchoscopy.

Purpose

- To detect or rule out structural and other abnormalities of the airways, bronchial tumors, or the presence of a foreign body.
- To obtain samples of lung secretions and tissues for analysis.
- To obtain samples of lung tissue for analysis.

How it works A thin fiber-optic tube with a light source is passed into the airways in the lungs (bronchi), allowing the doctor to see the tracheal and bronchial structures.

Preparation

- You must fast for eight to 12 hours prior to the procedure.

- You remove clothing above the waist and don a hospital gown.
- Atropine and codeine or other medication may be injected intramuscularly to dry up saliva and suppress coughing.
- A local anesthetic is sprayed into your mouth and/or nose, depending on which way the scope will be passed into your lungs (see figure 7.1). Alternatively, anesthesia is injected under your chin on both sides of your neck to numb the voice box area.

PATIENT TIPS

- If you must take medication during the fast, you may take it with small sips of water.
- Up to a week before the test, you should stop taking any medication, such as aspirin or coumarin (Coumadin), that may cause excess bleeding.

- Electrocardiography electrodes are placed on your chest for monitoring your heartbeat, a blood pressure cuff is placed on your arm, and an oximeter is attached to your finger, earlobe, or toe to measure oxygen saturation in your blood.
- A soft tube that delivers oxygen is inserted into your nose or mouth, and an intravenous (IV) infusion is placed on your arm in order to administer medications.

Test procedure

- The doctor inserts a long viewing tube, called a bronchoscope, through your nose or mouth. If it is introduced through your mouth, you are asked to hold a plastic mouthpiece called a bite block

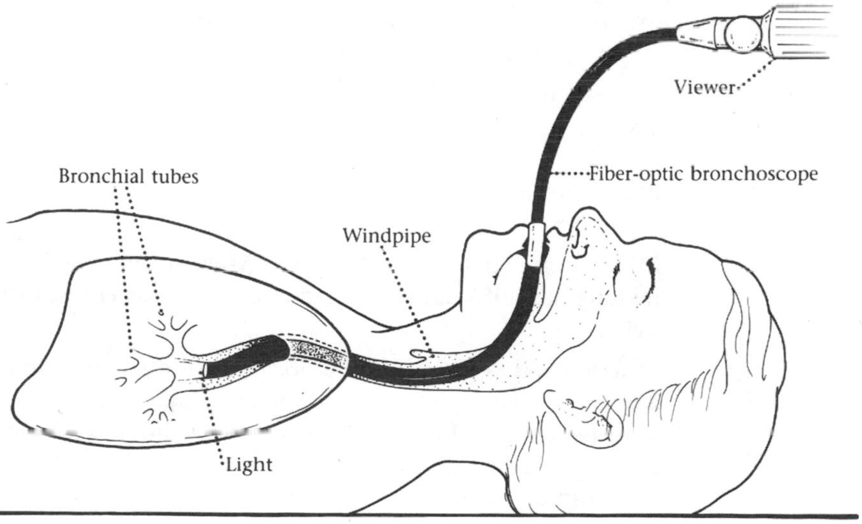

FIGURE 7.1 Bronchoscopy

This test entails inserting a viewing tube with magnifying and lighting devices through the mouth or nose and down the windpipe (trachea) and into the lung's bronchial tubes.

between your teeth, to prevent you from accidentally biting the tube. The bronchoscope is usually a flexible fiber-optic tube about the width of a pen. If a large foreign body must be removed or a large biopsy sample is required, the doctor may use a rigid bronchoscope—a hollow metal tube with a light source and a viewing device—which requires general anesthesia.

- Through the bronchoscope, the doctor inspects your voice box, windpipe, and the branches of the airways.
- Secretions from the lungs may be removed through the bronchoscope to clear the airways; the washings can be cultured or examined under a microscope.
- Bronchoalveolar lavage, in which a sterile saline solution is introduced into the lung through the bronchoscope and sucked back out, may be performed to diagnose infection or other conditions. Usually, the lavage is performed in the portion of the lung that looks abnormal on the chest X-ray.
- Bronchial brushing, in which a tiny brush on a long wire is introduced through the bronchoscope and rubbed against the airways or alveoli, may be used to obtain tissue samples from the lung. Samples are analyzed for the presence of fungi, bacteria, or other infectious agents, and for the prescence of abnormal cells.
- Tissue may also be removed (called endobronchial or transbronchial biopsy) with the help of tiny forceps. The lung has no pain sensation, but you may feel a tug when the tissue sample is removed. While the biopsy is performed, a fluoroscope, an X-ray device, may be used to visualize the lung. The picture, which is transmitted onto a TV monitor, helps the doctor guide the instruments.
- A needle may be inserted through the bronchoscope to puncture a lumph node and aspirate (withdraw) cells.
- Bronchoscopy may also be used to place radiation therapy catheters or stents.

After the test

- All monitoring equipment, the oxygen tube, and the IV infusion are removed.
- If the test included a biopsy, a chest X-ray is performed to make sure the lung has not been punctured and no air has entered the pleural cavity.
- If the test was performed under local anesthesia, you will be free to leave after sedation has worn off, which usually takes about two hours (you should have someone drive you home). If bronchoscopy was conducted under general anesthesia, you will be discharged to your hospital room or the recovery area.
- Avoid eating or drinking until the gag reflex returns, which may take two to four hours.
- You may experience hoarseness, mild fever, and coughing up small amounts of blood for about 24 hours. If you cough up large quanti-

ties of blood, have trouble breathing, have high fever, or experience pain, contact your doctor or go to a hospital emergency department immediately.

Factors affecting results Excessive coughing or gagging can interfere with obtaining adequate results or even prevent the test from being completed.

Interpretation Sometimes the doctor may establish or confirm the diagnosis simply by viewing the airways. In other cases, examinations of the tissue samples and secretions removed from the lung provide additional information.

Advantages

- The test is less invasive than surgical biopsy and can be performed on an outpatient basis.
- It requires only local anesthesia.
- It entails relatively low risk and little discomfort.
- It allows the doctor to view the airways directly.
- It produces reliable results.

Disadvantages

- It's more invasive than imaging techniques.
- The biopsy sample may be too small to diagnose some disorders, particularly noninfectious inflammatory lung diseases.
- The doctor can see only the airways, not the lung tissue itself.

The next step

- If the bronchoscopy renders a diagnosis, no further testing may be needed, and treatment can be started.
- If the bronchoscopy does *not* yield a diagnosis, further testing may be required, including surgical biopsy, needle aspiration of the lung, or further radiographic evaluation.

MEDIASTINOSCOPY

General information

Where It's Done	Who Does It	How Long It Takes	Discomfort/Pain
Hospital.	Doctor (chest surgeon) and surgical team.	1–2 hours.	Discomfort associated with general anesthesia and incision.
Results Ready When	**Special Equipment**	**Risks/Complications**	**Average Cost**
2 days.	Mediastinoscope, general anesthetic, and biopsy instruments.	Risks associated with surgery and general anesthesia.	$$

Other names Cervical or anterior mediastinoscopy.

Purpose

- To examine the mediastinum (the space between the lungs) if imaging techniques suggest that it contains an abnormality but cannot determine its nature.
- To diagnose sarcoidosis, cancers, tuberculosis, and other infections.
- To determine to what extent the cancer has spread (staging of lung or other cancer).

How it works

Fiber-optic technology allows direct viewing of the area between the lungs as well as removal of a biopsy sample.

Preparation

- Avoid eating or drinking for 12 hours before the test.
- You will receive general anesthesia. A soft breathing tube is usually inserted through your windpipe (called endotracheal intubation) to make sure you breathe properly during the procedure.

Test procedure

- A small incision is made through your skin and tissues, usually between the area of the collarbones.
- A mediastinoscope, a long tube with a light source, is introduced into the area between the lungs.
- The doctor examines the mediastinum through the viewing instrument and removes tissue samples (biopsy) from any suspicious areas.

After the test

After recovering from general anesthesia, a hospital stay of one to two days is typical. You should be able to return to regular activities within a few hours.

Factors affecting results

Accurate selection of the biopsy site.

Interpretation

The doctor observes the structures in the mediastinum. The biopsy sample removed during the procedure is examined under a microscope and provides additional information. A diagnosis may be suggested by the appearance of the mediastinum. Confirmation needs to be made pathologically. Biopsy material may also be sent for culture.

Advantages

The test allows the doctor to make definitive diagnosis of several disorders of the lung and chest.

Disadvantages

- It's invasive.
- It requires hospitalization.

The next step

- If a diagnosis is made by mediastinoscopy, decisions about treatment can be made.
- If a diagnosis is not made, further evaluation may be necessary, perhaps with other surgical biopsies.

NEEDLE BIOPSY OF THE LUNG

General information

Where It's Done	Who Does It	How Long It Takes	Discomfort/Pain
Hospital radiology department.	Radiologist and radiation technologist.	An hour or more, depending on the difficulty of reaching the right spot with the needle.	Stinging or burning associated with local anesthesia, discomfort from having to remain still, and a painful sensation when the pleura is penetrated by the needle.
Results Ready When	**Special Equipment**	**Risks/Complications**	**Average Cost**
2 days.	A long needle and an imaging device—ultrasound equipment, a fluoroscope, or a CT scanner.	Collapsed lung (20% of cases) or coughing up blood.	$$

Other names Fine-needle aspiration biopsy, transthoracic needle aspiration biopsy, transbronchial needle aspiration, and percutaneous needle aspiration.

Purpose To obtain a tissue sample to diagnose or rule out causes of localized lung masses, such as lung cancer or infection.

How it works Samples of cells or fluid are obtained for microscopic examination.

Preparation

- You must avoid eating and drinking for six to 12 hours before the procedure.
- You remove all clothing above the waist and don a hospital gown.
- Local anesthesia is applied to your skin and tissue under the skin.

Test procedure

- You lie on a scanning table on your stomach or back, depending on the location of the tissue to be biopsied.
- Local anesthesia is injected into the muscle of the chest wall.
- An imaging device such as a CT scanner or fluoroscope is used to guide appropriate placement of the needle.
- When the needle is about to penetrate the pleura, you are asked to hold your breath.
- Using a needle, the doctor aspirates (withdraws) a sample of tissue or fluid.
- The sample is sent to the laboratory for microscopic examination. A culture may be sent to detect infectious organisms (see chapter 4).

After the test

- A chest X-ray is taken to make sure you haven't developed pneumothorax (collapsed lung), which almost always goes away by itself but occasionally requires inserting a chest tube for drainage.
- You will remain in bed in the recovery area for up to three hours while your pulse, breathing, blood pressure, and temperature are monitored periodically.
- You are free to leave after the recovery period, but you should have someone drive you home. If there is a pneumothorax, observation in the hospital may be recommended.
- You may resume normal activities but should avoid heavy exertion for the first 24 hours.
- You may cough up small amounts of blood, but this should taper off and stop. If not, notify your doctor.
- Report to a hospital emergency department at once if you feel chest pain or have difficulty breathing.

Factors affecting results

- Accurate selection of the biopsy site.
- Ability to reach the abnormality with the needle.

Interpretation Examination of tissue samples obtained with this biopsy may help to detect infection, to diagnose lung cancer and determine its type, and to diagnose inflammatory disease.

Advantages It's less invasive than surgical lung biopsy.

Disadvantages

- It yields minute amounts of tissue compared with surgical lung biopsy.
- The part of the abnormality that is likely to be most helpful for diagnosis is sometimes missed.
- There are potential complications.

The next step

- If a diagnosis is made by needle biopsy, decisions about treatment can be made.
- If a diagnosis is not made, further evaluation with bronchoscopy or open surgical biopsies may be necessary.

THORACENTESIS

General information

Where It's Done	Who Does It	How Long It Takes	Discomfort/Pain
Hospital or doctor's office.	Doctor.	15–60 minutes.	Discomfort associated with local anesthesia.

Results Ready When	Special Equipment	Risks/Complications	Average Cost
1–2 days.	Needle, local anesthetics, and sometimes ultrasound or CT guidance equipment.	Collapsed lung, infection, or pain at the site of the test.	$$

Other names Pleural fluid "tap."

Purpose

- To determine the cause of abnormal accumulation of fluid in the pleural space.
- To drain large amounts of pleural fluid.

How it works A sample of the pleural fluid is analyzed in the lab for the presence of certain cells, sugar content, protein content, and other substances.

Preparation You remove all clothing from the waist up and don a hospital gown.

Test procedure

- The doctor examines your chest to locate excess pleural fluid. Ultrasound or a CT scan may be used if localization is difficult or if the amount of fluid is small.
- Local anesthesia is administered at the site of the test.
- Fluid from the pleural space is withdrawn with a long, thin needle inserted between the ribs (see figure 7.2).
- The sample is sent to a laboratory for analysis.

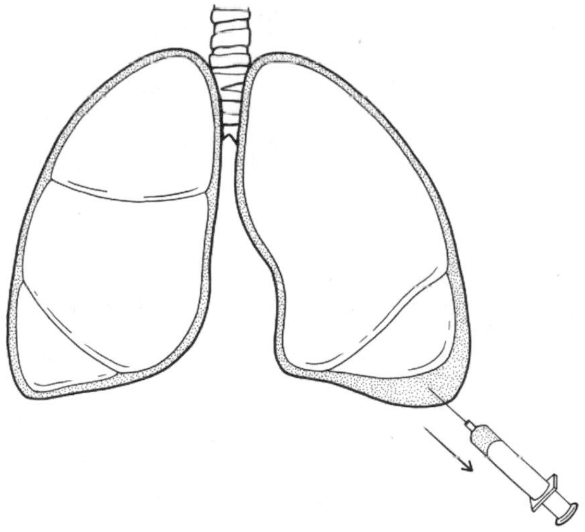

FIGURE 7.2 Thoracentesis

To do thoracentesis—or a pleural fluid tap—a thin, hollow needle is inserted between two ribs and into the space between the pleura, the membranes surrounding the lungs. If there is fluid in this space, a sample can then be withdrawn for laboratory analysis.

After the test

- Pressure is applied to the puncture site to prevent bleeding.
- An X-ray is taken to be sure the lung has not been punctured or collapsed (a condition called pneumothorax).

Factors affecting results Bleeding from the puncture site may interfere with analysis of the sample.

Interpretation The number and type of cells in the fluid, as well as the levels of glucose, acid, and various proteins, help establish whether the excess fluid is a result of infection, cancer, or other lung disease, or a complication of another disease such as congestive heart failure.

Advantages

- It's less invasive than open surgery.
- It's also easy to perform and minimally painful.

Disadvantage It doesn't always help diagnose disease inside the lung.

The next step

- If the pleural fluid analysis is diagnostic of the process causing it, treatment plans can be made.
- If the fluid is *not* diagnostic, further intervention—such as pleural biopsy, thoracoscopic evaluation, or lung biopsy—may be necessary.

THORACOSCOPY

General information

Where It's Done	Who Does It	How Long It Takes	Discomfort/Pain
Hospital.	Doctor (chest surgeon or pulmonary specialist) and surgical team.	2–4 hours.	Discomfort associated with general anesthesia; also chest discomfort after the procedure due to incision.
Results Ready When	**Special Equipment**	**Risks/Complications**	**Average Cost**
2 days.	Thoracoscope and surgical instruments; general anesthesia.	Risks associated with general anesthesia and surgery.	$$$

Other names Pleuroscopy.

Purpose

- To inspect abnormalities in the lung that require a surgical biopsy.
- To obtain lung tissue for examination to confirm or rule out lung diseases, including lung cancer.
- To investigate causes of unexplained fluid in the pleural cavity.

How it works A flexible tube that resembles a miniature telescope, a tiny camera, and surgical instruments are inserted through three tiny incisions in the chest wall, allowing the surgeon to view and take samples from the lungs.

Preparation

- Prior to the test, you will have a chest X-ray, electrocardiogram (if you are over age 35), and various blood tests. An arterial blood gas and a pulmonary function test may also be done.
- You must fast for 12 hours before the procedure.
- General anesthesia is administered, and preparations for chest surgery are made.

Test procedure

- The surgeon makes several incisions in your chest and inserts suction tubes that remove blood during the surgery.
- A bronchoscope is inserted into the airway to check for anatomical abnormalities (see the discussion of bronchoscopy above).
- A Y-shaped endotracheal tube with two inner tubes connected to a ventilator (breathing machine) is passed down the throat, and one end is inserted into each bronchus. The lung to be examined is allowed to partially deflate (during the procedure you will breathe through the other lung). This creates a space between the lung and chest wall that provides the doctor with a good view of the lung and inner chest structures.
- The thoracoscope, a viewing tube that has a light source and may be flexible or rigid, is inserted into the space between the lung and the chest wall. The camera displays the image on TV screens.
- The doctor examines the surface of the lung, makes a cut through the pleura, and removes tissue samples of the pleura and the lung. Biopsies can also be taken of any accessible structures and tissues.
- If a cancerous tumor is suspected, a biopsy sample is sent to the pathology lab for a "frozen section," the results of which are 95% accurate. If it is positive for cancer, open chest surgery may be performed to remove the malignancy and part or all of the lung. (The final pathology report takes three to seven working days.)

> **DID YOU KNOW?**
>
> In the early 1990s, thoracoscopy began replacing surgical lung biopsy in many cases, except when the patient is too ill to function temporarily on only one lung. Like open surgical lung biopsy, it requires hospitalization and general anesthesia, but the recuperation time is usually measured in days rather than weeks.

After the test

- The lung is reinflated, and two of the incisions are closed. A tube is placed in the third, which will remain in place for one to several days to remove air and fluids from the chest. When drainage of the fluid stops, the tube is removed.

- After one to two hours in the recovery room, you return to your hospital room for two to five days of recuperation.
- After discharge, refrain from lifting anything heavier than a phone book for two to three weeks.

Factors affecting results Accurate selection of the biopsy site.

Interpretation The doctor may make the diagnosis by observing the structures in the chest. The biopsy sample removed during the procedure is examined under a microscope and provides additional information. Additionally, cultures may be performed.

Advantages

- It requires a smaller incision than open lung biopsy, and a shorter recuperation time.
- It may provide definitive diagnosis.

Disadvantages

- It's invasive.
- It requires hospitalization of several days.
- It's usually used only to evaluate lesions that are close to the surface of the lung.
- It yields a smaller tissue sample than open lung biopsy.

The next step Treatment will be initiated if a disease is diagnosed.

OPEN LUNG BIOPSY

General information

Where It's Done	Who Does It	How Long It Takes	Discomfort/Pain
Hospital.	Doctor (chest surgeon and surgical team).	2–4 hours.	Discomfort associated with general anesthesia; chest discomfort afterward due to incision.
When Results Ready	**Special Equipment**	**Risks/Complications**	**Average Cost**
2 days.	Surgical instruments; breathing and suction tubes; general anesthesia.	Risks of surgery and general anesthesia (see chapter 5).	$$$

Other names Surgical lung biopsy.

Purpose

- To inspect abnormalities in the lung that require surgical biopsy.

- To obtain lung tissue for examination to confirm or rule out lung diseases, including cancer.
- To investigate causes of unexplained fluid in the pleural cavity.

How it works

- A sample of lung tissue is obtained for analysis in the laboratory for the presence of abnormal cells, infection, or inflammation.
- Prior to the test, you will have a chest X-ray, electrocardiogram, and various blood tests. An arterial blood gas and a pulmonary function test may also be done.

Preparation

- Avoid eating and drinking for 12 hours before the procedure.
- General anesthesia is administered and preparations are made for chest surgery (see chapter 5).
- A soft breathing tube is inserted through your windpipe (a procedure known as endotracheal intubation) to make sure you breathe properly during the procedure.

Test procedure

- An incision is made between two ribs near the breast bone.
- The abnormal area of the lung is identified.
- Small wedges of lung tissue are removed for microscopic and laboratory examination. A biopsy sample may be sent to the pathology lab for a frozen section. If the biopsy shows cancer, more extensive surgery may be performed to remove the tumor and all or part of the lung.
- A chest tube is placed in the pleural space to remove air and fluids, and will remain in place for several days. When drainage of air and fluids stops, the tube is removed.

> **DID YOU KNOW?**
>
> Improved imaging techniques and development of less invasive biopsy methods have greatly reduced the use of open lung biopsy.

After the test You will be taken to a recovery room for observation and to recover from anesthesia. Depending on the underlying illness, you will return to your hospital room for 3 to 7 days (average) of recuperation.

Interpretation The doctor may make the diagnosis by observing the structures in the chest. The biopsy sample will be studied microscopically; cultures may also be performed.

Advantages It provides definitive diagnosis of several disorders of the lung and chest.

Disadvantages

- It's invasive.
- It requires general anesthesia and several days of hospitalization.

The next step Treatment of underlying condition.

PULMONARY FUNCTION TESTS

General information

Where It's Done	Who Does It	How Long It Takes	Discomfort/Pain
Doctor's office, commercial pulmonary function laboratory, or hospital.	Doctor, respiratory therapist, or pulmonary lab technician.	20–45 minutes.	Test can be tiring.

Results Ready When	Special Equipment	Risks/Complications	Average Cost
Several hours to a few days.	Pulmonary function analyzer (usually includes a spirometer).	May aggravate symptoms of lung disease. Should not be performed in people with unstable asthma or respiratory distress, recent heart attack or unstable heart disease, pneumothorax, coughing up large amounts of blood, or active tuberculosis.	$

Other names Spirometry.

Purpose

- To assess the ability of the lungs to receive, hold, and use air.
- To evaluate the severity of lung disease.
- To distinguish between restrictive and obstructive lung disease.
- To monitor the course of lung disease.
- To monitor the effectiveness of treatment.

How it works The volume of air you exhale through a tube can be measured with a device called a spirometer, and is an indication of how well your lungs are functioning.

Preparation

- You must refrain from smoking or heavy eating for four to eight hours before the test.
- If possible, avoid using bronchodilators or other drugs for 24 hours prior to the test or as specified by your doctor before this test.
- Wear loose, comfortable clothing that doesn't restrict breathing.
- Your age, sex, height, and weight are recorded in order to calculate expected test values.
- A clip is placed on your nose to prevent the air from escaping through the nostrils.
- Loose-fitting dentures may be removed.

Test procedure

- You put a mouthpiece (made of cardboard or rubber, depending on the test) in your mouth and breathe normally while the technician makes sure the equipment is functioning properly (see figure 7.3).

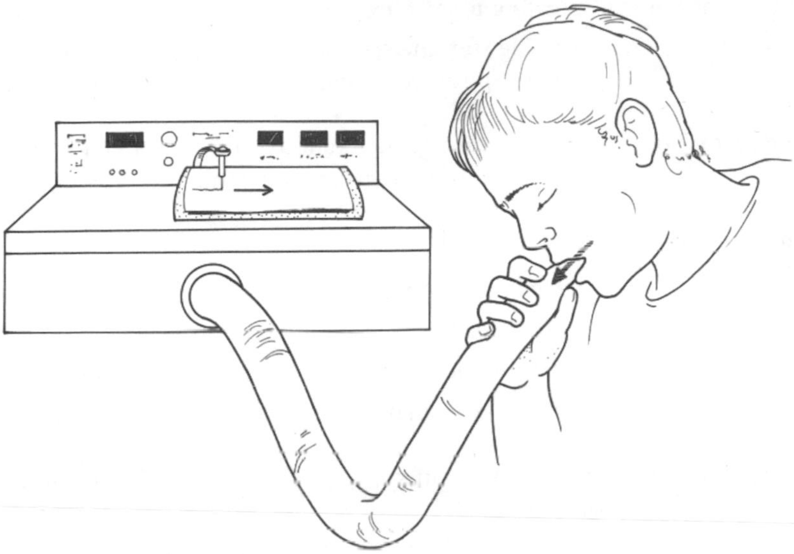

FIGURE 7.3 During pulmonary function tests (spirometry), the patient is asked to perform various breathing maneuvers by exhaling into a special mouthpiece attached to monitoring equipment.

- You perform various breathing maneuvers: taking a deep breath, holding it briefly, and forcefully blowing the air out through the mouthpiece, which is attached to a flexible tube that leads to the spirometer.
- These tests are usually repeated at least three times to make sure similar values are obtained at each attempt. Values that vary widely may indicate a technical problem.
- Various measurements are taken of the volume of air that you are able to inhale and exhale. The ability of your lungs to deliver oxygen to blood may be measured by inhaling one breath of air with a high concentration of carbon monoxide.

After the test The nose clip is removed, and you are free to leave.

PATIENT TIP

You may feel somewhat light-headed or dizzy after the test. If so, do not leave the test area alone until these symptoms disappear.

Factors affecting results

- Failure to follow instructions, such as not exhaling with maximum force.
- Anxiety or fatigue.
- Recent or current respiratory disease.
- Bronchodilators, sedatives, and other drugs that affect breathing or all body systems.
- Other procedures performed a few hours before the test, such as positive-pressure-breathing therapy.

- Time of day: pulmonary function tends to rise and then fall from morning to evening.
- Portable spirometers used at bedside tend to be less reliable than stationary spirometry equipment.

Interpretation Your test results, printed out as a table or a graph, are compared with average values for your age, sex, height, and weight.

Advantages

- It's noninvasive.
- It's reliable and reproducible.
- It produces few false-positive results.
- It provides information about pulmonary physiology.
- It provides a quantitative measure for the severity of lung disease.

Disadvantages Results may be affected by the patient's effort or understanding of instructions.

The next step The pulmonary test will be interpreted by your physician. Decisions regarding further evaluation or treatment can then be made.

BRONCHIAL CHALLENGE TEST

See also chapter 14

General information

Where It's Done	Who Does It	How Long It Takes	Discomfort/Pain
Doctor's office, commercial pulmonary function laboratory, or hospital.	Doctor, respiratory therapist, or pulmonary lab technician.	60 minutes to 2 hours.	Test can be tiring and can cause shortness of breath or other symptoms of lung disease in people with abnormally sensitive airways.
Results Ready When	**Special Equipment**	**Risks/Complications**	**Average Cost**
1–2 days.	Pulmonary function analyzer or spirometer, mouthpiece, nose clip, compressed gas nebulizers, compressed gas source, dosimeter, and various doses of methacholine solution.	Possible severe airway constriction. Should not be performed in people who have known severe asthma or whose pulmonary function measurements are significantly below normal.	$–$$

Other names Bronchial provocation test, bronchial inhalation challenge, methacholine challenge, and histamine challenge.

Purpose

- To detect asthma when it is suspected despite normal pulmonary function.
- To identify substances or exposures that trigger asthma attacks, particularly in people with occupational asthma.
- To evaluate the effectiveness of drugs in preventing airway constriction.

How it works The test replicates in a controlled setting the conditions in the environment that may be causing your airways to constrict.

Preparation

- Certain drugs, particularly bronchodilators, must be avoided prior to the test. Ask your doctor for instructions regarding specific medications.
- Do not smoke or take caffeine for six hours before the test.
- Avoid exercise and exposure to cold air for two hours before the test.

PATIENT TIP

Caffeine is found not only in coffee and tea but also in chocolate, cola drinks, and in some aspirin-combination analgesic products. These should all be avoided prior to the test because caffeine can affect test results.

Test procedure

- Baseline pulmonary function tests are performed using a spirometer (see above).
- If it is necessary to test the effectiveness of a drug in preventing airway constriction, you will receive the drug before continuing the test.
- You breathe in aerosolized methacholine through a nebulizer for about two minutes. Then, after a 30-second wait, you exhale forcefully through the mouthpiece. Methacholine is a histamine, a substance released in an allergic response. In the test, it simulates the conditions in the airways after exposure to an allergy-causing substance.
- Other substances suspected of causing airway constriction, such as chemicals in the workplace, may be used in subsequent tests (see also chapter 14). If your symptoms seem to worsen with cold air exposure, a controlled amount of cold air may be pumped into your mouthpiece instead. If exercise is suspected of triggering asthma, you will be instructed to exercise.
- Spirometry tests are repeated.
- The tests may be repeated with higher concentrations of methacholine, colder air, or after more strenuous exercise.

After the test

- You remove the nose clip, replace the dentures if necessary, and are free to resume normal activities.
- You may wheeze or cough for 30 to 60 minutes after the test, and may need a bronchodilator to decrease symptoms.

Factors affecting results

- Failure to follow instructions, such as not holding your breath or exhaling with maximum force.
- Anxiety or fatigue.
- Recent or current chest infection, a cold, or other respiratory disease.
- Bronchodilators, sedatives, and other drugs that may affect breathing.
- Other procedures, such as positive-pressure-breathing therapy, performed a few hours before the test.

Interpretation The results before and after the challenge (the tested exposure) are compared. If your lung function dropped 20% or more after exposure to cold, exercise, methacholine, or to whatever substance is used for the test, your airways are abnormally sensitive to these exposures. It is likely that in normal circumstances, that exposures or various substances that trigger allergic reactions may cause your airways to narrow and trigger asthma attacks. Diagnosis of asthma, however, can only be made after test results are correlated with your symptoms, because abnormal sensitivity of the airways may be present in various disorders, including, among others, chronic obstructive pulmonary disease, bronchiolitis, and cystic fibrosis.

Advantages It's highly reliable.

Disadvantages

- There is a risk of causing severe airway constriction.
- Results can only be interpreted in the light of symptoms.

The next step Based on the test results, your doctor may be better able to decide if treatment is needed or to adjust your treatment.

PEAK FLOW MEASUREMENT

General information

Where It's Done	Who Does It	How Long It Takes	Discomfort/Pain
At home, in a hospital, or virtually anywhere.	Patient.	Less than 1 minute.	None.

Results Ready When	Special Equipment	Risks/Complications	Average Cost
Immediately.	Peak flow meter.	May make you feel temporarily out of breath, but no real risk.	$ (only cost of meter).

Other names Peak expiratory flow.

Purpose To monitor the condition of the airways in order to monitor asthma, help predict an asthma attack, and determine when medication or emergency care is needed. Because it is a self-test, it can be done at virtually any time.

How it works The flow of air you are able to generate forcefully into a closed cylinder is an indication of whether or not your airways are constricted.

Preparation Avoid eating a heavy meal for about three hours before taking the test.

Test procedure

- Insert the mouthpiece of the peak flow meter between your teeth, and make sure your lips form a tight seal.
- Exhale strongly, with the greatest possible force.
- Repeat the maneuver at least twice, until results vary by no more than 10%.
- Record the maximum flow rate shown on the meter.

After the test If results are within 20% of your normal capacity, no special care is necessary (see Interpretation below).

Factors affecting results

- Insufficient effort on your part during the test.
- Lack of a tight seal over the mouthpiece.
- Improper handling of the peak flow meter (most devices must be held horizontally to achieve accurate measurements).

Interpretation Compare the measurements with your usual results. If they drop 20% below your average, follow your doctor's orders for taking medication or getting medical help.

DID YOU KNOW?

Peak flow measurement is a simple test that asthmatics can do to monitor themselves, thus enabling them to take preventive medication and perhaps avoid the need for emergency medical care. It is recommended for all asthmatics, and in particular for the following persons:

- People who experience severe asthma attacks with little warning.
- Those who require daily, high-dose, or low-dose inhaled corticosteriods.
- Those with wide variations (20% or more) in the peak flow rate.
- Home peak flow meters are easy enough to use that they can be used for children with asthma. Many models are small, lightweight (less than 3 ounces) cylinders that can be carried in a purse or briefcase.

Advantages

- You and your physician may be able to use peak flows to help you monitor your asthma.
- It's quick, inexpensive, and noninvasive.
- It provides valuable information for asthmatics.

Disadvantages It's reliable only if performed properly.

The next step You take your medication if it is indicated.

MOUTH PRESSURE TEST

General information

Where It's Done	Who Does It	How Long It Takes	Discomfort/Pain
Doctor's office, commercial pulmonary function laboratory, or hospital.	Doctor, respiratory therapist, or pulmonary lab technician.	5–10 minutes.	None.
Results Ready When	**Special Equipment**	**Risks/Complications**	**Average Cost**
Immediately to 1–2 days.	Electronic manometer equipped with a flexible hollow tube ending in a rubber mouthpiece, and a nose clip.	None.	$

Other names Maximum inspiratory pressure/maximum expiratory pressure or MIP/MEP.

Purpose To assess the functioning and strength of respiratory muscles when they are suspected of causing symptoms arising from the respiratory system, or if pulmonary function tests show small lung volumes.

How it works Air pressure, determined by the force with which you inhale and exhale, is recorded by a device called a manometer and reflects the strength of your respiratory muscles.

Preparation

- You put on a nose clip to prevent air from escaping through your nostrils.
- Loose-fitting dentures may have to be removed.

Test procedure

- You insert the mouthpiece between your teeth, seal your lips tightly around it, take a deep breath, and then exhale, blowing the air out as forcefully as possible. The test also requires a forceful inhalation manueuver.

- The technician records the pressure measurements shown on the manometer.
- The test is repeated three or four times to ensure that measurements are accurate.

After the test After removing the nose clip and replacing dentures if they were removed, you are free to return to previous activities.

Factors affecting results

- Failure to inhale or exhale with maximum effort.
- Lack of a tight seal over the mouthpiece.

Interpretation Weak muscles may prevent the lungs from functioning properly.

Advantages The test is quick, inexpensive, and noninvasive.

Disadvantages It detects poor function of respiratory muscles but not its cause.

The next step

- If results are abnormal, tests aimed at detecting the cause of muscle weakness may be performed.
- If results are normal, other causes of small lung volume besides neuromuscular problems will be pursued.

PULMONARY EXERCISE TESTING

General information

Where It's Done	Who Does It	How Long It Takes	Discomfort/Pain
Doctor's office, commercial pulmonary function laboratory, or hospital.	Respiratory therapist or pulmonary lab technician, under the supervision of a doctor.	1–2 hours.	A high level of exertion; people may find the test intimidating.
Results Ready When	**Special Equipment**	**Risks/Complications**	**Average Cost**
Several days.	Bicycle ergometer or treadmill, oxygen and carbon dioxide analyzers, mouthpiece and nose clips, ECG equipment, pulse oximeter, sphygmomanometer, and a wave-form analyzer or computer to process signals from measuring devices.	May aggravate symptoms of the underlying lung or heart disease. Should not be done in people with unstable asthma, chest pain, high blood pressure, or heart failure that cannot be controlled with drugs, nor in people with high fever and several other lung or heart abnormalities.	\$–\$\$

Other names Incremental exercise testing or cardiopulmonary stress test.

Purpose

- To detect an abnormality causing unexplained shortness of breath or inability to exercise. In particular, to determine whether the shortness of breath and inability to exercise is due to a heart or lung problem.
- To identify the cause of shortness of breath not revealed by pulmonary function tests, electrocardiogram, or other procedures.
- To detect lung disease that is apparent only during exercise.
- In people seeking disability evaluation, to determine the level of physical exertion they are able to achieve.

How it works Your ability to exercise under controlled conditions is an indication of heart and lung fitness and capacity. It can be measured using equipment that records your heart rate, blood pressure, and respiration.

Preparation

- Wear loose-fitting, comfortable clothing and tennis or other comfortable shoes for pedaling on an exercise bike or walking on a treadmill.
- Avoid heavy meals for at least two hours before the test.
- Your medical history, height, and weight are recorded and used to calculate the workload you are expected to achieve during the test.
- ECG electrodes are attached to your chest (the area may be shaved if necessary), a blood pressure cuff is placed on your arm, and a pulse oximeter is placed on your finger, ear, or nose.
- A clip is placed on your nose to prevent air from leaking through the nostrils.
- You are given supporting headgear to keep the mouthpiece in place during the test.

Test procedure

- You insert the mouthpiece between your teeth and make sure your lips form a tight seal (loose-fitting dentures may have to be removed).
- You start pedaling on a stationary bicycle at a given rate, or start walking on the treadmill.
- After two or three minutes, the workload is increased. The increases continue and are intended to bring you to the point of maximal exercise capacity within eight to 12 minutes.
- You stop exercising when you cannot reach maximal exercise capacity, cannot continue due to exhaustion, or because of medical reasons—for example, if the ECG shows an abnormality.
- The ECG recording is performed continuously during the test, and your blood pressure and the amount of oxygen in your blood are monitored.

- Measurements taken during the test include heart rate, breathing rate, oxygen uptake by the lungs, and the concentration of oxygen and carbon dioxide in the exhaled air. A sample of arterial blood may be drawn to determine the amounts of various gases it contains (see the description of arterial blood gases below).

After the test

- You slow down gradually to let your heart rate and breathing return to normal.
- All equipment that was attached to your body is removed, except the blood pressure cuff.
- Blood pressure is measured until it returns to normal.

Factors affecting results

- Failure to apply maximum effort during the test.
- Lack of a tight seal over the mouthpiece.
- Medications or the presence of disease.
- Ability to complete the test.

Interpretation

The doctor analyzes your oxygen consumption, carbon dioxide exhaled, and other measurements obtained during the test; correlates them with values expected for a person of your age, height, weight, and sex; and tries to establish the cause of any limitation in your ability to exercise. In disability evaluations, specific jobs are assigned levels of oxygen consumption that a worker must be able to achieve comfortably in order to be judged able to perform those jobs.

Advantages

- It's noninvasive.
- The risk of serious complications is extremely low (lower than in a cardiac stress test) because these patients normally do not have heart disease.

Disadvantages

- It cannot be performed in people who are unable to exercise.
- It detects the existence of a problem but not its cause.

The next step

- An abnormal test result may help your doctor decide which system (lungs, heart, or other) should be further evaluated.
- A normal test indicates that your lungs are not the source of the shortness of breath or inability to exercise.

BODY PLETHYSMOGRAPHY

General information

Where It's Done	Who Does It	How Long It Takes	Discomfort/Pain
Doctor's office, commercial pulmonary function laboratory, or hospital.	Doctor, respiratory therapist, or pulmonary lab technician.	20 minutes.	Some people feel claustrophobic, and some are uncomfortable breathing against a closed shutter.

Results Ready When	Special Equipment	Risks/Complications	Average Cost
Immediately to 1–2 days.	Body plethysmograph, or "body box," pneumotachograph, shutter, transducers, mouthpiece, nose clip, and oscilloscope.	None.	$–$$

Other names Airway resistance or thoracic gas volume.

Purpose

- To measure the volume of air in the lungs.
- To diagnose lung disease or assess its severity.
- To determine whether the airways are obstructed and to what extent.

How it works The test is conducted inside a tightly sealed box where changes in air pressure and volume as you inhale and exhale can be measured and compared to normal values for someone of your age, sex, height, and weight.

Preparation

- Avoid eating heavy meals for three hours before the test.
- Wear comfortable clothing that doesn't restrict breathing.
- Loose-fitting dentures may be removed.
- A clip is placed over your nose.

Test procedure

- You sit inside a plethysmograph, a glass-walled, airtight box about the size of a refrigerator, and insert the mouthpiece into your mouth with your lips sealed around it.
- The door of the plethysmograph is closed and tightly sealed.
- You breathe quietly through the mouthpiece, then are instructed to pant lightly. While you are panting, place your palms flat on your cheeks to make sure the air you exhale is leaving your mouth and not filling your cheeks instead.

- As you perform various breathing exercises, the pressure in the breathing tube and in the box are recorded.
- You will be talked through the test by a technician who is usually sitting right next to the plethysmograph.

After the test You remove the nose clip and exit the plethysmograph. You replace dentures if necessary, and are free to leave.

Factors affecting results

- Lack of a tight seal over the mouthpiece.
- Bulging of the cheeks during breathing out.

Interpretation Pressure of the exhaled air against the shutter and changes in lung volume are used to evaluate the ability of your lungs to fill up with air, and to assess the flow of air through the airways.

Advantages It's noninvasive.

Disadvantages It detects a problem but doesn't identify its cause.

The next step Test results should help your doctor more precisely understand your pulmonary physiology.

OXYGEN SATURATION

General information

Where It's Done	Who Does It	How Long It Takes	Discomfort/Pain
Doctor's office, commercial pulmonary function laboratory, hospital, or home.	Doctor, respiratory therapist, pulmonary lab technician, or patient.	About 1 minute.	None.
Results Ready When	**Special Equipment**	**Risks/Complications**	**Average Cost**
Immediately.	Pulse oximeter.	None.	$ ($$ if done on a treadmill).

Other names Pulse oximetry.

Purpose To evaluate how well the lungs are providing oxygen to the blood during rest, exercise, or a medical procedure.

How it works Oxygen concentration determines the color of the blood, which in turn determines the refraction of light that passes through the skin. A device called an oximeter analyzes the refraction to determine the blood's oxygen saturation: Well-oxygenated blood is bright red, while blood carrying less oxygen is darker.

Preparation None.

Test procedure

- The probe is attached to your finger, earlobe, or toe.
- The probe emits a light signal, which passes through the finger, earlobe, or toe.
- Because some people have poor blood oxygenation only during activity, the test may be performed while you are exercising on a stationary bicycle or treadmill.

PATIENT TIPS

Ask about the following in advance so you can be prepared:

- If exercise will be involved, wear comfortable walking or running shoes or sneakers, and loose-fitting shorts or exercise pants.
- If a finger probe will be done, do not wear nail polish.

After the test

- The clip is removed, and you are free to return to previous activities.
- After exercise, cool down gradually by walking or pedaling slowly for a few minutes. Your pulse and blood pressure may be monitored during this time until they return to normal.

Factors affecting results

- Poor circulation in the fingers, toes, or earlobe.
- Bright external light.
- Smoking can affect blood oxygenation.

Interpretation It is considered abnormal if oxygen saturation declines by more than 5% during exercise or sleep. Normal resting oxygen saturation is usually greater than 90%.

Advantages It's noninvasive, quick, and simple.

Disadvantages It has limited diagnostic value because it evaluates only oxygen saturation.

The next step Measurement of oxygen saturation will help your doctor evaluate the severity of your disease, and will determine if you need supplemental oxygen.

ARTERIAL BLOOD GASES (ABG)

General information

Where It's Done	Who Does It	How Long It Takes	Discomfort/Pain
Doctor's office, commercial pulmonary function laboratory, or hospital.	Doctor, respiratory therapist, or pulmonary lab technician.	5–10 minutes.	Puncture can be painful.

Results Ready When	Special Equipment	Risks/Complications	Average Cost
Minutes.	Blood gas syringe and needle, and blood gas analyzer.	Can cause injury to the artery (rarely).	$

Other names None.

Purpose To evaluate the lungs' ability to provide blood with oxygen and remove carbon dioxide, and to measure the acidity of the blood.

How it works The blood's acidity and concentrations of various gases in the blood can be measured in the laboratory and compared with normal values to determine how well the lungs are working.

Preparation

- The person performing the test may first check your circulation by pressing on the radial and ulnar arteries of your wrist. When the arteries are pressed, the palm will turn white; when they are released again, they will become pink and flush. Failure to flush within 5 seconds indicates decreased blood flow.
- If this test indicates that the artery on the wrist cannot be used as a puncture site, blood may be drawn from an artery elsewhere in the body.

Test procedure

- The site to be punctured is scrubbed clean, and a blood sample is drawn from the artery in a needle puncture.
- The blood sample is analyzed in a laboratory for the presence of oxygen and carbon dioxide and for pH.

After the test

- After the needle is removed from the artery, you are instructed to compress the puncture site with a sterile gauze for at least five minutes—or longer if you have clotting problems, are taking anticoagulant therapy, or are taking aspirin or an aspirinlike medication.
- A bandage is placed over the puncture site and should be kept in place for 30 to 60 minutes.

Factors affecting results

- Hyperventilation (from pain or anxiety).
- Cigarette smoking.
- Carbon monoxide inhalation.

Interpretation Abnormal measurements may signal the presence of various disorders including lung disease.

Advantages It provides immediate and accurate assessment of gases in the blood and blood acidity.

Disadvantages It's invasive.

The next step Your doctor will make an assessment of your lungs based on the ABG results. Treatment, including oxygen therapy, may be decided.

8

Robert M. Donaldson Jr, MD

The Digestive System

Tests Covered in This Chapter

The case of Ray O., a 69-year-old retiree:

> *I went for a routine rectal exam and sigmoidoscopy, as I do every year. Although my previous exams hadn't shown anything unusual, this time the doctor spotted a small, flat tumor. She tried to remove it through a colonoscope, but she couldn't, so I ended up having surgery. During the colonoscopy, however, she did find two polyps—growths that can sometimes develop into colon cancer—and she removed both of them.*

The Tests In sigmoidoscopy, a viewing tube inserted through the rectum allows the doctor to view the rectum and the lower part of the colon. In colonoscopy, a longer, flexible tube is used to view the entire colon.

The Outcome Ray's surgery successfully removed the tumor; he then underwent six weeks of radiation treatment and six months of chemotherapy. According to his doctor, he is a walking advertisement for the benefits of colon cancer screening. As in Ray's case, the most common abnormality found with sigmoidoscopy is a precancerous polyp that hasn't yet produced any symptoms.

Ray's two follow-up exams showed everything to be okay, although the radiation therapy did cause some inflammation of the colon that will eventually go away. He will continue to have annual colonoscopies for the next several years. After that, should no new polyps or cancers arise, the test will be repeated every two or three years.

INTRODUCTION

In the digestive system, food is broken down into components that can be absorbed by the body and used to produce energy and build tissues. Part of the digestive process is mechanical (grinding the food and moving it through the digestive tract), and the rest is chemical (mixing food with digestive juices and other substances).

The digestive tract is a hollow tube, 25 to 30 feet long, that starts at the mouth and ends with the anus. The food is chewed and cut into smaller pieces in the mouth and descends through the throat into a muscular tube called the esophagus. The esophagus leads to the stomach, a pear-shaped organ that churns the food and secretes gastric acids and enzymes that aid digestion.

The stomach empties into a relatively thin tube called the small intestine. The esophagus, stomach, and duodenum (the upper part of the small intestine) are referred to as the upper digestive tract. The lower digestive tract includes the rest of the small intestine and the large intestine. The large intestine consists of the 3-foot-long colon and the rectum, which is about 6 to 8 inches long and 3 to 4 inches wide. The intestines are also referred to as the bowels.

Food is propelled through the digestive tract by coordinated muscular contractions in a process known as peristalsis. In the small bowel, digestion is completed, and the nutrients and water that can be used by the body are absorbed. Undigested food passes through the colon, which absorbs the remaining water and expels solids through the rectum.

Other major organs of the digestive system include the liver, pancreas, and gallbladder. The liver is a large organ that lies in the upper right part of the abdomen. Its function is so complex that it is sometimes referred to as a chemical factory. It produces bile salts, enzymes, acids, and numerous other substances that aid digestion and play a regulatory role in body processes. It screens poisons or breaks them down and removes the waste in the bile.

The pancreas, a gland that lies beneath the stomach, produces powerful enzymes that aid in digestion and hormones that play an essential role in metabolism.

The gallbladder is a small sac located beneath the liver. Its main function is to store bile, which is required for digesting fats. The bile is transported through thin tubes, called bile ducts, that start inside the liver and connect it to the gallbladder. A large bile duct connects the gallbladder to the duodenum.

Disorders of the digestive system may result from infection, inflammation, tumors, other structural abnormalities, and disruption of the immune system. These disorders are usually grouped according to the organ they affect (see the accompanying box).

Common Digestive Disorders

- Esophagus: gastroesophageal reflux, cancer of the esophagus, esophageal diverticula
- Stomach: stomach cancer, gastritis, ulcers
- Duodenum: ulcers
- Small intestine: malabsorption syndromes, intestinal obstruction, vascular disease
- Colon: colon cancer, ulcerative colitis, diverticulitis
- Liver: hepatitis, cirrhosis, fatty liver disease, liver cancer (hepatoma)
- Gallbladder: gallstones, cholecystitis
- Pancreas: cancer, pancreatitis
- Rectum: cancer, hemmorhoids, anal fissure
- Other disorders: infections, appendicitis, Crohn's disease, peritonitis

HOW YOUR DOCTOR DIAGNOSES A DIGESTIVE DISORDER

Approaches to diagnosis of digestive system disorders vary because the system includes many organs and can give rise to numerous symptoms (see the accompanying box). Your doctor will start by taking a detailed medical history and doing a physical examination. He or she will pay close attention to your symptoms. For example, if your main complaint is abdominal pain, the most common symptom arising from the digestive system, the doctor will ask you about the location of the pain. Other questions about the pain may include the following:

- *To where does the pain radiate?* For example, pain caused by stones in the gallbladder may radiate to the chest, where it may be mistaken for a heart attack, while some ulcers may cause pain that radiates to the back.
- *Is the pain steady or cyclical?* For example, ulcer pain tends to be cyclical: it is relieved by eating but then may wake you up in the middle of the night. In contrast, pain caused by cancer is more likely to be continuous.
- *Is the pain crampy?* This kind of pain may signal intestinal obstruction because it can be caused by expansion of the smooth muscles trying to overcome the obstruction.

Other symptoms that accompany the pain may offer important clues. For example, if there is pain in the lower abdomen and changes in bowel movements, an abnormality in the large intestines is probably present. A combination of pain and fever signals inflammation and warrants immediate medical attention.

Another major diagnostic clue is bleeding from the digestive tract. The type of bleeding provides clues about its origin. For example, bright red blood in the vomit usually comes from the upper diges-

Signs and Symptoms of Digestive Disorders

- Abdominal pain
- Nausea and vomiting
- Heartburn and indigestion
- Bleeding from the digestive tract (vomiting blood or passing blood in the stool)
- Constipation
- Diarrhea
- Difficulty swallowing
- Jaundice
- Weight loss
- Intestinal gas

tive tract, which includes the duodenum. Blood darkens while it remains in the stomach; blood from the small intestine only reaches the stomach if there is a small bowel obstruction. With respect to blood passed in the stools, bright red blood comes from the lower digestive tract, and black, tarry blood from the upper. Sometimes the blood in stools is present in such small amounts that it cannot be seen with the naked eye. This so-called occult blood can be detected only with a special test.

During the physical examination, the doctor will look for tenderness in the abdomen. If it is located in the lower right part, it may signal appendicitis, and in the upper right part, gallstones or inflammation in the gallbladder. The doctor will also check the size of the liver and spleen, since these organs are often enlarged in gastrointestinal disorders. He or she will then feel for masses caused by tumors, large cysts, or impacted stool. The groin and the part of the neck behind the collarbone will be examined for signs of malignant tumors that may spread there from the abdomen. A digital rectal exam is usually part of the examination, particularly if there are changes in bowel movements or anemia, which may be caused by bleeding from the digestive tract. During the rectal exam, the doctor feels for masses in the rectum and, in males, the prostate.

If ulcerlike pain is your only symptom and there is no evidence of bleeding or other abnormalities, the doctor may prescribe treatment without ordering any imaging procedures. Tests will be ordered later if the treatment produces no relief. If, however, a serious disorder is suspected, tests may be ordered immediately.

The results of diagnostic tests and procedures must always be correlated with your symptoms because the abnormalities they reveal are not necessarily related to your disease. In fact, abnormalities in the digestive system are very common and often produce no symptoms. For example, although gallstones may cause abdominal pain, they are very common and often produce no symptoms. Even if gallstones are detected, they may not be responsible for the symptoms that prompted your visit to the doctor.

The doctor usually starts by ordering noninvasive tests, such as ultrasound or computed tomography (CT) scanning. CT scans, which reveal tumors less than an inch in diameter that cannot be felt by your doctor, are one of the major advances in the diagnosis of digestive system disorders in the past 15 to 20 years. Results of imaging tests are interpreted by a radiologist, who communicates his or her conclusions to your doctor.

If these tests do not lead to a diagnosis, endoscopy, a test that allows the doctor to look inside the digestive tract, may be performed. As thin, flexible viewing tubes have been developed and intravenous tranquilizers have made the test easier on patients, endoscopy has become more common. It also makes it possible to take a biopsy of tissues or to sample digestive fluids.

Angiography, in which a contrast dye is injected through tubes introduced into a major blood vessel, is usually the last test to be performed because it involves some risk.

If infection of the digestive tract is suspected, tests that detect infectious organisms may be performed on stools or, less commonly, blood (see chapter 22). If the infection affects the liver, liver function tests may be ordered. In the case of hepatitis, tests that determine its cause and type may be indicated. When the infection leads to abscesses of the liver or other organs, a needle aspiration may be performed to determine which type of bacteria is causing the abscess, so that appropriate antibiotics can be prescribed.

ABDOMINAL X-RAY

General information

Where It's Done	Who Does It	How Long It Takes	Discomfort/Pain
Hospital, doctor's office, or commercial X-ray facility.	Radiologist or X-ray technician.	No longer than 1 minute.	None.
Results Ready When	**Special Equipment**	**Risks/Complications**	**Average Cost**
Within 1 hour in urgent situations; within 48 hours if there is no emergency.	X-ray machine (portable or stationary).	Risks associated with exposure to radiation, although the doses are very small.	$

Other names Plain abdominal films, abdominal radiography, and KUB.

Purpose

- To determine the cause of acute abdominal pain, especially in cases of a swallowed foreign object, suspected intestinal obstruction, or a suspected perforation in the digestive tract.

- To examine the urinary tract when a kidney disorder is suspected (in which case it is referred to as KUB, which stands for kidneys, ureters, and bladder).

How it works X-rays reveal the shape of organs, foreign bodies, and the air that fills the abdominal cavity when there are holes in the walls of the digestive tract. The distribution of abdominal gases within the bowels helps reveal obstruction: the bowel will be dilated with gases up to the point of, but not beyond, the obstruction.

Preparation You remove your clothing and jewelry and don a hospital gown.

Test procedure

- The technician positions you against the X-ray machine.
- You are asked to take a deep breath and hold it while an X-ray of your abdomen is taken from the front.
- Additional X-rays may be taken from different angles. A chest X-ray may also be taken because pain in the lower part of the lungs due to lung disease may be mistaken for abdominal pain. Also, "free" air present in the abdomen (and not in the bowel where it belongs) rises to the area just below the diaphragm and is often easy to detect on a chest X-ray taken in the standing position.
- If you are unable to stand, the X-ray is performed while you are lying on one side. In this case, you will be asked to remain in this position for at least five minutes before the picture is taken to allow the "free" air to move up to the elevated side of the abdomen.
- Occasionally, a dilute contrast material is used if small bowel obstruction is suspected (see the description of contrast X-rays of the digestive tract below).

After the test

- You get dressed and are free to leave.
- The film is processed in a developing machine, and X-ray pictures are produced.

Factors affecting results

- Metal jewelry or belts may cover up structures in the abdomen.
- Moving or breathing during the test may distort the image.

Interpretation The X-ray is analyzed for the presence of abnormalities, including holes or obstructions in the various organs of the digestive tract.

Advantages

- The test is simple, quick, and noninvasive.
- It's also inexpensive and widely available.

Disadvantages

- It entails exposure to a small amount of radiation.

- If an obstruction is found, contrast dye X-rays may be required to determine its precise location.
- It may detect obstruction in the intestines but not its cause.

The next step Depending on the findings, contrast X-rays or other imaging studies, sigmoidoscopy, or colonoscopy may be recommended.

ABDOMINAL ULTRASOUND

For a full description of this test, see chapter 3.

Other names Abdominal ultrasonography.

Purpose

- To make an initial assessment of abnormalities in the gallbladder, bile ducts, liver, pancreas, spleen, digestive tract, and abdominal cavity. These abnormalities may include gallstones, cysts, tumors, abscesses, inflammation, enlargement, or changes in body tissues.
- To diagnose the presence of fluid in the abdomen, known as ascites.

> **DID YOU KNOW?**
>
> Ultrasound has now virtually replaced cholecystography as the best initial test for gallstones.

Preparation

- For ultrasound of the liver, gallbladder, pancreas, or digestive tract, you will be asked to fast overnight or for at least six hours prior to the test, which reduces bowel gas that can obscure the image and keeps the gallbladder filled with bile, making it easier to visualize its contents.
- For ultrasound of the stomach, duodenum, or small bowel, you may be given water to drink immediately before the test because these organs are better visualized if they are filled with fluids. A water enema may be used to fill the colon with fluids.
- You remove your clothing before the test and don a hospital gown.

Variations In a new approach known as *endoscopic ultrasound,* ultrasound is combined with endoscopy. In this case, a miniature ultrasound probe attached to a viewing tube called an endoscope is inserted into the digestive tract (see the description of esophagogastroduodenoscopy below). The method makes it possible to sweep the ultrasound probe over the organ that needs to be examined with minimal interference of other tissues or gas. It is particularly valuable in detecting abnormalities in organs such as the pancreas, which are difficult to examine with regular ultrasound because they are largely covered by the bowel.

Interpretation The abdominal ultrasonogram is assessed for the size, shape, and composition of different structures. In cirrhosis of the liver, ultrasound may detect changes in the way blood passes through the large vessels entering or leaving the liver. In people with jaundice, it can determine whether the disorder is caused by a blocked bile duct or by disease of the liver cells. Gallstones produce characteristic shadows on a sonogram and can be detected in the gallbladder with near-perfect accuracy.

The next step

- If liver or pancreatic disease is suspected, a CT scan may identify abnormalities not seen by ultrasound.
- If disease of common duct of gallbladder is suspected, ERCP may be necessary.

CONTRAST X-RAYS OF THE DIGESTIVE TRACT

General information

Where It's Done	Who Does It	How Long It Takes	Discomfort/Pain
Hospital, doctor's office, or commercial X-ray facility.	Radiologist.	30–60 minutes.	Many people find the barium drink or meal unpleasant; some discomfort associated with the need to assume various positions required for taking the X-rays and with having an enema.
Results Ready When	**Special Equipment**	**Risks/Complications**	**Average Cost**
Within 1 hour in urgent situations; otherwise, within 24–48 hours.	Contrast material (barium), X-ray machine, and fluoroscope.	Risks associated with radiation, particularly during pregnancy; the barium may accumulate and block the intestines if it is not removed within a day or two.	$$

Other names Gastrointestinal (GI) series; this test may include barium swallow or esophagram, upper gastrointestinal (GI) series, small bowel series (enteroclysis or small bowel enema), and colon films or barium enema.

Purpose

- To detect abnormalities in the esophagus that may be causing difficulty swallowing (barium swallow or esophagram).
- To look for the cause of stomach pain or discomfort, bloating, or belching; to detect strictures, hernia, pouches, or tumors in the esophagus; or to detect ulcers and other inflammatory conditions in the lining of the esophagus, stomach, or duodenum (upper GI series).

- To detect abnormalities of the small bowel lining, including Crohn's disease, abnormal pouches (diverticula), and tumors (enteroclysis or small bowel enema).
- To detect polyps and tumors of the colon and rectum, and to assess the type, extent, and severity of inflammatory bowel disease (colon films or barium enema).

How it works Since barium, the contrast dye used in this test, cannot be penetrated by X-rays, the cavities of organs that are filled with the dye show up on X-ray film as having a sharp, white outline, making it possible to detect structural and tissue abnormalities that cannot be seen on regular X-rays.

Preparation

- Adults should have a light, liquid meal the evening before the test and avoid food and drink after midnight. Children should have nothing to eat for four hours before the test.
- If a small bowel enema is included in the examination, a laxative or enema is given on the day before the test to clear any feces from the colon.
- If the lower GI series is performed, you may have only clear liquids starting at lunchtime on the day before the test. A drug that triggers diarrhea and rapidly cleanses the bowel is also given.
- Prior to the test, you remove all clothing and don a hospital gown.

PATIENT TIP

Clear liquids include black tea or coffee, broth or bouillon, plain jello, strained fruit juice, popsicles, water, carbonated sodas, and fruit ices, but not milk or cream.

Test procedure

- For an X-ray of the upper digestive tract, you are given a barium solution to drink. For a small bowel series, the radiologist merely follows the passage of swallowed barium along the small bowel. For a procedure called enteroclysis, or small bowel enema, barium is steadily pumped through a flexible tube that opens into the beginning of the small bowel. When the examination involves the colon and rectum, a barium enema is given.
- Once the barium is given, you are secured to a table that can be tilted to propel the barium to the appropriate part of your digestive tract. The X-rays are then taken while you are asked to keep still.
- The doctor examines your digestive organs with the help of a fluoroscope, which produces a continuous moving image. The doctor also pushes on your abdomen as part of the examination.

- If you are having a double-contrast X-ray, air is introduced into the colon during the barium enema. The air helps the barium coat the colon wall, making it possible to see small polyps and cancers.
- After the barium is expelled, X-rays may be repeated to see if the dye has been trapped by any tissues, which may signal an abnormality.
- If X-rays of the entire digestive tract are required, the barium enema is usually done first. The colon is then cleansed of barium residues, and the rest of the X-rays are done the following morning.

After the test

- You may receive a mild laxative to purge your body of barium.
- Your stools may be light-colored and chalky for one to three days after the test.

Factors affecting results

- Presence of food in the stomach or bowel.
- Movements during the test.

Interpretation

The contrast X-ray images are examined for abnormalities that may signal disease.

Advantages

- It provides a better view of abdominal organs than regular X-rays.
- It's less expensive and less invasive than endoscopy.

Disadvantages

- It entails exposure to radiation.
- There is a risk of adverse reactions to the contrast dye.

The next step

- Upper endoscopy and biopsy of the gastric antrum may be necessary to rule out the presence of *H. pylori*, bacteria that are associated with ulcers and that should be eradicated with antibiotics.
- Ulcers in the stomach may require upper endoscopy and biopsy to rule out gastric cancer.
- Others conditions may require an examination of stools for parasites or other infectious organisms.
- Still other conditions, such as the presence of polyps or other growths, may require sigmoidoscopy or colonoscopy and a biopsy to obtain an actual tissue sample for diagnosis.

CHOLECYSTOGRAPHY

General information

Where It's Done	Who Does It	How Long It Takes	Discomfort/Pain
Hospital, doctor's office, or commercial X-ray facility.	X-ray technician.	1 minute to see the gallbladder (same as plain film of abdomen). To see the gallbladder empty into the duodenum may require several films at 15-minute intervals.	None.

Results Ready When	Special Equipment	Risks/Complications	Average Cost
Within 1 hour in urgent situations; otherwise, within 24–48 hours.	Tablets containing the contrast material and an X-ray machine.	Risks associated with radiation, particularly during pregnancy; adverse reactions to the contrast dye.	$$$

Other names Oral cholecystography or gallbladder series or X-ray.

Purpose To detect gallstones or cholecystitis—an inflammation of the gallbladder—especially when a person has pain of unknown cause in the upper right abdomen.

DID YOU KNOW?

Cholecystography is now rarely performed because it has been largely replaced by ultrasound of the gallbladder.

How it works A special contrast dye is swallowed and fills the gallbladder, making it possible to detect gallstones and other abnormalities that cannot be seen on regular X-rays.

Preparation

- On the evening before the test, you take the contrast dye tablets and then fast until after the test.
- Some radiologists recommend eating a high-fat lunch on the day before the test and a fat-free dinner that evening to stimulate emptying of the gallbladder and its refilling with contrast dye. However, other radiologists believe this practice has no bearing on the effectiveness of the test.
- Prior to the test, you remove all clothing and don a hospital gown.

Test procedure

- X-rays are taken of the gallbladder, which is now filled with contrast dye.
- Every time an X-ray picture is taken, you will be instructed to breathe in and remain still. The X-rays may be repeated several times at 15-minute intervals to monitor the emptying of the gallbladder.

After the test

- You dress and are free to leave.
- If the gallbladder is not clearly seen on the X-ray, the test may be repeated the next morning after a double dose of dye tablets.

Factors affecting results

- Movement during the test.
- Failure to take a full dose of dye tablets.
- If your bowel does not absorb the contrast material, the gallbladder may not be visualized on X-ray films.

Interpretation The doctor examines the X-ray film, called a cholecystogram, for evidence of disease. Gallstones usually show up as dark spots against a bright background. If the gallbladder is sluggish or infected, other abnormalities of shape or structure may be detected.

Advantages

- It provides a better view of the gallbladder than regular X-rays.
- It also demonstrates radiolucent gallstones not seen on plain films of the abdomen.

Disadvantages

- It entails exposure to radiation.
- There is a risk of adverse reactions to the contrast dye.

The next step The gallbladder and bile ducts are often better seen with invasive procedures such as endoscopic retrograde cholangiopancreatography (ERCP).

COMPUTED TOMOGRAPHY (CT) SCAN OF THE ABDOMEN

General information

Where It's Done	Who Does It	How Long It Takes	Discomfort/Pain
Hospital or commercial X-ray facility.	A technician. Results are interpreted by a radiologist.	45 minutes to 1 hour.	Lying on a hard surface can cause discomfort in people with back problems, the contrast dye can cause a hot flush, and some people may experience anxiety during the test.
Results Ready When	**Special Equipment**	**Risks/Complications**	**Average Cost**
Within 1 hour in urgent situations; otherwise, within 24–48 hours.	CT scanner.	Risks associated with radiation, particularly during pregnancy; adverse reaction to contrast dye.	$$$

Other names Computed axial tomography of the abdomen.

Purpose

- To search for the cause of abdominal pain when simpler, less expensive tests fail to explain the symptom.
- To detect small tumors that cannot be found with other imaging methods.
- To detect cysts and abscesses.
- To evaluate the spread of cancer.
- To detect and evaluate liver disorders, including cirrhosis and fatty liver disease.
- To look for enlarged lymph nodes in the abdomen.

> **DID YOU KNOW?**
>
> The CT scan, which may be used as the initial method of diagnosis or to clarify results of other imaging tests, is one of the major ways of examining the digestive system. It is particularly valuable in examining the liver and pancreas, which are not penetrated by contrast dyes used for the imaging of the digestive tract.

How it works CT scan technology involves taking X-ray pictures of thin slices of an organ and using computers to combine these pictures into a high-resolution image, making it possible to detect even minor abnormalities (for more on CT scanning, see chapter 3).

Preparation

- If no contrast dye is used, avoid eating for two hours before the test.
- If a contrast dye is used, avoid eating for four hours before the test and drink lots of fluids on the day before the test to prevent dehydration.
- If you are 60 or older, or have atherosclerosis (clogged arteries), diabetes mellitus, or kidney disease, a blood test for serum creatinine will be performed first to determine whether the dye can be safely used.
- Children and some adults may require a sedative before the test.
- You remove all clothing and don a hospital gown.

Test procedure

- About one hour prior to the test (the timing varies with the suspected diagnosis), you may be asked to drink about 15 ounces (450 mL) of a barium solution to provide an outline of the digestive tract. In addition, contrast dye may be injected into your vein to highlight the major blood vessels in the examined area.
- You lie flat on your back on a table that is slowly moved through the hollow center of the CT scanner, a large structure equipped with an X-ray device.
- You are instructed to remain still and to hold your breath for several seconds as each picture is taken.

After the test

- In the rare event that you develop an adverse reaction to the dye, its symptoms are treated.
- You are free to dress and leave.

Factors affecting results

- Moving or breathing during the pictures may cause the images to be blurred.
- Image quality is higher in heavier people because layers of fat separating the organs sharpen the image.

Interpretation The doctor studies the images for abnormalities that may signal disease within the abdomen.

Advantages

- It provides high-quality pictures that make it possible to identify abnormalities 1 to 10.5 inches in diameter.
- It produces a better image of muscles and other soft tissues than conventional X-rays.

Disadvantages

- It's expensive and time-consuming.
- It can be uncomfortable.
- It entails greater radiation exposure than regular X-rays.
- It detects the existence of an abnormality but does not establish a definitive diagnosis.

The next step Treatment, usually surgical, if gallstones or other abnormalities are found.

RADIONUCLIDE SCANNING OF THE DIGESTIVE SYSTEM

General information

Where It's Done	Who Does It	How Long It Takes	Discomfort/Pain
Hospital or commercial X-ray facility.	Doctor or lab technician.	30–60 minutes for first scan; scans may be repeated several hours later.	Minor pain after radioactive material is injected; minor discomfort while assuming various positions required for imaging.

Results Ready When	Special Equipment	Risks/Complications	Average Cost
30–60 minutes.	Radioactive material (most commonly, technetium) and gamma scintillation camera.	Risks associated with exposure to radiation are minimal, but the test should not be performed during pregnancy.	$$$ (Cost varies greatly, depending on the individual procedure.)

Other names Gastrointestinal (GI) radionuclide imaging or GI scintigraphy.

Purpose

- *Liver scan.* To evaluate liver function by measuring how well it takes up and secretes the radioactive material. The scan may also be used to determine whether a spot detected in the liver by another procedure is a malignancy or a hemangioma (a collection of blood vessels). The spleen may also be examined, in which case the test is referred to as liver-spleen scanning.
- *Gallbladder or biliary scan.* To detect cholecystitis, an inflammation of the gallbladder, and to ascertain whether the bile ducts are open and functioning.
- *Stomach scan or gastric emptying.* To detect the cause of unexplained nausea, vomiting, bloating, or weight loss. The test helps determine whether these symptoms occur because the stomach doesn't empty properly, which may be due to mechanical obstruction, neuromuscular diseases, or disorders such as anorexia nervosa or depression. The condition (stomach not emptying properly) is also common in those who have had diabetes for a number of years.
- *Esophagus scan.* To measure the emptying rate of the esophagus. In cases of heartburn and regurgitation lasting at least one month, to look for gastroesophageal reflux, a disorder in which food and fluids back up from the stomach into the esophagus.
- *Abdominal scan.* To locate the site of bleeding into the digestive tract.

How it works

- A minute amount of radioactive material (radionuclide) is introduced into the body and taken up by the organ to be examined.
- A scanning camera called a gamma scintillation camera picks up the gamma rays emitted by the radionuclide and produces an image (for more information on radionuclide scanning, see chapter 3).

Preparation

- Depending on the organ examined, you may be asked to fast for two to 12 hours prior to the test.
- For the gastric-emptying study, you may wear your street clothes. For others, you remove all clothing and don a surgical gown.

Test procedure

- The radionuclide is introduced into your body by injection into your vein (liver, gallbladder, or abdomen scan); alternatively, you may be asked to drink a radioactive solution (esophagus scan) or eat a meal containing a radionuclide (gastric-emptying scan). For a scan to detect the site of rectal bleeding, a sample of your blood may be drawn, mixed with the radionuclide, and reinjected.
- You are positioned in front of the scintiscanner and asked to remain still while the picture is taken. If organ function is being evaluated,

the picture may be taken repeatedly at certain intervals. Scans of the stomach, for example, are performed at 15- to 30-minute intervals to assess the emptying rate of the stomach by measuring the amount of radionuclide that remains inside. For detecting bleeding in the digestive tract, which may be intermittent and can be missed on a single scan, the scan may be repeated periodically over a period of up to 24 hours.

After the test You get dressed and are free to leave.

Factors affecting results

- Residual radioactive substance from another medical procedure performed shortly before the scan.
- Movement during the test.

Interpretation The image allows a gross evaluation of the size, shape, and location of the organ. By following the movement of the radionuclide, your doctor can also evaluate whether the organ is functioning properly. For example, if the radionuclide is present only in a portion of a biliary duct, the duct may be blocked or not functioning properly. Or, if the bile ducts and the gallbladder cannot be visualized within 40 minutes of the radionuclide injection, an impaired liver may be blocking the radioactive material. The functioning of the esophagus is assessed by the speed with which it transports the radionuclide. Gastroesophageal reflux can be diagnosed when the radionuclide is shown to back up from the stomach into the esophagus.

Advantages

- It entails minimal exposure to radiation.
- Adverse reactions to radionuclide material are extremely rare.

Disadvantages It detects an abnormality but not its cause.

The next step

- Esophageal or gastric motility studies may define a functional cause of impaired emptying. Upper endoscopy may define a structural cause. Esophagoscopy may demonstrate whether reflux is associated with inflammation of the lower esophagus.
- If bleeding in the digestive tract is detected, an arteriogram may be ordered to pinpoint the exact source and location.
- If the common bile duct, but not the gallbladder, fills with the radionuclide in a patient with acute pain, a diagnosis of acute cholecystitis is virtually certain.

ABDOMINAL ANGIOGRAPHY

General information

Where It's Done	Who Does It	How Long It Takes	Discomfort/Pain
Hospital.	Radiologist assisted by X-ray technician.	30–90 minutes.	Discomfort associated with having an artery punctured and lying on a hard table; there may be a burning sensation when the contrast dye is injected.

Results Ready When	Special Equipment	Risks/Complications	Average Cost
Within 1 hour in urgent situations; otherwise, within 24–48 hours.	Fluoroscope, angiographic catheter and wires, X-ray machine, and contrast dye.	Risks associated with exposure to radiation, particularly during pregnancy; adverse reaction to the contrast dye, including kidney failure; bleeding at the puncture site; perforation of the artery; injury to the nerves; and blood clots that may form on the catheter and travel through the bloodstream.	$$$

Other names Celiac and mesenteric arteriography.

Purpose

- To diagnose blood vessel disease in the small and large intestine. Specifically, to look for a narrowed or blocked artery that may be causing pain because of an inadequate oxygen supply to the abdomen.
- To look for abnormalities in blood vessels of the liver or spleen, and to investigate the cause of increased pressure in the portal vein, the blood vessel entering the liver from the digestive organs.
- To determine whether a tumor has invaded or encased blood vessels, which helps to determine whether the tumor is operable.
- To locate the site of bleeding or an aneurysm in the digestive tract.
- As treatment, to help deliver drugs directly into liver tumors or to plug intestinal bleeding sites with artificial clots.

How it works

- Contrast dye injected into the bloodstream fills blood vessels, making it easier to visualize the vessels and the blood flow on moving X-rays.
- Be sure to tell the doctor of any allergies, especially to seafood or iodine. Otherwise, you may suffer an adverse reation to the dye.
- About one in ten patients has an adverse reaction to the dye when it is injected, becoming nauseated and possibly vomiting.

Preparation

- You consume only clear liquids for six to eight hours before the test.
- You remove all clothing and don a hospital gown.

Test procedure

- About 30 minutes before the test, you are given a sedative and a painkiller, which will leave you drowsy but able to converse.
- You lie down, and an intravenous line is attached to your arm to prevent dehydration and give drugs during the test if necessary. Your heart rate and pulse are monitored during the test.
- Anesthetic is injected at the site where the catheter is to be inserted.
- A small incision is made in the groin or thigh, and a thin catheter is inserted into a major artery in the abdomen and guided with the help of a fluoroscope toward the area to be examined.
- A contrast dye is injected through the catheter, and the doctor views the arteries while moving and still pictures (angiograms) are made for later study and interpretation.

After the test

- The catheter is removed, pressure applied to the puncture site until bleeding stops, and a bandage applied.
- You will be instructed to stay in bed for about four hours, with your legs straight. A small sandbag is usually placed over the incision for a few hours to prevent bleeding.
- Your vital signs—heart and breathing rate, blood pressure, and temperature—are monitored at regular intervals for at least four hours, and the puncture site will be examined for signs of bleeding or swelling.
- If your condition remains stable and without bleeding, you can then sit up, stand, and walk for about 15 to 30 minutes. If there is no bleeding after that, outpatients can usually leave the testing center but must be driven home.
- Before you go home, a doctor or nurse should show you how to apply pressure to stop any bleeding at the incision site. Any bleeding that lasts more than a few minutes requires emergency medical attention.
- You should refrain for a few days from overexerting the leg in which you have an incision.
- In the first few hours after the test, you will be given apple juice, water, or other clear fluids. Drink as much as you can to speed the kidney's removal of the dye from your body.

DID YOU KNOW?

Abdominal angiography is now performed less frequently because in many cases it has been replaced by less invasive procedures (such as ultrasound, CT scanning, and ERCP) that make it possible to detect tumors and other abnormalities directly. However, it may still be performed when it is necessary to actually visualize the blood traveling through the arteries and veins of the abdomen, or to provide greater anatomical detail than these other tests can provide.

Factors affecting results

- Movement during the X-rays may cause blurred images.
- Obesity and failure to fast before the test may obscure the X-rays.
- Sometimes it is impossible to place the catheter into a specific artery that needs to be examined.

Interpretation The doctor examines the angiogram for signs of disease. Normally, the arteries should be smooth and taper gradually as they branch. Narrowing, irregular borders, or bulging of the arteries may signal abnormalities. In particular, pressure exerted on the arteries may suggest the presence of tumors in the area.

Advantages The test provides an excellent view of the arteries in the abdomen.

Disadvantages

- It's invasive.
- It entails risks of bleeding or abnormal clotting.
- It also entails exposure to radiation.
- Some people experience adverse reactions to the dye.

The next step Angiography is usually the last in a series of diagnostic procedures. Surgery, laparoscopy, upper endoscopy, or colonoscopy may be required to treat any lesions that are found.

ESOPHAGOGASTRODUODENOSCOPY (EGD)

General information

Where It's Done	Who Does It	How Long It Takes	Discomfort/Pain
Hospital or outpatient endoscopy suite.	Doctor (gastroenterologist or gastrointestinal surgeon), helped by an endoscopy assistant.	About 10 minutes, plus preparation time; a little longer if a biopsy is done.	Anesthetic spray may have an unpleasant taste. Discomfort associated with swallowing the endoscope and with having air pumped into the stomach.
Results Ready When	**Special Equipment**	**Risks/Complications**	**Average Cost**
Immediately for visual findings; within 24–48 hours for biopsy results.	Fiber-optic endoscope and light source.	Perforation of esophagus or stomach, bleeding, aspiration of gastric juices into the lungs, infection, abdominal pain, and transient fever.	$$–$$$ (Cost varies depending upon extent of test.)

Other names Upper gastrointestinal (GI) endoscopy or esophagoscopy (if esophagus alone is examined).

Purpose

- To examine the inner lining of the esophagus, the stomach, and the duodenum when there are such unexplained symptoms as difficulty swallowing, diarrhea or heartburn that is not promptly relieved by drugs, persistent nausea or vomiting, vomiting blood or bloody stools, loss of appetite and weight loss, or chest pain in the absence of heart disease.
- To confirm suspected cancer of the esophagus or stomach.
- To perform a biopsy of the gastric antrum in order to identify *H. pylori* as a cause of peptic ulcer or gastritis.
- To perform a biopsy of the small bowel in cases of suspected malabsorption syndrome.
- As treatment, to control bleeding, remove polyps, dilate narrowed passages, or remove a foreign body.

How it works

- A fiber-optic viewing instrument called an endoscope is introduced into the digestive tract, allowing the doctor to view the organs of the digestive system directly.
- The endoscope has side channels that can be used to withdraw fluids, pump in air, or introduce brushes, snares, small forceps, or other devices required for obtaining tissue samples.

Preparation

- Avoid taking aspirin and other nonsteroidal anti-inflammatory drugs for one week before the test because these can cause inflammation of the stomach lining as well as increasing the risk of bleeding.
- If the test is performed on an outpatient basis, you must arrange in advance to have someone drive you home afterward.
- Avoid ingesting food and drink for eight hours before the procedure.
- You remove all clothing above the waist and don a hospital gown. Dentures must be removed as well.

Test procedure

- Your throat is sprayed with a local anesthetic to suppress the gag reflex, and you receive a sedative intravenously. You may drift off to sleep during the procedure.
- A plastic mouthpiece called a bite block is placed between your teeth to prevent you from accidentally biting the endoscope.
- You are asked to swallow the endoscope, a thin, flexible tube. The device is then guided through the esophagus and, if necessary,

PATIENT TIP

Some people fear choking on the endoscope or being unable to breathe, but there is no such danger because the device does not enter the trachea (windpipe) or interfere with the passage of air.

the stomach and duodenum while the doctor watches its progress through a tiny camera in the scope. The image may also be displayed on a TV monitor.

- Air may be blown through the endoscope into the bowels in order to dilate them and make viewing easier.
- If a sample of tissue or digestive fluid is required, the doctor may perform an *endoscopic biopsy* using tiny tools within the scope (see Variations).
- When the examination is complete, the endoscope is gradually removed from your digestive tract.

Variations While biopsies of the upper digestive tract are mostly performed during endoscopy, tissue samples from the small bowel may also be obtained using a tube that is similar to an endoscope but has no viewing lens (hence, the procedure is called a *"blind" small bowel biopsy*). The instrument is guided through the digestive tract with the help of a fluoroscope, a small X-ray machine held over the patient's abdomen. The blind biopsy allows the doctor to reach farther into the small bowel than is possible with EGD and to collect a larger piece of tissue.

After the test

- You are taken to the recovery room, and your vital signs—heart and breathing rate, blood pressure, and temperature—are monitored.
- Once the sedation wears off, which usually takes about an hour, you are free to dress and have someone take you home.
- Avoid eating and drinking until the gag reflex returns, which may take two to four hours.
- Because of the amount of air instilled into your stomach, you may experience excessive belching and flatulence for the next 24 hours. You may also experience discomfort in the throat for a few days.
- Let your doctor know immediately if you have severe abdominal pain or blood in the stools after this test.

Factors affecting results

- Uncontrolled bleeding in the digestive tract and the presence of blood, food, or antacids in the stomach may interfere with the examination.
- As is true for all endoscopic procedures, lack of cooperation on your part will interfere with the test.

Interpretation The doctor studies the lining of your digestive tract for abnormalities such as ulcers, erosions, polyps, tumors, or bleeding sites. Fluids and tissue samples obtained during the procedure are sent to a laboratory for analysis. They may be examined for the presence of infectious organisms (such as the bacterium *Helicobacter pylori*, believed to be responsible for at least some ulcers), inflammation, or cancerous cells.

Advantages

- The test provides a direct view of the lining of the bowels.
- It also makes it possible to perform a biopsy without surgery.

Disadvantages

- It's invasive and somewhat uncomfortable.
- It's also expensive.
- It makes it possible to see the inside of the digestive tract, but it does not allow viewing of solid organs such as the liver, abnormalities within the wall of the digestive tract, or the abdominal cavity outside the stomach and intestines.

ENDOSCOPIC RETROGRADE CHOLANGIOPANCREATOGRAPHY

General information

Where It's Done	Who Does It	How Long It Takes	Discomfort/Pain
Hospital or doctor's office.	Doctor (gastroenterologist).	30 minutes to 2 hours, depending on the extent of the exam and the difficulty in getting a catheter into the desired duct.	Discomfort associated with swallowing the endoscope and having air instilled into the stomach and duodenum.
Results Ready When	**Special Equipment**	**Risks/Complications**	**Average Cost**
Within 1 hour in urgent situations; otherwise, within 24–48 hours.	Endoscope, contrast dye, fluoroscope, and X-ray machine.	Inflammation of the pancreas, infection, and complications of EGD (see above). When performed by a skillful endoscopist, complications occur in about 1% of cases.	$$–$$$ (Cost varies depending on whether therapy is added.)

Other names None.

Purpose

- To detect obstructions of the bile ducts such as tumors, gallstones, and abnormal narrowings known as strictures, which may be causing pain and/or jaundice.
- To diagnose or rule out cancer or other diseases of the pancreas when a CT scan or ultrasound fails to detect abnormalities or produces uncertain results.
- To find the cause of recurrent inflammation of the pancreas when it can't be determined by other tests.
- To evaluate the pancreas before surgery is performed.

- As treatment, to remove stones from the bile ducts, dilate narrow ducts, unblock obstructions caused by tumors, or open up the muscular ring at the point where the common bile duct empties into the duodenum.

How it works

- A combination of endoscopy and contrast X-rays allows the doctor to view the main pancreatic duct and the common bile duct directly and to examine smaller ducts with contrast X-rays.
- ERCP is ordered after less invasive imaging procedures, such as CT scanning or ultrasound, have failed to lead to a definitive diagnosis.

Preparation

- Same as for EGD (see above). You may wear a T-shirt under your hospital gown if you wish.
- If you are at a high risk of certain types of heart disease, you may be given antibiotics to prevent infection because bacteria may be introduced into the bloodstream during the procedure and infect the lining of the heart. You may also be given antibiotics if your bile ducts are blocked.

Test procedure

- Your throat is sprayed with a local anesthetic to suppress the gag reflex, and you receive a sedative intravenously.
- A plastic mouthpiece called a bite block is placed between your teeth to prevent you from accidentally biting the endoscope.
- You lie on your side on an X-ray table. Grounding pads may be placed under your buttocks to protect you against an electrical shock from the X-ray equipment.
- A regular X-ray may be performed first.
- You are asked to swallow the endoscope, a flexible tube about 2½ feet long and ⅓ of an inch in diameter. The device descends through the digestive tract into the duodenum while the doctor watches its progress through a tiny camera in the scope. The image may also be displayed on a TV monitor and a fluoroscope.
- Throughout the procedure, excess saliva is suctioned from your mouth, fluids are administered intravenously, and your blood pressure and oxygen levels are monitored.

PATIENT TIPS

Although most people are able to swallow the endoscope without problems or discomfort, anxiety and the gag reflex keep others from being successful on the first try. The more attempts you have to make, the harder it is and the more likely that your throat will become sore. Try to relax and remember these tips:

- Be sure to breathe evenly.
- Tuck your chin into your chest.
- Most important, *swallow.* Because your throat has been numbed, you may not feel yourself swallow; nevertheless, make the same effort.

- Once the endoscope reaches the duodenum, a cannula (small tube) is threaded through the endoscope and into the opening of the ampulla of vater in the duodenum. Contrast dye is then injected through the cannula into the common bile duct and sometimes into the pancreatic duct.
- You may be given an injection of glucagon to calm your stomach, or of mylicon, an antigas medication.
- X-rays of the ducts are then taken.
- Air may be blown through the endoscope into the bowels in order to dilate them and make viewing easier.
- Tissue samples may be obtained for biopsy with the help of forceps or brushes passed through the endoscope.
- Gallstones may be removed, or a stent (a tubular structure that supports or widens a duct) may be inserted to allow drainage of a duct.

After the test

- Same as for EGD (see above). After the gag reflex returns, consume only clear liquids for 24 hours.
- If the ERCP was performed as part of treatment, you may be required to stay overnight in the hospital or to stay in an area where you have ready access to an emergency room in case of complications.
- If you received the antinausea medication atropine, you may experience a rapid heart rate, blurred eyesight, hives, dry mouth, or urinary retention. Contact your doctor immediately if you experience any of these symptoms.
- The procedure sometimes results in a bout of pancreatitis, an inflammation of the pancreas that can bring on significant pain. At the first sign of abdominal or back pain, contact your doctor.

Factors affecting results

- Same as for EGD (see above).
- A pancreatic or bile duct distorted by disease may be impossible to fill with contrast dye for an X-ray.

Interpretation

During the visual exam, the doctor may discover tumors, swelling, reddening, pus, or bleeding. Contrast X-rays may reveal stones and structural abnormalities. Laboratory analysis of biopsy samples can help detect infection and inflammation or establish the diagnosis of cancer.

Advantages

- The test provides a direct view of parts of the pancreatic and bile ducts.
- It makes it possible to perform a biopsy and certain treatments without surgery.

Disadvantages

- It's more invasive than CT scanning and more expensive than ultrasound.
- It may cause discomfort.

- It entails a small exposure to radiation.

The next step

- Surgical or laparoscopic treatment may be necessary.
- Further clarification with mesenteric angiography may be recommended.

SIGMOIDOSCOPY

General information

Where It's Done	Who Does It	How Long It Takes	Discomfort/Pain
Hospital or doctor's office.	Doctor (many primary care physicians are qualified to perform sigmoidoscopy but do not usually do biopsies). Also gastroenterologists and gastrointestinal surgeons.	10–30 minutes.	Discomfort associated with having endoscope inserted into the rectum and having air instilled into the bowel.
Results Ready When	**Special Equipment**	**Risks/Complications**	**Average Cost**
As soon as the test is over; if biopsies are taken, they require 48–72 hours for analysis.	Sigmoidoscope and light source.	Perforation of the rectum or colon in 1 of about 5,000–7,000 people, bleeding, infection, and pain in the lower bowels.	$$

Other names Flexible fiber-optic sigmoidoscopy or proctosigmoidoscopy.

Purpose

- As a screening test, to look for colorectal cancer or for polyps that may increase the risk of such cancer (see chapter 2).
- To look for fissures and hemorrhoids, to establish the cause of persistent bloody diarrhea, and to diagnose inflammatory bowel disease.

How it works A flexible or rigid viewing instrument called a sigmoidoscope is inserted into the rectum and part of the colon, allowing the doctor to view the lining of these organs directly.

DID YOU KNOW?

Improvements in viewing instruments have made this test much more compfortable for patients. Most doctors use a soft, flexible tube that is less than half an inch in diameter. For sigmoidoscopy, which examines the lower third of the colon, the tube is about 2 feet long; for colonoscopy (see below), it is about twice that length. Rigid sigmoidoscopy is mainly used to examine hemorrhoids and abnormalities in the anus.

Preparation

- You may be instructed to give yourself an enema and/or a laxative at home, or this may be done at the testing site.
- If you are at a high risk of heart disease, you may be given antibiotics to prevent infection, since there is a small risk that infectious organisms from the bowels may penetrate the bloodstream as a result of this procedure and may travel to the heart.
- You remove all clothing and don a hospital gown.
- Sedatives or anesthetics are usually not required.

Test procedure

- You lie on your side on the examination table, and the doctor inserts a gloved finger into your rectum to perform a digital exam.
- A viewing tube called a sigmoidoscope is lubricated and inserted into the rectum. Flexible sigmoidoscopes may be advanced up to about 25 inches into the colon.
- Air may be introduced to dilate the bowels, but in smaller quantities than during colonoscopy.
- Tissue samples for a biopsy or stool samples may be collected if necessary during the procedure. They are removed with the help of special forceps and suction devices introduced through special channels in the sigmoidoscope.

> **PATIENT TIP**
>
> If you are extremely anxious about this procedure, discuss it with your doctor ahead of time. You can be given a sedative, but you will have to arrange to have someone drive you home afterward.

After the test

- You get dressed and are free to leave. You may pass a great deal of gas after the test.
- Let your doctor know immediately if you experience abdominal pain or bleeding from the rectum. If a biopsy was performed, small amounts of blood in the stool can be expected but should not continue to appear for more than one to two hours.

Factors affecting results

- Stool in the bowels.
- Lack of patient cooperation.

Interpretation

The doctor studies the lining of your colon and rectum and looks for abnormalities, particularly polyps and bleeding sites. Any stool and tissue samples obtained are sent to a laboratory to be examined for the presence of infectious organisms, inflammation, or cancerous cells.

Advantages

- The test provides a direct view of the bowels.
- It makes it possible to perform a biopsy without surgery.

- It can be readily performed in a doctor's office without major preparation.

Disadvantages

- It's uncomfortable.
- It's somewhat invasive, although less so than EGD, ERCP, or colonoscopy.

The next step Colonoscopy if an abnormality is found; possible biopsy.

COLONOSCOPY

General information

Where It's Done	Who Does It	How Long It Takes	Discomfort/Pain
Hospital or outpatient endoscopy suite.	Doctor (gastro-enterologist, some gastrointestinal surgeons) and endoscopy assistant.	20–90 minutes, depending on the time needed to reach the colon and whether additional procedures, such as polyp removal, are involved.	Discomfort associated with having the colonoscope inserted into the rectum and colon and having air instilled into the bowel.
Results Ready When	**Special Equipment**	**Risks/Complications**	**Average Cost**
Immediately; 48–72 hours for analysis of biopsy samples.	Colonoscope and light source.	Perforation of the colon or rectum in 0.01% to 0.5% of cases, bleeding, infection, dehydration from excessive use of laxatives.	$$–$$$

Other names Lower endoscopy.

Purpose

- To evaluate tumors, narrowing of the colon, or ulcers found on contrast X-rays.
- To diagnose inflammatory bowel disease.
- To look for a cause of chronic diarrhea after less invasive tests have failed to clarify its origin.
- To establish the cause of gastrointestinal bleeding, especially in the presence of iron deficiency anemia.

PATIENT TIP

Doctors have different opinions as to when colonoscopy is appropriate, and some experts believe the procedure is overused. If your doctor suggests this test, ask why it is necessary and whether a diagnosis can be established with simpler methods.

- To rule out or diagnose malignancy in people with a family history of colon cancer or familial polyposis.
- To examine the colon of people who have undergone treatment for cancer or inflammation.
- As part of treatment, to remove colon polyps, stop bleeding, dilate narrowed passages, or remove a foreign body.

How it works A viewing instrument called a colonoscope is inserted into the colon through the rectum, allowing the doctor to view the large intestine directly. (For more on GI endoscopy, see the discussion of esophagogastroduodenoscopy above.)

Preparation

- Refrain from eating food and consume only clear liquids on the day before the test. If your exam is scheduled for the morning, consume nothing after midnight. If it is scheduled for the afternoon, follow instructions for taking your laxative.
- You will be given a special laxative (such as Phospho-Soda) to take with large quantities of water and clear liquids the day before the test. In addition, you may be given an enema on the morning of the examination.
- Avoid taking iron supplements, aspirin, and other nonsteroidal anti-inflammatory drugs for five days before the test to reduce the risk of bleeding.
- If the test is performed on an outpatient basis, you must arrange in advance to have someone drive you home afterward.
- Immediately before the test, you will be asked to remove all clothing and don a hospital gown.
- If you are at a high risk of certain types of heart disease, you may be given antibiotics to prevent infection, since there is a small risk that infectious organisms from the bowels may penetrate the bloodstream as a result of this procedure and may travel to the heart.

Test procedure

- A nurse will set up an IV line so you can be given a sedative, and will clip an oximeter on your finger to monitor the level of oxygen in your blood.
- You lie on your side on the examination table with your knees bent, and the doctor examines the rectum with a gloved finger (see figure 8.1).
- The doctor then inserts a lubricated colonoscope (a flexible endoscope about 4 feet long) into your rectum and guides it through the colon. Occasionally, a fluoroscope may be used to guide the colonoscope.
- Air may be blown into the bowels in order to dilate them, provide a better view of the lining, and make it easier to advance the colonoscope. (If the air makes you extremely uncomfortable, it can be

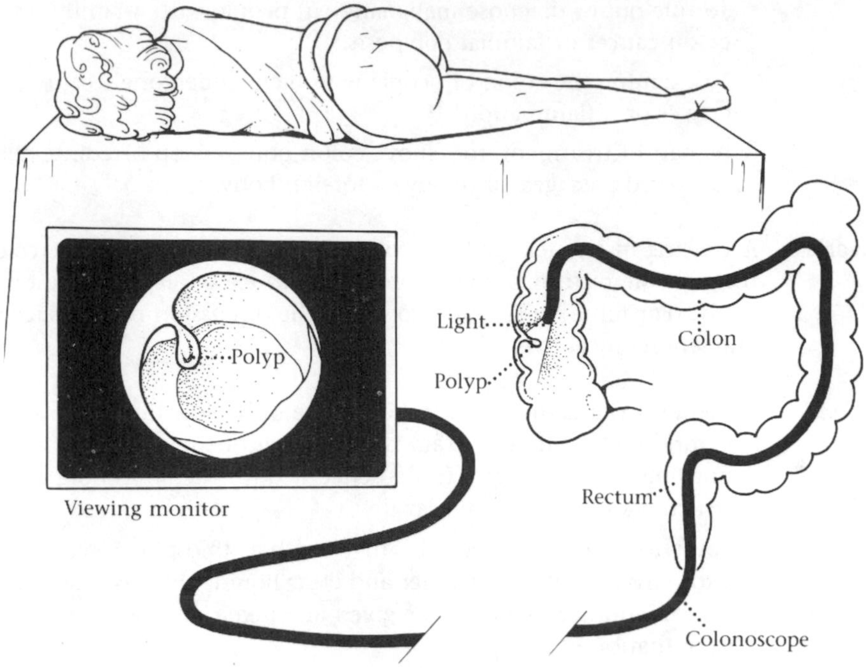

FIGURE 8.1 Colonoscopy entails inserting a flexible viewing instrument called a colonoscope into the colon, or large intestine, via the anus and rectum. During the examination, the patient usually lies on an examination table with one leg extended and the other bent at the knee. The colonoscope's special fiber-optic devices allow the doctor to view the inside of the colon; biopsy specimens and minor surgical procedures, such as the removal of small polyps, also can be done during colonoscopy.

removed.) A water jet may be used to remove solid stool or thick mucus from the lining of the colon. Blood and liquid feces may be removed from the bowels with a suction device.

- If the image obtained through the colonoscope is transmitted onto a monitor, you may be able to watch the procedure yourself. You may also be able to converse with the doctor during the test although you will be under mild sedation.
- You may have a feeling of distension and have an urge to defecate or pass gas. You may experience pain as the colonoscope is guided along the loops of the colon, but the pain is usually brief and can be somewhat alleviated by breathing slowly and deeply. While people often dread colonoscopy, many find the procedure less unpleasant than they feared.

- Tissue samples may be obtained from the lining of the colon with the help of forceps or brushes introduced through special channels inside the colonoscope. Likewise, polyps may be cauterized using electrical current and a special snare or forceps.

After the test

- Your vital signs—heart and breathing rate, blood pressure, and temperature—are checked, and you remain in the recovery area until the sedation wears off, which usually takes about an hour.
- You may pass large amounts of gas for several hours.
- Rest in bed for the remainder of the day.
- Drink only clear liquids (and no alcohol) for the next 24 hours.
- Do not take aspirin or aspirin substitutes or lift more than 5 pounds for one week.
- Let your doctor know immediately if you don't feel well or if you notice or experience significant bleeding from the rectum, severe abdominal pain or distension, black stools, or fever.

Factors affecting results

- Even small amounts of stool, blood, or mucus in the bowels may obscure the lens of the colonoscope.
- Lack of cooperation on your part will interfere with the test.

Interpretation

The doctor studies the lining of your bowels for abnormalities, including polyps, changes in color, bleeding sites, ulcers, tumors, abnormal pouches, and strictures (narrowed areas). Tissue samples obtained during the procedure are sent to a laboratory to be examined for the presence of infectious organisms, inflammation, or cancerous cells.

Advantages

- The test provides a direct view of the bowels.
- It makes it possible to perform a biopsy or remove polyps without surgery.

Disadvantages

- It's invasive.
- It involves unpleasant preparation and discomfort.
- It's also expensive and time-consuming.

The next step

If a tumor is found, biopsy, bone scans, CT scans, and treatment may be recommended.

LAPAROSCOPY

General information

Where It's Done	Who Does It	How Long It Takes	Discomfort/Pain
Hospital operating room.	Doctor (general surgeon or gastrointestinal surgeon).	30–60 minutes depending on complexity.	Discomfort associated with minor surgery.

Results Ready When	Special Equipment	Risks/Complications	Average Cost
Within 24–48 hours.	Veres needle, gas insufflator, laparoscope, and light source.	Injury or perforation of bowels, liver, spleen, ovary, gallbladder; bleeding; infection; rupture of aorta; pain in the abdomen and shoulder.	$$$

Other names Peritoneoscopy or peritoneal endoscopy.

Purpose

- To establish the cause of fluids in the abdomen.
- To examine and biopsy the liver, particularly if liver cancer is suspected.
- To determine the stage of cancer of an abdominal organ.
- As treatment, to remove the gallbladder.

How it works A rigid viewing tube called a laparoscope is inserted into the abdomen, allowing the doctor to view internal organs directly.

DID YOU KNOW?

Laparoscopy is a versatile procedure for which new uses are regularly being found. It is most commonly used to remove gallbladders and to examine female reproductive organs; less often, to diagnose diseases of the digestive system. Laparoscopy is currently being used on an experimental basis to remove the appendix and even the colon.

Preparation

- You should avoid taking aspirin and other nonsteroidal anti-inflammatory medications for several days before the test.
- Blood tests will be performed to be sure there is no infection.
- If general anesthesia is to be used, an electrocardiogram and a chest X-ray will usually be ordered first.
- Avoid ingesting food and drink for at least eight hours before the procedure.
- The part of the abdomen on which the procedure will be performed may need to be shaved.

- You will be instructed to empty your bladder before the test.
- If local anesthesia is to be used (it usually is), you will receive a mild sedative.
- You remove all clothing and don a hospital gown.

Test procedure

- You are placed on your back on the operating table.
- A special needle, known as the Veres needle, is inserted into your abdomen in the area of the navel, and air is pumped through it so that abdominal organs are easier to visualize. The needle is then removed.
- A small incision is made, and the laparoscope is introduced into the abdominal cavity. If you are not under general anesthesia, you may be asked to perform simple maneuvers during the procedure to facilitate a better view of certain abdominal structures.
- A tissue sample may be removed from the liver or other abdominal organs with the help of forceps or special instruments passed through the laparoscope.
- Once the exam is completed, the laparoscope is removed and the incision is closed with small stitches.

After the test

- Your vital signs—heart and breathing rate, blood pressure, and temperature—will be checked, and you will be observed in the recovery area for at least several hours, depending on your general condition and the extent of the procedure performed.
- You may have pain in the abdomen and right shoulder for a day or two.
- Avoid drinking carbonated beverages for about two days, as they may adversely interact with the gases introduced into your abdomen during the procedure.

Factors affecting results

- The procedure may be difficult to perform in obese people.
- Lack of cooperation on your part will interfere with the test.

Interpretation The doctor examines the appearance of abdominal organs for signs of disease, including tumors, adhesions, abscesses, foreign bodies, and inflammation. If cancer is present, the doctor can determine how far the malignancy has spread. Fluids and tissue samples are sent to the laboratory for analysis.

Advantages

- The test provides a direct view of abdominal organs from the outside.
- It makes it possible to perform a biopsy without major surgery.

Disadvantages It's invasive and uncomfortable.

The next step Additional treatment as indicated.

ESOPHAGEAL MANOMETRY

General information

Where It's Done	Who Does It	How Long It Takes	Discomfort/Pain
Hospital or doctor's office.	Nurse, supervised by gastroenterologist.	20–90 minutes.	Discomfort associated with having a catheter inserted through the nose.

When Results Ready	Special Equipment	Risks/Complications	Average Cost
Within 1 hour if urgent; otherwise, within 24–48 hours.	Manometry probe, pressure transducer, and polygraph.	Minor risk associated with insertion of a catheter through the nose, including bleeding.	$$–$$$

Other names Esophageal motility study.

Purpose

- To measure the pressure in the esophagus in cases of chronic heartburn or chest pain when there is a suspicion of gastroesophageal reflux, a disorder in which stomach acids regurgitate into the lower part of the esophagus.
- To detect the cause of difficulty swallowing when imaging tests have revealed no mechanical obstruction.
- To evaluate the function of the esophagus in disorders such as scleroderma, in which general muscle weakness may prevent the esophagus from contracting properly.

> **DID YOU KNOW?**
>
> While gastroesophageal reflux is fairly common, manometry is not done in every suspected case. Contrast X-rays and endoscopy are usually performed first, and treatment is prescribed. Only if treatment fails to relieve the symptoms are manometry and pH monitoring likely to be ordered in an attempt to establish a definitive diagnosis.

How it works The muscles of the esophagus must contract and relax normally in order to carry food from the throat to the stomach and prevent acids from backing up from the stomach into the esophagus. The amplitude and duration of contractions can be measured with a pressure transducer introduced into the esophagus.

Preparation

- You are instructed to refrain from consuming food and drink for at least eight hours before the test.
- You slip a hospital gown over your shirt or blouse.

Test procedure

- Your blood pressure and pulse are taken, and a local anesthetic is sprayed into your throat.
- You sit up straight and bring your chin down to your chest. A manometry probe—a long, thin, soft tube about the size of a pencil—is introduced through your nostrils and guided down the esophagus into the stomach (alternatively, it may be inserted via the mouth).
- You recline on your left side. After a baseline reading of the pressure in the stomach, the probe is slowly withdrawn, less than ¼ of an inch at a time, until it reaches the upper esophagus. At each point, you swallow a small amount of water, wait 30 seconds, and then swallow water again. After the second swallow, the probe measures the pressure in the esophagus and the amplitude and duration of contractions. Since the adult esophagus averages 15 inches long, the procedure takes at least an hour.
- If you have chest pain that is not due to heart disease, certain maneuvers may be performed to trigger the pain and look for its nature and cause.

After the test If you are not having a pH test (see below), you are free to return to previous activities.

Factors affecting results None.

Interpretation Information from the pressure transducer is translated into tracings that resemble an electrocardiogram; these are read by a gastroenterologist and may reveal various abnormalities in esophageal contractions. Contractions that are too long or too powerful may lead to spasms, difficulty swallowing, and pain. When they are too weak, the esophagus may not be closed off effectively, causing gastric juices to flow back and leading to gastroesophageal reflux.

Advantages The test may help explain the cause of chest pain, heartburn, or difficulty swallowing when other tests fail to lead to a diagnosis.

Disadvantages

- It's expensive.
- It's unpleasant, although less so than endoscopy.
- A high rate of false-negative results is possible.

The next step In the majority of cases, esophageal manometry is followed immediately by pH testing.

pH TESTING

General information

Where It's Done	Who Does It	How Long It Takes	Discomfort/Pain
Hospital or doctor's office.	Nurse, supervised by a gastroenterologist.	Can last 12–24 hours.	Discomfort associated with having a catheter inserted through the nose.

Results Ready When	Special Equipment	Risks/Complications	Average Cost
Within an hour if urgently needed; otherwise, within 24–48 hours.	pH electrode and meter.	Minor risks associated with inserting catheter through the nose, including bleeding.	$

Other names None.

Purpose Same as for esophageal manometry (see above).

How it works pH testing detects acidity in the esophagus, which may signal that the muscles are not functioning properly, allowing the acids to regurgitate from the stomach. While manometry evaluates muscle function directly, the pH test establishes whether the function is adequate for keeping gastric acid out of the esophagus.

Preparation

- If possible, avoid ingesting antacids, nitrates, calcium channel blockers, pain medications, and anticholinergic drugs for 24 hours prior to the procedure.
- Do not consume food and drink for at least eight hours before the test.

Test procedure

- If pH testing follows esophageal manometry, it is performed after the manometry probe is removed. A pH probe, a thin tube with a miniature pH meter at the tip, is introduced through your nose into your esophagus. A series of tests is then performed.

  Acid clearance test. A small dose of hydrochloric acid, which is similar to the normal stomach acid, is injected through the probe into the esophagus. You are asked to swallow every 30 seconds until the acidity disappears, which should normally take at least 15 swallows. If the pH is still low after 15 or so swallows (meaning that the level of acidity in the esophagus is still high), you may have a disorder in which the movements of the esophagus are disrupted.

  Bernstein test (acid perfusion test). Small amounts of liquid are infused through the probe, and you are asked whether you experience chest pain or discomfort. You will receive infusions of both hydrochloric acid and regular salt water, but you won't be told which is which.

If you experience chest pain or heartburn in response to the acid but not the salt water, you may have an inflamed esophagus. If both acid and salt water produce pain, your esophagus is probably overly sensitive. If neither produces pain, your symptoms are probably not due to esophagal inflammation caused by reflux of acid from the stomach.

Standard acid reflux test (SART). The pH in your esophagus is measured while you are asked to perform several maneuvers, such as bearing down as if having a bowel movement, or drawing your knees to the chest. The maneuvers may be performed while you are standing or lying on your back, abdomen, or right or left side. The pH is measured before and after infusion of hydrochloric acid. If acid is detected in any of the positions, you may have gastroesophageal reflux.

- After the initial series of tests, acidity in your esophagus may be monitored via the probe for another 12 or 24 hours, during which time you may have to stay in the hospital (you may be able to walk around if portable equipment is used). The acidity is continuously recorded on a paper strip while you are asked to record any symptoms you experience. The episodes in which acidity is detected are then correlated with your symptoms. Your diet will be restricted to foods that will not neutralize acidity, and you may not smoke or drink coffee or alcohol during the monitoring.

After the test You are free to return to previous activities.

Factors affecting results

- Failure to observe dietary and other restrictions during the monitoring.
- Results may be distorted if the tip of the pH meter becomes coated with mucus.

Interpretation A drop below the normal pH of 4 signals the presence of acid. The measurements are valuable in correlating subjective symptoms with objective measurements of acidity. If acidity corresponds with chest pain in at least three-quarters of the episodes, the pain is highly likely to be caused by the acid as a result of reflux.

Advantages The test may help explain the cause of chest pain, heartburn, or difficulty swallowing when other tests fail to lead to a diagnosis.

Disadvantages

- It's expensive and time-consuming.
- It's unpleasant, although less so than endoscopy.
- Hospitalization may be required.
- A high rate of false-negative results is possible.

The next step Treatment with medications.

ANORECTAL MANOMETRY

General information

Where It's Done	Who Does It	How Long It Takes	Discomfort/Pain
Hospital or doctor's office.	Doctor (gastroenterologist).	30–90 minutes.	Discomfort associated with having a probe inserted into the rectum.

Results Ready When	Special Equipment	Risks/Complications	Average Cost
Immediately.	Manometry probe or balloon manometry system, and pressure transducer.	Allergic reaction to the latex manometry balloon.	$$

Other names Anal rectal motility.

Purpose

- To evaluate the functioning of the anal canal, usually to diagnose the cause of chronic constipation or fecal incontinence.
- To confirm suspected cases of Hirschsprung's disease, in which a defect in the nerves supplying the colon causes chronic constipation.
- To confirm the cause of fecal incontinence when it is suspected that surgery or disease has injured the nerves or muscles in the anus, or when diabetes may have resulted in impaired sensation in the rectum.
- As treatment for fecal incontinence, to retrain anal muscles to contract more forcefully.

How it works A probe inserted into the anal canal measures the pressure exerted by the sphincter muscles that ring the canal and, by relaxing and contracting, control bowel movements.

Preparation

- You may be given an enema to clear any feces from the rectum.
- Children and very anxious individuals may be given a sedative.
- You disrobe and don a hospital gown.

Test procedure

- You recline on an examining table while the doctor examines your rectum with a gloved finger.
- The manometry probe, a thin tube of soft plastic or rigid metal, is inserted into your rectum about 4 inches and then slowly withdrawn halfway. As the probe is withdrawn, the transducer continuously records the pressure at different points. The measurements help locate anal sphincters, muscle rings that close the anus when they contract. Alternatively, the pressure may be measured with a balloon manometry system, a hollow metal cylinder to which three balloons are attached.

- You are asked to squeeze the anus as forcefully as possible, while pressure in the sphincters is recorded.
- A balloon at the tip of the probe is inflated, and you are asked to report whether you have a sensation that your rectum is full and you feel an urge to defecate.

After the test You are free to return to previous activities.

Factors affecting results

- Pressure in the rectum decreases somewhat with age.
- On average, the pressure is slightly higher in men than in women.

Interpretation Higher-than-normal pressure in the rectum may lead to constipation, while pressure that is too low may cause fecal incontinence. Measurements made at different points in the rectum help locate any problem in the functioning of the rectal muscles or nerves. Abnormal reflexes in the rectum may also signal disease. For example, internal sphincters should relax when the rectum is full. Failure to relax when the rectum is dilated with a balloon may indicate Hirschsprung's disease.

Advantages

- It's safe.
- It may sometimes eliminate the need for a muscle biopsy.

Disadvantages It's uncomfortable.

The next step Treatment as indicated.

NEEDLE BIOPSY

General information

Where It's Done	Who Does It	How Long It Takes	Discomfort/Pain
Hospital. May be performed in a doctor's office, but this practice is controversial.	Gastroenterologist or intervention radiologist.	30–60 minutes.	Moderately uncomfortable during needle insertion.

Results Ready When	Special Equipment	Risks/Complications	Average Cost
Usually in a few days, but can be sooner in some cases.	Biopsy needles with syringes, specimen collection containers, and sometimes an imaging device (ie, ultrasound or CT scan).	Bleeding (aspirin increases bleeding risk), leakage of bile, and injury to internal organs or blood vessels.	$$

Other names Fine-needle biopsy, liver biopsy (if a sample of liver tissue is obtained), and pancreatic biopsy (if a sample of the pancreas is obtained).

Purpose

- To confirm the diagnosis of liver cirrhosis and, if possible, establish its cause.
- To diagnose other liver disorders, including chronic hepatitis and cancer.
- To detect the cause of liver enlargement when less invasive tests fail to find a cause.
- To examine a suspected growth of the pancreas detected on a CT scan.

How it works

- For organs, primarily the liver and pancreas, that lie outside the digestive tract and cannot be reached with endoscopy, diagnosis can sometimes be made by extracting a tissue sample via a fine needle and sending it to a laboratory to be analyzed for signs of abnormalities, including infection, inflammation, and cancer.

Preparation

- Do not consume food and drink for at least 12 hours before the test.
- You will be asked to empty your bladder immediately before the test.
- You remove your clothing and don a hospital gown.

Test procedure

- You lie on your back on a table, and local anesthetic is injected at the site of the needle puncture.
- The biopsy needle is inserted into the organ to be biopsied. Ultrasound equipment or a CT scan may be used to guide placement of the needle.
- You may be asked to exhale and hold your breath when the needle is inserted to reduce the risk of a punctured lung.
- Suction is applied to the syringe, and a thin wedge of tissue is aspirated (withdrawn) through the needle, a procedure that lasts about 1 second.
- The needle may be inserted at several sites to obtain samples from different parts of the organ.

After the test

- Pressure is applied to the puncture site to control bleeding, and an adhesive bandage is placed over it.
- Your heart and breathing rate, blood pressure, and temperature are monitored in a recovery area until it is certain you have no complications.
- You are instructed to stay in bed for 24 hours. If a liver biopsy was performed, you will have to lie on your right side for the first two hours.
- Consume only clear liquids for several hours, then full liquids for 12 to 24 hours.

- Nearly half of patients have pain after the test, usually in the right shoulder, which may last one to two days.

Factors affecting results

- Failure to fast before the test.
- Obesity.

Interpretation The tissue sample is stained with various dyes and examined under a microscope. Abnormal patterns observed in the sample may be characteristic of various conditions, including infection, inflammation, and cancer.

Advantages It provides a tissue sample without surgery.

Disadvantages

- It's invasive.
- It yields minute amounts of tissue compared with a biopsy performed during surgery. As a result, the abnormality or the part of the abnormality that is likely to be most revealing for diagnosis may be missed.

The next step Possible surgical exploration and treatment.

PARACENTESIS

General information

Where It's Done	Who Does It	How Long It Takes	Discomfort/Pain
Hospital or doctor's office.	Doctor.	5–20 minutes for diagnostic purposes; longer for treatment.	Mild local pain.
When Results Ready	**Special Equipment**	**Risks/Complications**	**Average Cost**
24–72 hours.	Needle, syringe, and catheter; collecting bottles.	Needle injury to internal organs or blood vessels, bleeding, swelling, infection, and drop in blood pressure when large amounts of fluids are removed rapidly.	$$

Other names Ascites fluid "tap," abdominal paracentesis, and peritoneal fluid analysis.

Purpose

- To establish the cause of abnormal fluid accumulation in the abdomen that has been detected by physical examination or X-rays.
- As treatment, to remove fluid from the abdomen, relieving discomfort and restoring the ability to eat and function normally.

How it works The cause of ascites (the accumulation of fluid in the spaces between tissues and organs in the abdomen) may be determined on the basis of its composition. For example, the presence of bacteria or large amounts of infection-fighting immune cells may signal infection, while blood in ascites may be caused by trauma or cancer. Sometimes, ascites may contain cancer cells.

Preparation

- Do not consume food and drink for at least 12 hours before the test.
- You will be asked to empty your bladder immediately before the test.
- You remove your clothing and don a hospital gown.

Test procedure

- You lie on your back on an examining table as local anesthesia is given and a needle is inserted into the abdomen.
- Using a CT scan or abdominal ultrasound for guidance (particularly if you have only a small amount of fluids), the doctor inserts the needle into the peritoneal space, the area surrounding the intestines and other abdominal organs, and draws a sample of fluids.
- If you have only a small amount of fluid, the doctor may ask you to get on your hands and knees to allow the fluid to collect at the front of the abdomen. If you have a large amount of fluid, the doctor may replace the syringe with connecting tubes that will drain the fluids into vacuum bottles.

After the test

- A pressure dressing is applied to the puncture site and checked for leakage. If fluid is leaking, lie on your back until it stops.
- Your heart and breathing rate, blood pressure, and temperature will be monitored periodically for two or three hours. If a large amount of fluids was removed, your blood pressure will be measured frequently.

Factors affecting results

- Abdominal scars may sequester fluid, making it difficult to obtain a sample.
- Bile, urine, feces, or blood from the puncture site or from punctured blood vessels may interfere with analysis of the sample.

Interpretation Cloudy fluid may indicate a bacterial infection, while bloody fluid may be caused by cancer or inflammation of the pancreas. A high protein level may signal infection or cancer; glucose levels that are less than half the plasma levels may signal infection; a high concentration of amylase (an enzyme secreted by the pancreas) indicates disease of the pancreas; and high levels of white blood cells may be due to infection, cancer, or inflammation of the pancreas.

Advantages

- It's usually simple and safe.
- It's less invasive than surgery.
- It relieves pressure in the abdomen.

Disadvantages

- There is a risk of infection.
- It doesn't provide as much information as laparoscopy or biopsy.

The next step Treatment of diagnosed condition.

STOOL FAT

General information

Where It's Done	Who Does It	How Long It Takes	Discomfort/Pain
Hospital, doctor's office, commercial laboratory, or patient's home.	Lab technician.	72 hours.	Collecting stools is unpleasant.
Results Ready When	**Special Equipment**	**Risks/Complications**	**Average Cost**
24–48 hours.	Applicators and screw-cap containers.	None.	$$

Other names Fat balance study.

Purpose To diagnose diseases, including Crohn's disease, chronic inflammation of the pancreas, and cystic fibrosis, in all of which fat is poorly absorbed from the diet.

How it works If your digestive system is functioning properly, most fat from the diet is absorbed by the small bowel. Fat found in large amounts in the stool may indicate an abnormality in the lining of the small bowel, or in bile acids or enzymes secreted by the pancreas.

Preparation

- Following the instructions of a dietitian, eat a diet containing about 100 grams of fat a day for three days before the test and during the time stool is collected. You should, however, avoid mineral oil, which is not absorbed by the intestines.
- Make sure the stool samples are not contaminated by oily materials such as creams and lubricants.

Test procedure

- You are instructed to collect all the stools you pass during 72 hours.
- Keep the stools in the refrigerator in tightly sealed containers during the collection period.
- At the end of the 72 hours, you bring the stools to a laboratory where they are examined for fat content.

After the test You are free to return to previous activities.

Factors affecting results

- The amount of fat in your diet.
- Mineral oil taken by mouth.
- Debris other than feces, such as toilet paper, in the collection container.

Interpretation Excretion of more than 6 or 7 grams of fat a day in the stool is considered abnormal.

Advantages It's a noninvasive, reliable test for malabsorption.

Disadvantages

- It provides no explanation for the presence of fat in the stool.
- It's unpleasant.

The next step Since it is impossible to know whether excessive fat excretion is caused by a disease of the small bowel, pancreas, or liver, tests evaluating these organs must be ordered to clarify the cause of the abnormality. These include a GI series with small bowel visualization and enteroscopic study of the small bowel, with biopsy if indicated.

OCCULT BLOOD IN STOOL

General information

Where It's Done	Who Does It	How Long It Takes	Discomfort/Pain
Hospital, doctor's office, commercial laboratory, or patient's home.	Lab technician.	A few minutes required to collect stool specimens.	Collecting stools is unpleasant.
Results Ready When	**Special Equipment**	**Risks/Complications**	**Average Cost**
Immediately.	Applicator, screw-cap containers.	None.	$

Other names Fecal occult blood test (FOBT)

Purpose

- To detect occult blood (blood present in amounts too small to be seen with the naked eye) resulting from bleeding in the digestive tract, which may be caused by a variety of disorders, including ulcers, gastritis, dilated or twisted veins, inflammatory bowel disease, hemorrhoids, polyps, or cancer.

DID YOU KNOW?

The lining of the gastrointestinal tract has a vast surface, equivalent to the area of a tennis court. As a result, it is prone to disruptions that often cause bleeding.

- To screen people without symptoms for premalignant growths in the colon or rectum and for colorectal cancer (see chapter 2).

How it works Occult blood can be detected with the help of various methods in which the stools are treated with special chemicals. While it is normal for people to shed less than half a teaspoon of blood a day in the digestive tract, significant amounts of occult blood in stools may indicate bleeding in the stomach or bowels.

Preparation For three days before the test and during the testing period, you will be instructed to observe at least some of the following (the instructions may vary depending on the testing method used):

- Avoid taking vitamin C or eating large amounts of foods, such as citrus fruits, that contain this vitamin.
- Eat a diet that contains no red meat or fruits and vegetables rich in an enzyme called peroxidase—turnips, horseradish, artichokes, mushrooms, radishes, broccoli, bean sprouts, cauliflower, apples, oranges, bananas, cantaloupes, and grapes.
- Eat high-fiber foods (such as beans and vegetables) to increase the bulk of stools.
- Avoid antacids, steroids, and nonsteroidal anti-inflammatory drugs such as aspirin.
- Avoid substances, such as alcohol, that irritate the bowels and stomach.
- Avoid iron supplements.
- If your gums have a tendency to bleed, try not to brush your teeth for three days before the test.

Test procedure

- You collect stools in a clean plastic container for three consecutive days and then use the application stick supplied to smear a dab of each specimen on a special card.
- You bring the stool specimens to a laboratory to be analyzed for occult blood.

DID YOU KNOW?

A positive test for occult blood, even at high levels, does not necessarily signal cancer. It may be caused by numerous other disorders (see below) or by extraneous factors. When bleeding is detected, further tests are performed to determine its cause after extraneous factors are excluded.

After the test You are free to return to previous activities.

Factors affecting results

- False-negative results may be caused by vitamin C, antacids, or stool samples that have dried more than 7–10 days on the card.

- False-positive results may be caused by peroxidase-rich foods in the diet (see Preparation), iron supplements, alcohol or certain drugs that irritate the lining of the bowels, blood from the gums or hemorrhoids, menstrual blood, or watery stools.
- Eating beets or other reddish foods may turn the feces red but will not cause false-positive results.

Interpretation Various methods may be used to analyze stools for occult blood, some of which detect only the presence of blood, while others also measure its amount. When occult blood is detected, unrelated factors, such as bleeding gums, will be ruled out before further tests are ordered.

Usually, stools are tested for occult blood at home with the help of a self-test kit. If this produces positive results, stool specimens are collected again and sent directly to a laboratory for analysis.

Advantages Noninvasive.

Disadvantages

- It's unpleasant.
- It detects occult blood in stools but not its cause.
- False-positive results are common with some testing methods and may cause unwarranted anxiety about cancer and lead to unnecessary further tests.
- False-negative results are common with some testing methods and may miss disease in its early stages.

The next step Contrast X-rays and endoscopic visualization of GI tract to find source of bleeding.

LIVER FUNCTION TESTS

General information

Where It's Done	Who Does It	How Long It Takes	Discomfort/Pain
Hospital, doctor's office, or commercial laboratory.	Doctor, nurse, or lab technician.	Less than 5 minutes.	Minor discomfort associated with drawing blood.
Results Ready When	**Special Equipment**	**Risks/Complications**	**Average Cost**
24–48 hours.	Syringe and needle and equipment required to analyze blood samples.	Negligible.	$

Other names Liver battery or liver profile.

Purpose To assess liver function and diagnose diseases of the liver and bile system.

How it works Abnormal levels of various substances in the blood may indicate that the liver or other organs are not functioning properly. The most commonly measured substances include alkaline phosphatase (ALP), alanine aminotransferase (ALT), aspartate aminotransferase (AST), bilirubin, and gamma glutamyl transferase (GGT).

Preparation Usually, you will be requested to refrain from consuming food and drink for at least eight hours prior to the test.

Test procedure Blood is drawn from a vein in your arm and analyzed for the levels of various substances.

After the test You follow the standard procedure after a venipuncture (see chapter 4), and you are free to leave.

Factors affecting results

- ALP levels may be increased or decreased by certain drugs. They may also be increased in healthy people in the following situations: pregnancy, during period of rapid bone growth in puberty, chronic alcoholism, while healing from a bone fracture, after excessive consumption of vitamin D, and from consuming food, especially fatty foods, too soon before the test.
- ALT levels may be increased as a result of muscle trauma, obesity, and certain drugs.
- AST levels may be increased by regular drinking, trauma, surgery, and certain common drugs.
- Bilirubin levels may be increased by a large number of drugs, including certain antibiotics and birth control pills, and may be abnormally high as part of an adverse reaction to a blood transfusion.
- GGT levels are increased by alcohol, certain medications (particularly antiepileptic drugs), infectious mononucleosis, and eating large amounts of simple carbohydrates. They are also increased in infancy.

Interpretation The tests may be ordered separately, but they often provide useful information when used in combination. For example, in acute viral hepatitis with jaundice, ALT and AST levels are increased as well as bilirubin levels, while in Gilbert's syndrome, a liver disorder that produces similar symptoms, only bilirubin is high. Individual tests may also signal the possibilities described below.

- Increased levels of ALP (an enzyme that is produced in several body organs, including the liver and bones) may signal various abnormalities, particularly diseases of the liver or bones, including obstruction of bile ducts, cirrhosis of the liver, hepatitis, cancer metastases to the liver or bone, diabetes, Paget's disease, osteomalacia, and rickets.
- Decreased ALP levels may signal an underactive thyroid gland, malnutrition, vitamin D deficiency, or pernicious anemia, requiring further

tests. However, ALP levels may be altered by many harmless factors that must be taken into account to prevent unnecessary testing.

- ALT (also referred to as serum glutamic pyruvic transaminase, or SGPT) is an enzyme that may be released into the bloodstream in increased amounts when the liver is damaged by inflammation or other abnormalities.
- AST (also referred to as serum glutamic oxaloacetic transaminase, or SGOT) is an enzyme produced in various organs, including the heart, liver, and skeletal muscle. Increased levels may signal a variety of disorders, including a heart attack; but levels that are exceptionally high—over 500 units—usually indicate liver disease and/or shock.
- Bilirubin is a waste product of red blood cells that is processed in the liver. An excess in the blood can cause a yellowish color (jaundice) in the skin and the whites of the eyes. The levels may be increased as a result of hepatitis, bile duct inflammation, cirrhosis of the liver, liver cancer, and other types of liver disease, as well as by alcoholism, infectious mononucleosis, anorexia, fasting for 36 hours or more, pernicious anemia, pulmonary embolism, and congestive heart failure.
- GGT is an enzyme that is present in bile but also found in blood. Increased GGT levels can signal obstruction of bile ducts, cancer of the liver or pancreas, inflammation of the pancreas, cirrhosis, and hepatitis. Since alcohol increases GGT levels, the enzyme may be measured to monitor abstinence in recovering alcoholics.

Advantages It's noninvasive.

Disadvantages It detects the presence of an abnormality but not its cause.

The next step Liver biopsy, imaging studies, or treatment may be recommended depending on the diagnosis.

Richard J. Robbins, MD

9 The Endocrine System

Tests Covered in This Chapter

The case of Maryanne D., 30, a mother of two boys:

When I was nine months pregnant, I weighed 208 pounds. Four months later, I was down to 117 pounds. I had lost so much weight that people thought I must be on drugs! I also had a rapid heart rate and I felt warm a lot. I was very hyper, yet tired all the time. My gynecologist thought that I was suffering from an overactive thyroid gland and referred me to an endocrinologist, who diagnosed me with Graves' disease. At the time, I knew nothing about it; I've sure learned a lot about it since.

Graves' disease is a form of hyperthyroidism caused by a disturbance in the immune system. The body generates antibodies that mistake the thyroid for a foreign body. They stimulate the thyroid gland to enlarge and to secrete too much thyroid hormone, which increases the body's metabolism rate. That caused me to burn calories faster than normal and accounted for my weight loss.

The Tests Maryanne first had blood tests to measure the levels of several thyroid hormones. Although these T_3, T_4, and TSH tests don't specifically diagnose Graves' disease, they do indicate hyperthyroidism. These were followed by a thyroid scan and an iodine uptake test, which helped confirm the diagnosis of Graves' disease. For these, Maryanne was given a small dose of radioactive iodine, which the thyroid gland incorporates into thyroid hormone. The doctor can actually see this on the scan and calculate how much of the dose the thyroid gland takes up.

The Outcome For the first year, Maryanne took two antithyroid drugs to control her body's production of thyroid hormone. Then she had radioactive iodine therapy, in which she was given an oral dose of radioactive iodine. This essentially destroys the thyroid and slows down the rate at which it secretes thyroid hormones.

For the next four years Maryanne was relatively normal. Then she developed *hypo*thyroidism—an *under*active thyroid, a fairly common problem with Graves' disease sufferers. She was put on a synthetic thyroid hormone, which she will probably take for the rest of her life. Her thyroid function is now completely normal.

INTRODUCTION

The endocrine system is a complex network of glands that produces hormones and releases them into the bloodstream so that they can influence tissues throughout the body. These hormones are chemical messengers that affect every organ in your body. Endocrine glands also send signals to other endocrine glands, resulting in complex interactions.

Normally these hormones maintain a delicate balance within the body's complex metabolic processes. When that balance is upset by the overproduction or underproduction of even a single hormone, the results can be dramatic, even life-threatening. In one disorder alone, Cushing's syndrome, the consequences of the overproduction of cortisol by the adrenal gland can include bone pain, depression, fungal infections, high blood pressure, increased facial hair, muscle wasting, a "moon face" appearance, thinning of skin (leading to stretch marks and easy bruising), weakness, and weight gain.

The major endocrine glands include the hypothalamus, pituitary gland, thyroid gland, parathyroid glands, adrenal glands, pineal gland, thymus gland, pancreas, testes, and ovaries.

By secreting various hormones, the hypothalamus and the pituitary gland control many normal functions, including sleep, appetite, temperature, sexual maturation, and reproduction. The hypothalamus, located at the base of the brain, is connected by blood vessels to the nearby pituitary gland. The hormones they control include those described below.

Growth hormone (somatotropin). Promotes protein building in cells and other functions that stimulate muscle and bone growth through childhood and adolescence.

Oxytocin. Starts uterine contractions in childbirth and promotes milk release during breast-feeding.

Prolactin. Stimulates milk production for breast-feeding.

Vasopressin or antidiuretic hormone (ADH). Helps maintain the body's fluid balance and blood pressure by preventing the kidneys from excreting too much water and by causing small blood vessels to constrict.

The tropic hormones (those that stimulate other glands to produce hormones), including the following:

ACTH (adrenocorticotropic hormone). Stimulates adrenal gland secretion of corticosteroids, aldosterone (a salt-retaining hormone), and weak androgens.

FSH (follicle-stimulating hormone). Responsible for production of sperm in males and stimulation of the follicles in the ovary that produce the ova (eggs).

LH (luteinizing hormone). Stimulates the secretion of the male sex hormone testosterone and the female sex hormone estrogen. In women, stimulates the release of an egg from the ovary (ovulation) each month.

MSH (melanocyte-stimulating hormone). Controls the production of pigment cells in skin.

TSH (thyrotropin). Stimulates the thyroid gland to secrete the hormone thyroxine.

The butterfly-shaped thyroid gland lies at the front of the neck, just below the Adam's apple, over the windpipe. Its main function is to convert tyrosine (an amino acid) and iodine into the hormones thyroxine and triiodothyronine, which regulate the body's metabolism. Thyroxine, the more abundant of the two, is necessary for normal development through infancy and childhood.

The thyroid gland also produces calcitonin, a hormone that is thought to act in conjunction with parathyroid hormone (see below) to regulate the level of calcium in the body.

Located on the side and back of each thyroid wing are the parathyroid glands, which regulate the level of calcium and phosphorus in the blood by secreting parathyroid hormone.

The adrenal glands sit on top of each kidney. The outer part of each gland, called the adrenal cortex, is responsible for the production of male (androgens) and female (estrogens) sex hormones, as well as hormones (aldosterone and cortisol) that regulate metabolism and fluid balance. The inner part is the adrenal medulla, which produces epinephrine (adrenaline) and norepinephrine, hormones that control blood pressure and heart rate and the so-called stress response.

The role of the tiny, pinecone-shaped pineal gland, which is located deep within the brain, is only now becoming understood. The pineal gland secretes the hormone melatonin, which is thought to suppress the brain's electrical activity, thus facilitating sleep. It is also involved in regulating diurnal (light–dark) body cycles.

The thymus gland produces a type of lymphocyte that is necessary for the proper functioning of the body's immune system. It gradually disappears after puberty, but lymphocytes continue to be produced by the spleen and lymph glands.

Note: Disorders of the pancreas (which secretes insulin) and the testes and ovaries (which secrete sex hormones) are discussed in chapters 19 (Diabetes), 10 (The Male Reproductive System), and 11 (The

Female Reproductive System), respectively. Other endocrine-related disorders are included in chapters 20 (Hypertension) and 25 (Pregnancy).

HOW YOUR DOCTOR DIAGNOSES ENDOCRINE SYSTEM DISORDERS

The wide variety and sheer number—literally scores—of symptoms that can be produced by hormone imbalances make diagnosing endocrine disorders a challenge. The symptoms of hormone disorders are too numerous to include here, but some of them occur in specific constellations that give the first clue to the problem. For example, the classic combination of excessive thirst, frequent urination, and unexplained weight loss invariably points to diabetes.

If your doctor suspects a hormone imbalance, he or she may make a preliminary diagnosis or refer you directly to an endocrinologist, a specialist in endocrine disorders. In either case, the first steps will be to take a careful family and medical history, including your symptoms, and to conduct a thorough physical examination. These will probably be followed by a blood test to measure levels of hormones or related molecules that show changes when an endocrine problem exists. Although a simple blood test may be sufficient in some cases, hormones exhibit certain characteristics and interrelationships that have led to the development of more complex testing. Three key aspects of hormone behavior that help explain endocrine testing are described below.

Hormone Level Cycles

Daily (diurnal) changes. Some hormones such as cortisol, which is made by the adrenal glands, have a characteristic daily (diurnal) pattern. Levels are highest in the early morning—from about 5 AM to 8 AM—and lowest in the evening—from about 8 PM to 2 AM.

Rapid pulses. Many hormones are released from their glands in a pulsatile pattern. For example, your growth hormone level may be 2 nanograms per milliliter of blood at 9 AM, but can then shoot up to 12 ng/mL at 9:30 AM and be back down to 2 at noon.

Changes related to stress. Many hormone levels change after strenuous exercise, in response to pain, and as a result of illness. These conditions may increase or decrease certain hormone levels for several hours.

Changes following eating. Some hormone levels change dramatically after the ingestion of a meal. These changes may differ, depending on the content of the meal.

Binding Proteins

Carrier proteins provide a large reservoir of hormones that can be considered held in reserve. A small percentage of many hormones diffuse away from the carrier proteins, and are thus "free" hormones, which can then diffuse into cells in various tissues. The total level of a hormone in the blood (those bound to carrier proteins plus those that are free) may therefore not always reflect the true "free" levels that determine the actual activity.

Interaction of Different Hormones (Feedback Regulation)

Virtually all hormones control and are controlled by other hormones. One gland, the pituitary, operates as a master gland in that it regulates the activity of many other glands. When the levels of estrogen from the ovary are low, the pituitary secretes gonadotropins (leutinizing hormone—LH—and follicle-stimulating hormone—FSH) to stimulate more estrogen production. In normal menopause, for example, estrogen levels are low and LH and FSH levels are high. A low estrogen level associated with normal LH and FSH levels indicates a problem involving the pituitary gland because the LH and FSH levels normally should be elevated under those circumstances.

Testing Procedures

These aspects of the endocrine system explain some of the testing procedures, such as 24-hour hormone level estimates, used in diagnosis. For example, the hormone cortisol has both a diurnal and a pulsatile pattern. Any single blood test may not accurately reflect the overall pattern. In this situation, your endocrinologist may ask you to collect a 24-hour urine sample for measurement of the total daily production.

To test the responsiveness of certain endocrine glands, it is sometimes necessary to block the production of a feedback hormone or administer a stress to activate an endocrine gland. These tests, called suppression and stimulation tests, usually involve administration orally or by injection of a drug or other substance that stimulates or suppresses hormones, followed by blood drawings at set intervals to measure the hormone levels over time.

The main types of endocrine tests are blood tests, urine tests, function tests, stimulation and suppression tests, structural tests, and pathology studies. Blood and urine testing are discussed in chapters 4 and 12. Function tests directly monitor the functioning of different glands through the use of radioactive materials and imaging procedures. Structural tests such as magnetic resonance imaging (MRI), magnetic resonance angiography (MRA), CT scans, ultrasound, and X-rays allow the doctor to visually inspect internal structures of the body and are covered, along with imaging tests, in chapter 3. Biopsies, needle aspirations, and other pathology tests are covered in chapter 4.

The following section lists the major endocrine disorders, arranged by the glands that control them, and the tests used to diagnose them. These tests are then listed in alphabetical order and described briefly in table 9.1.

TABLE 9.1 Tests for Endocrine Disorders

The following are brief descriptions of tests used to diagnose disorders of the endocrine glands. More complete descriptions of blood tests can be found in chapter 4 under venipuncture (the method used to draw a blood specimen from a vein); of urine tests, in chapters 4 and 12; and of CT scans, MRI scans, and X-rays, in chapter 3.

Name of Test	Type of Test/Comments
1,25 and 25 (OH) vitamin D	Blood tests used to diagnose calcium imbalance problems.
24-hour urine collection for calcium	Urinalysis. Normal values are based on average calcium intake of 600–800 mg/day. Results are altered by taking diuretics. See chapters 4 and 12.
24-hour urine collection for metanephrine, norepinephrine, or urine catecholamines	See chapters 4 and 12.
24-hour urine collection for vanillylmandelic acid (VMA)	Urinalysis. Diet restrictions (no coffee, tea, bananas, etc) and drug restrictions before test. See chapters 4 and 12.
Adrenocorticotropic hormone (ACTH) level	Blood test. Samples drawn between 6 AM and 10 AM.
Alkaline phosphatase level	Blood test. Results can be elevated in diseases of bone or liver. A specific bone alkaline phosphatase can also be obtained.
Androstenedione level	Blood test. Normal results lower in postmenopausal women than in men and adult premenopausal women.
Angiograms	Used to screen for cysts, tumors, or change in shape of endocrine glands. Direct injection of dye into an artery to define all of the smaller arteries in an individual endocrine gland.
Antimicrosomal antibody	Blood test. An antithyroid antibody.
Antithyroglobulin antibody	Blood test. An antithyroid antibody.
Bone biopsy	Used in evaluation of thin bones to determine underlying disease or rate of bone formation. See chapter 13.
Calcitonin level	Blood test for certain thyroid tumors.
Calcium level	Blood test that measures bound and free calcium.
Cosyntropin or cortrosyn (ACTH) test	Stimulation test that requires an overnight fast. Test begins at 8 AM with a blood test for cortisol. Then cosyntropin is injected intravenously and blood samples are drawn 30 minutes and 60 minutes later to measure cortisol levels.
CT scan	Involves IV injection of a contrast agent and multiple X-rays combined by a computer. See chapter 3.
Dexamethasone test	A suppression test in which the drug dexamethasone is given in the evening to suppress secretion of ACTH (adrenocorticotropic hormone), which normally stimulates the adrenal gland to secrete cortisol. Normally, a blood test done the next morning following the drug dose should show decreased levels of cortisol.
Dual photon absorptiometry	A type of bone X-ray. See chapter 26.
Fine-needle aspiration	Used to evaluate types of cells in thyroid nodules. See chapter 4.

Follicle-stimulating hormone (FSH) level	Blood test. Normal levels the same for men and premenopausal women. Can surge during mid–menstrual cycle. Higher after menopause.
Free thyroxine index (EFT, T_7, FTI)	Blood test. Calculation depends on both the T_4 and T_3 resin uptake results, which can be influenced by pregnancy, contraceptive pills, and other factors.
Glucagon test	Stimulation test used to bring on a discharge of catecholamines in a person with pheochromocytoma.
Glucose tolerance test	Stimulation test. See chapter 19.
Growth hormone level	Blood test that requires fasting. Stress can affect the results.
Hypertonic saline test	Used for diabetes insipidus.
IGF-I (somatomedin C) level	Blood test. Overnight fasting before test. Normal values depend on age and sex. Higher values during normal puberty.
Insulin tolerance test	Stimulation test in which a dose of insulin is given intravenously. Blood is drawn before and every 15 minutes after the insulin dose for 90 minutes. Blood is tested for glucose, growth hormone, cortisol, and prolactin. In normal circumstances, the test causes hypoglycemia, which is usually treated with dextrose (a kind of sugar).
Iodine uptake test	See below for a full description.
Ionized calcium level	Blood tests that measure only free calcium level.
LHRH test	Stimulation test of ability of the pituitary to produce LH and FSH. Involves rapid IV injection of LHRH, then blood sampling. Rise in LH and FSH peak at 30 to 60 minutes following injection. Response in women varies with phase of menstrual cycle.
Luteinizing hormone (LH) level	Blood test. Normal levels the same for men and premenopausal women. Can surge during mid–menstrual cycle. Variable results during pregnancy and higher after menopause.
Metyrapone test	Stimulation/suppression test in which metyrapone is given with a snack at midnight the night before the test. Can cause nausea. Blood sample is taken at 8 AM the next morning. The test causes decrease in cortisol levels, which causes increase of ACTH levels.
MRI scan	Radio-frequency waves are reflected by tissues in a strong magnetic field. See chapter 3.
Osteocalcin level	Blood test that is a measure of bone formation.
Parathyroid hormone level	Blood test.
Petrosal sinal catheterization	Involves the insertion of IV catheters that are positioned on each side of the pituitary glad. Blood is withdrawn and tested for ACTH. Used in evaluation of Cushing's syndrome when diagnosis is complicated.
Phentolomine test	Test used to lower blood pressure in a person with pheochromocytoma.
Phosphorus level	Blood test.
Prolactin level (PRL)	Blood test. Influenced by estrogens and many other medications. Fasting required before test. The sample can be drawn at any time during the day. Results are higher in pregnant and breast-feeding women.
PTH-related peptide (PTH-RP)	Blood test that measures a calcium-elevating hormone (overproduced by some cancers).
Selective vein catheterization	Angiography test that measures cortisol and/or aldosterone or catecholamines. See chapter 3.

(continued next page)

TABLE 9.1 (continued)

Name of Test	Type of Test/Comments
Serum aldosterone	Blood test. Diuretics, antihypertensive drugs, some hormone medications, and licorice should be avoided 2–4 weeks before tests. A normal sodium diet should be ingested for 2–4 weeks before tests. Normal values are different depending on your position (supine or upright) when the sample is drawn. Levels may be low in diabetics.
Serum cortisol	Blood test. Normal values will be higher for samples taken at 8 AM than for those taken at 8 PM.
Serum dehydroeipandrosterone sulfate (DHEA-S) level	Blood test. Made by adrenal cortex.
Serum epinephrine (adrenaline)	Blood test.
Serum norepinephrine	Blood test.
T_3 resin uptake	Blood test. An estimate of thyroid-binding proteins, not a measure of T_3 levels. Results are affected by pregnancy, oral contraceptives, and other medications.
Thyroid binding globulin	Blood test. Levels rise during pregnancy.
Thyroid function tests	A group of tests that measure thyroid hormones as part of the standard workup for suspected thyroid problems. They include T_4, T_3, and TSH tests.
Thyroid scan	Generates a picture of thyroid function. See below for a full description.
Thyroid stimulating hormone (TSH)	Blood test.
Thyroid ultrasound (echo)	Generates a picture of thyroid density based on the penetration of sound waves.
Thyroid uptake	Measures the ability of the thyroid to take up iodine. See below for a full description.
Thyrotropin (TSH) level	Blood test.
Thyroxine (T_4)	Blood test.
TRH test	A stimulation test in which a dose of TRH is rapidly given by IV. Blood is drawn before and at 30 minutes after the dose. May cause flushing, nausea, and an urgent need to urinate. Blood is tested for TSH, which should rise somewhat. Results are low in hyperthyroidism, elevated in hypothyroidism.
Triiodothyronine (T_3)	Blood test. Results are higher in childhood and during pregnancy.
Urinary nephrogenous cyclic AMP	Urinalysis that estimates the action of parathyroid hormone.
Vasopressin challenge	A stimulation test in which the drug desomopressin acetate (DDAVP) is injected, which stimulates water conservation by the kidney.
Water deprivation test	Used to evaluate excessive thirst and urination. Individuals with diabetes insipidus (deficiency of ADH) will not be able to conserve water after an 18-hour period of dehydration.

COMMON DISORDERS OF THE ENDOCRINE SYSTEM AND THEIR DIAGNOSIS

Disorders of the Thyroid Gland

Thyrotoxicosis. General term for severe hyperthyroidism that refers to the collection of symptoms and physical changes, regardless of the cause. Characterized by nervousness, weight loss, diarrhea, heat intolerance, palpitations, insomnia, and weakness.

Caused by: Excess thyroid hormone production leading to increased metabolism.

Tests: Free thyroxine (T_4) index, free T_3 level, radioactive iodine uptake, and TRH test.

Graves' Disease. The most common cause of thyrotoxicosis; may be an autoimmune disease. Characterized by the above symptoms plus bulging eyes (exophthalmus), lymph system swelling, and blurred or double vision, and skin problems.

Caused by: Excess thyroid hormone production, often following an infection or physical or emotional stress, including pregnancy.

Tests: Free thyroxine (T_4) index, free T_3 level, radioactive iodine uptake, and TRH test.

Thyroid Storm. Life-threatening, uncontrolled hyperthyroidism characterized by high fever, fast heart rate, dehydration, low or very high blood pressure, decreased mental ability, and heart failure.

Caused by: Usually occurs when an individual with thyrotoxicosis is suddenly stressed.

Tests: Free thyroxine (T_4) index, free T_3 level, radioactive iodine uptake, and TRH test.

Hypothyroidism. Underactivity of the thyroid gland characterized by cold intolerance, tiredness, weight gain, sleepiness, and constipation.

Caused by: Removal of all or part of the thyroid gland, an overdose of antithyroid medication, atrophy of the thyroid gland, or inability of the pituitary gland to produce thyroid-stimulating hormone (TSH).

Tests: T_4, T_3RU, TSH level, CT scan of hypothalamus and pituitary (if TSH is not elevated).

Myxedema Coma. Most severe form of hypothyroidism. In addition to those listed above, symptoms include hypothermia, shallow breathing, low blood pressure, altered mental state, and dehydration.

Caused by: Same as above.

Tests: Same as for hypothyroidism, plus arterial blood gas, kidney, heart, and liver tests.

Thyroid Nodules and Cancer. Characterized by lump or cysts in the thyroid gland that may be the underlying cause of goiter.

Caused by: May simply be areas of underactivity, but in 15% to 20% of cases may be malignant tumors.

Tests: Thyroid scan, thyroid function tests, fine-needle aspiration, ultrasound, calcitonin, and thyroglobulin.

Goiter. An enlarged thyroid.

Caused by: Benign nodules (see above), inefficient thyroxine production, or inflammation or overstimulation by thyroid-stimulating hormone (TSH). May be an autoimmune disease.

Tests: Thyroid function tests and ultrasound.

Disorders of the Pituitary Gland

Acromegaly. Enlargement of all the tissues in the body, especially the bones of the face, jaw, hands, and feet.

Caused by: Oversecretion of growth hormone and insulinlike growth factor-I (IGF-I).

Tests: GH level, MRI scan of pituitary, thyroid tests, IGF-I test, hand/foot X-rays, and glucose tolerance test.

The Amenorrhea/Galactorrhea Syndrome. The cessation of the menstrual cycle (amenorrhea) or the production of milk not related to childbirth (galactorrhea).

Caused by: Oversecretion of the hormone prolactin.

Tests: Prolactin level, MRI scan of pituitary, and thyroid tests.

Cushing's Disease. Characterized by redistribution of fat to the face and trunk, and rapid protein breakdown.

Caused by: (Usually) the oversecretion of ACTH (adrenocorticotropic hormone) by a benign pituitary tumor. Less commonly due to adrenal tumors or cancer.

Tests: ACTH level, MRI scan of the pituitary gland, blood glucose check for diabetes, prolactin level, dexamethasone suppression, 24-hour urine collection (free cortisol test), petrosal sinus cathertization.

Hypogonadism. Delayed sexual maturation, or loss of libido or function of the ovary or testes.

Caused by: Underproduction of FSH (follicle-stimulating hormone) and/or LH (luteinizing hormone).

Tests: LH level, FSH level, MRI, and prolactin level.

Hypothyroidism. See thyroid disorders above.

Caused by: (Sometimes) underproduction by the pituitary gland of TSH, which normally stimulates the thyroid gland.

Tests: TSH level, MRI, prolactin level, and free thyroxine (T_4) index.

Disorders of the Adrenal Gland

Addison's Disease. Underactivity of the adrenal glands, causing gastrointestinal symptoms (nausea, vomiting, pains, etc), weakness, dizziness or fainting, darkening of the skin, and problems coping with physical stresses such as an infection. May be life-threatening if untreated.

Caused by: (Usually) autoimmune destruction of the adrenal gland.

Tests: Cortisol level, ACTH level, and cortrosyn stimulation test.

Conn's Syndrome (Primary Hyperaldosteronism). Causes high blood pressure and lowered potassium levels, disrupting the body's biochemical balance and normal muscle functioning.

Caused by: (Usually) small tumors of the adrenal glands that produce too much aldosterone, a salt-retaining hormone.

Tests: Serum aldosterone, hematocrit measurement, potassium level, sodium level, plasma renin studies, and plasma aldosterone level.

Cushing's Syndrome. Symptoms are indistinguishable from those of Cushing's disease.

Caused by: Oversecretion of cortisol by the adrenal gland, most often due to a benign adrenal tumor.

Tests: Serum cortisol, metyrapone test, dexamethasone suppression test, 24-hour urine collection (free cortisol), CT scan or MRI of adrenal glands, and DHEA-S level.

Drug-related Temporary Adrenal Insufficiency. Underactivity of the adrenal gland, due to chronic suppression of ACTH production. Sudden cessation of steroids used for treating other diseases may cause symptoms of Addison's disease (see above) or atrophy of the adrenal gland. This is the most common type of adrenal insufficiency.

Caused by: Long-term use of steroid medication for other conditions, such as arthritis or asthma.

Tests: Cortisol level, ACTH level, and cortrosyn stimulation test.

Pheochromocytoma. Characterized by high blood pressure and sudden spells of severe headaches, palpitations, a "sense of doom," and sweating.

Caused by: An adrenal gland tumor that causes release of excessive epinephrine (adrenaline) and norepinephrine.

Tests: Serum epinephrine, serum norepinephrine, 24-hour urine collection for vanillylmandelic acid (VMA), metanephrine, normetanephrine, phentolamine test, glucagon test, abdominal CT scan, and adrenal vein catheterization studies.

Disorders of the Parathyroid Gland and Mineral Metabolism

Hyperparathyroidism (Hypercalcemia). Overproduction of parathyroid hormone that results in elevated blood calcium levels, weakness, constipation, nausea, and kidney stones.

Caused by: Usually due to a single benign tumor.

Tests: Calcium level, phosphate level, PTH level, 1,25 OH vitamin D level, 24-hour urine collection (for calcium).

Parathyroid Hormone Deficiency (Hypoparathyroidism). Rare condition in which low level of calcium in the blood produces muscle spasms, seizures, and thin bones.

Caused by: Occasionally results after thyroid or parathyroid surgery or in association with an autoimmune disorder.

Tests: Calcium level, phosphate level, calcitonin level, and vitamin D levels.

IODINE UPTAKE AND THYROID SCAN

General information

Where It's Done	Who Does It	How Long It Takes	Discomfort/Pain
Nuclear testing section of a hospital.	Radiologist, nurse, or nuclear medical technician.	About 1 hour total, spaced over 2 days.	Minor discomfort during injection; some discomfort from neck hyperextension during the scan.
Results Ready When	**Special Equipment**	**Risks/Complications**	**Average Cost**
Within 1 week.	Radioisotope and gamma scintillation camera.	Rare risk of radioisotope overdose.	$$

Other names Radioactive iodine uptake, RAIU, and radioiodine thyroid uptake and/or scan.

Purpose

- To determine the size, structure, and function of the thyroid gland.
- To diagnose the cause of an overactive thyroid gland.
- To evaluate thyroid nodules for activity, inactivity, and malignancy.
- The scan alone may be used to determine the extent of thyroid cancer.

How it works These two tests, which are almost always done together, are based on the fact that iodine is taken up easily by the thyroid gland (which converts it to hormones) but only minutely by other body tissues. By tagging iodine or a similar substance with a radioisotope, it is possible to measure the amount absorbed by the thyroid gland (the uptake study) or, by using a gamma scintillation camera, to actually see the thyroid tissue (the scan).

Preparation

- Your physician will give you a list of drugs (including thyroid hormones) as well as foods containing iodine (such as shellfish) to avoid during the week before the test.
- Blood samples for thyroid function tests will be drawn before the injection.
- You may have a thyroid ultrasound exam before (or after) the scan.
- If you are to take radioactive iodine in oral form, you will be asked to fast for anywhere from two to 12 hours before the test.
- For day two of the test, wear a loose-fitting T-shirt to make hyperextending your next as comfortable as possible.

Test procedure

- You will be given a small dose of radioactive iodine, orally or by injection.
- You will return in two, six, or 24 hours (or at each of these times) to check the uptake of the iodine.
- A stationary probe (which doesn't generate, but only measures, radioactivity) will be aimed at your neck and the amount of uptake recorded.
- For the scan, a radioisotope is injected into the vein on the inside of your elbow.
- You will lie on your back on a table while your head is stretched backward and your neck hyperextended. A pillow is placed under your neck to make this more comfortable.
- A gamma scintillation camera detects the radioisotope that collects in your thyroid gland over 20 to 30 minutes, and produces an image on a screen. Photographs can also be taken for further analysis.
- The time needed to produce the pictures depends on how long it takes the isotope to travel to the thyroid. More time may be necessary if special views of the thyroid are taken.

After the test You are free to leave and resume normal activities.

Factors affecting results Failure to refrain from using iodine-containing compounds and foods.

Interpretation The results of the uptake test are expressed as the percentage of the dose taken up by the thyroid gland. A low uptake usually indicates that you have an underactive thyroid gland or are taking too much thyroid supplement. A high intake indicates an overactive thyroid gland.

Advantages The test effectively assesses the anatomy of and measures the function of the gland.

Disadvantages It entails low-level exposure to a radioactive substance.

The next step The test is considered definitive, and treatment can begin.

Robert M. Weiss, MD ■ Kevin R. Anderson, MD

10 The Male Reproductive System

Tests Covered in This Chapter

The case of Roberto B., 48, an advertising photographer:

My first wife didn't want children. At the time, in my twenties, I thought I didn't either, so I had a vasectomy. That was 24 years ago. I also believed I would be married to the same women for the rest of my life.

But the marriage failed and we divorced. I recently married another woman and we would like to have a child. The doctor who performed the vasectomy made it clear beforehand that the chances of successfully reversing it would be minuscule. But my wife and I decided to investigate the possibility anyway.

My new doctor explained that while surgery to reverse the vasectomy would most likely be successful, the number of healthy sperm I produced would be extremely low. A month after the surgery, I saw a fertility specialist who magnified a slide of my semen on a TV monitor: I could see some of the sperm actually move! Unfortunately, they were moving very slowly, so the doctor suggested that my wife and I explore in vitro fertilization.

The Tests Before the vasovasostomy (surgery to reverse the vasectomy by reconnecting the severed ends of the vas deferens), Roberto's doctor injected saline solution into the end of the vas that travels to the penis to be sure there was no obstruction. Had there been one, caused perhaps by scar tissue, surgery would have been pointless. A semen analysis was performed afterward to check the structure and motility (ability to move) of the sperm.

The Outcome Roberto decided to see another doctor who pointed out that it takes three to 12 months after a vasovasostomy for new sperm to grow and enter the semen. This meant that the sperm present in Roberto's semen at the time of his test had actually matured *before* the operation. Roberto and his wife decided to continue trying for a pregnancy before relying on in vitro fertilization. The operation paid off; after six months, the wife had conceived.

INTRODUCTION

The organs of the male urogenital system represent an intricate interrelationship between the organs that carry urine out of the body and those that are used for sexual pleasure and procreation. They include the following:

- *Prostate,* which produces the enzyme prostatic acid phosphatase and secretes fluids that form a part of the semen.
- *Seminal vesicles,* which release fluid for the semen.
- *Penis,* the major male sexual organ, which transports and releases urine and semen from the body via a narrow tube called the urethra.
- *Testicles* (also called testes, or testis in referring to one), which produce sperm and the male sex hormones, including testosterone.
- *Epididymides,* a pair of long coiled tubes (each called an epididymis) in which sperm mature.
- *Vasa deferentia,* a pair of muscular tubes (each called a vas deferens) that transport sperm from the testicles to the urethra.

Reproduction requires that a male sex cell (called a spermatozoan, or sperm) units with an egg produced by a female. Sperm are formed in the testicles beginning at puberty. Each testicle is an egg-shaped organ suspended inside a sac (the scrotum) from a cord containing blood vessels and a vas deferens.

DID YOU KNOW?

Sperm are microscopically tiny, about 0.002 of an inch long. An average ejaculation contains about 100 million of them, but only half to three-quarters of them have the ability to swim. Of these, few—perhaps 1,000—survive the journey to the egg. Once one has fused with the egg, the outer shell of the egg hardens within seconds so that no other sperm can penetrate it.

The sperm travel from the testicles to the epididymis, where they finish maturing and are stored. Just before ejaculation, the sperm travel from the epididymis through the vas deferens to the seminal vesicles, where fluid is added to the sperm, forming part of the semen. This mixture, also called ejaculate, then travels to the urethra. As the urethra passes through the prostate gland, additional seminal fluid is secreted into the mixture. The semen is then ejaculated from the penis during orgasm.

REPRODUCTIVE SYSTEM DISORDERS AND SYMPTOMS

A wide range of disorders, from inflammation to tumors to impotence, can affect various parts of the male reproductive system. The most common ones are described below, along with the tests used to help identify them.

Epididymis

Epididymitis. Inflammation and enlargement of the epididymides, usually caused by infection, sexually transmitted disease, or tuberculosis. Characterized by scrotal and groin pain, fever, pus in urine, and problems urinating.

Tests: Doppler ultrasound (to differentiate it from testicular torsion) and testicular scan (see chapter 3).

Tumors of Epididymis. Benign or cancerous lump that can be felt or may not show symptoms.

Tests: Ultrasound.

Testes and Surrounding Area

Spermatocele. Sperm-filled swelling above and behind the testicles that may appear as a cystlike lump.

Tests: Transillumination and ultrasound.

Testicular Torsion. Twisting of the testicle on the cord that suspends it within the scrotum and that contains its blood supply. Characterized by sudden severe pain, nausea, and vomiting, accompanied by general swelling and tenderness of the scrotum. Requires immediate medical treatment to prevent loss of the testicle.

Tests: Color Doppler ultrasound (to differentiate it from epididymal disorders and orchitis).

Torsion of Appendix Testis. A twist of a small appendage on the testis that results in a pea-sized blue dot and pain that is not as severe as that of testicular torsion.

Tests: Color Doppler ultrasound and transillumination.

Testis Tumor. Benign or cancerous growth that results in chronic tenderness, swelling, or a lump.

Tests: Blood test for alpha-fetoprotein and beta-human chorionic gonadotropin (a hormone), ultrasound, and possible CT scan to check for cancer spread.

Orchitis. Inflammation of the testicles causing pain and inflammation.

Tests: Ultrasound.

Hydrocele. Fluid around the testis that may produce no symptoms or be felt as a dull pain, lump, or heaviness in the scrotum.

Tests: Ultrasound and transillumination.

Varicocele. A common abnormality caused by a distended (varicose) veins in the scrotum. Sometimes described as the scrotum feeling like a bag of worms, it is a cause of male infertility that may be correctable with surgery.

Tests: Usually only a physical exam, but Doppler ultrasound may be used if the varicocele is small.

Penis

Priapism. Prolonged erection associated with extreme pain.

Tests: Test for arterial blood gases (see chapter 4).

Penile Cancer. Cancer that may cause no symptoms or may result in local infection.

Tests: Biopsy (see chapter 4).

Balanoposthitis (Balanitis). Inflammation of the foreskin and glans of the penis that produces mild pain and redness of the foreskin.

Tests: Fungal smear (see chapter 22).

Impotence. An inability to achieve or maintain an erection. The problem may be psychological, although the majority of cases are thought to be due to a variety of physical causes, including nerve damage related to diabetes, vascular disease, high blood pressure, chronic alcoholism, prolonged heavy smoking, and hormonal abnormalities.

Tests: Penile/brachial index, carvernosometry, cavernosonography, and sleep test for impotence (RIGI scan).

Phimosis. Tightness of the foreskin of an uncircumcised penis, which may be due to infection. It may cause pain, difficulty urinating, and the inability to retract the foreskin, or it may produce no symptoms.

Tests: None other than a physical exam.

Paraphimosis. In contrast to phimosis, the foreskin of an uncircumcised penis stays retracted, or pulled back, resulting in pain and swelling of the penis.

Tests: None other than a physical exam.

Retrograde Ejaculation. Failure of the neck of the bladder to close during ejaculation, causing semen to spill back into the bladder instead of traveling to the tip of the penis. A cause of infertility.

Tests: Urinalysis to identify sperm in the urine.

Disorders of the Prostate

Acute Prostatitis. Acute inflammation of the prostate, which causes burning on urination, pain, pus in the urine, fever, urinary obstruction, and retention of urine.

Tests: Urinalysis (see chapter 4).

Chronic Prostatitis. Long-term prostate inflammation that results in the same symptoms as the acute form, minus the fever.

Tests: Urinalysis.

Benign Prostatic Hyperplasia (BPH). Enlarged prostate, a very common condition in men as they age, which results in a slow urine stream, straining during urination, an urgent need to urinate, and multiple nighttime voidings.

Tests: Rectal exam, PSA blood test, prostate ultrasound, voiding cystourethrography (test of residual urine left after urination—see chapter 12).

Prostate Cancer. Cancerous growth in the prostate that may have no symptoms or have the same symptoms as benign prostatic hyperplasia.

Tests: PSA blood test, ultrasound, and biopsy.

Hematospermia. Blood in the semen, causing it to appear pinkish.

Tests: None other than a physical exam.

Other Disorders

Infertility. Defined as the inability to conceive after one year of trying. About 30% of infertility problems originate with the man, about 30% originate with the woman, and about 40% are the result of a combination of factors.

Tests: Sperm count, semen analysis, physical exam for varicocele, and vasogram.

HOW YOUR DOCTOR DIAGNOSES REPRODUCTIVE SYSTEM DISORDERS

If you suspect that you have an infection, you may seek treatment from your family practitioner or internist. If your problem is more complicated, you may be referred to a urologist, a doctor who specializes in problems of the male reproductive system and in diseases of the urinary tract in both sexes. If infertility is your problem, you may see a urologist, or possibly an endocrinologist.

In addition to a thorough physical exam, your doctor will rely on your history of symptoms and complaints to provide the first clues about the nature of your problem. Some of the most common questions a doctor asks are the following:

- Does it hurt or burn when you urinate?
- Do you feel an urgency to urinate?
- Do you have to strain to urinate?
- Do you urinate in the middle of the night?
- Have you noticed a strong odor or any blood or other discoloration in your urine?
- Do you have sexual problems?
- Do you wake up with an erection?

If you are having problems conceiving, your doctor may ask the following questions:

- How long have you been trying?
- How often do you and your partner have intercourse?
- Have you ever fathered a child?
- Do you have a history of sexually transmitted disease?
- Are you a heavy user of alcohol or illicit drugs (especially marijuana) or a heavy smoker?

Your answers to these questions may lead your doctor to ask more detailed questions. In replying to these inquiries, you should answer honestly and thoughtfully, without being embarrassed. Although most people are not used to talking about these subjects, physicians—especially urologists—deal with them every day.

Physical Exam

The causes of many male reproductive complaints can often be determined during a physical examination. After pressing on your abdomen, testes, and penis, your doctor will give you a digital rectal exam to check for an enlarged or painful prostate. This entails inserting a lubricated, gloved finger into your rectum. If you are over 50, you should have a rectal exam annually (Note: The American Cancer Society recommends annual exams beginning at age 40. Certainly, if many of your relatives have prostate problems, you should have an annual rectal exam starting at age 40). You may find the physical exam slightly uncomfortable, but it will be much easier if you try to relax and breathe deeply.

Test for PSA

Some physicians check for prostate cancer with a blood test that measures the prostate-specific antigen (PSA) in the blood (also see chapters 2 and 4). The value of this test is controversial: men with benign prostatic hyperplasia (BPH)—a noncancerous condition—may have high PSA levels (a false-positive result) while some with prostate cancer have normal levels (false-negative). This is problematic, because a positive test may cause needless worry and lead your doctor to recommend a prostate biopsy (the removal of a small piece of the gland to check for cancer). While a biopsy can confirm prostate cancer, it is an invasive test that can cause infection and should not be performed unless absolutely indicated. An important factor is that prostate cancer is often very slow growing and may not require treatment.

Despite the controversy, however, the PSA test is the most reliable test for prostate cancer available, and most physicians use it, especially when symptoms of prostate disease are present.

Other Tests

Blood and urine testing for hormones and other chemicals (see chapter 9 and table 10.1), as well as ultrasound and other noninvasive imaging tests (see chapter 3 and tables 10.2 and 10.3) may be sufficient—along with a physical exam—to diagnose problems with the male reproductive organs.

In addition to prostate abnormalities, ultrasound can delineate other reproductive structures that may cause complaints. The other imaging tests—such as contrast radiography, in which a contrast dye is injected and an X-ray taken—may also assist the physician in determining the problems in the reproductive system, especially if they are caused by blockages.

Infertility and Impotence

Because so many conditions can cause infertility and impotence, urologists often consult other specialists when testing for these problems. For example, to identify the cause of impotence, it is helpful to know whether a man experiences erections during sleep (a normal occurrence). If so, this may indicate that his problem is primarily psychological, not physical, in origin. This can be determined with a sleep study called a nocturnal penile tumescence test, which is usually performed in a sleep physiology laboratory.

Simple tests such as semen or blood analysis (see tables 10.4 and 10.1) often reveal why a man is infertile. For more difficult cases, however, an endocrinologist (a physician who studies the production and effects of hormones) may be consulted to determine if a subtle hormonal disorder is the culprit.

TABLE 10.1 Blood Tests

Test	Use
BUN creatinine	Since these chemicals are usually removed by the kidneys, high levels in the blood indicate impaired kidney function.
Calcium, phosphorous	High levels indicate bone, kidney, or metabolic disease.
Alpha-fetoprotein	Measures levels of an antigen that may be elevated by some tumors in the testicles.
Beta-human chorionic gonadotropin	Measures levels of a hormone that may be elevated by some tumors in the testicles.
Prostate specific antigen (PSA)	Measures levels of an antigen that may be elevated by prostate cancer.
Electrolytes	Levels of these substances, including sodium, potassium, chloride, bicarbonate, calcium, and phosphate, may be altered in a variety of disorders, including kidney problems (see chapter 4).
Erythropoietin, renin	Levels of these hormones are altered by kidney problems.
LH, FSH, testosterone, prolactin	LH (leuteinizing hormone) instructs the testicles to produce the male sex hormone testosterone, while FSH (follicle-stimulating hormone) controls the cells that manufacture sperm. Fertility depends on normal levels of these three hormones. An excess of the hormone prolactin also affects fertility, as can a lack of LH-releasing hormone, which stimulates production of LH.

TABLE 10.2 Imaging Tests*

Test	Use
Excretory urography	Contrast dye and radiography (X-ray) show kidneys, ureters, bladder, and surrounding structures.
Computed tomography (CT)	Noninvasive technique that shows relationships of internal structures. Used to evaluate tumors or for guidance during biopsies.
Magnetic resonance imaging (MRI)	Noninvasive technique that shows relationship of internal structures without X-rays. Used when CT scan does not confirm diagnosis.
Ultrasound	Noninvasive diagnostic tool for studying the genitourinary tract without X-rays. May be transurethral (through the urethra), transabdominal (through the abdomen), or transrectal (through the rectum). Doppler ultrasound evaluates blood flow and effectively diagnoses fluid collection, obstruction, abscesses, and dilated ureters.

* See also chapters 3 and 12.

TABLE 10.3 Contrast X-ray Studies*

Test	Use
Retrograde pyelography	Contrast dye is injected and X-rayed, usually to identify ureteral strictures or blockage, and tumors.
Cystography	Contrast dye is injected and X-rayed to study the bladder.
Retrograde urethrography	Contrast dye is injected and X-rayed to study the urethra.
Voiding cystourethrography	Contrast dye is injected and X-rayed to detect urine backup into the kidneys, delineate the urethra, and determine whether the bladder empties after urination (see chapter 12).

* See also chapter 3.

TABLE 10.4 Infertility Tests

Test	Use
Semen analysis	Evaluates semen volume and pH, and sperm count.
Postcoital test (PCT)	Determines sperm motility in normal mucus from partner's cervical mucus (see chapter 11).
Mixed erthrocyte-spermatozoa antiglobulin reaction (MAR test)	Checks for antisperm antibodies by mixing sperm with sensitized red blood cells and antihuman IgG antiserum. Men and women may possess antibodies. Test is used if sperm count is normal but postcoital test result is poor, indicating that the woman may have antibodies to her partner's sperm.
Sperm agglutination tests (GAT, TSAT, TAT)	Checks for antisperm antibodies in blood of either partner or in sperm.
Sperm cervical mucus contact (SCMC) test	Sperm is mixed with preovulatory cervical mucus to see if antisperm antibodies are present in genital secretions.

TESTICULAR BIOPSY

General information

Where It's Done	Who Does It	How Long It Takes	Discomfort/Pain
Surgical facility, out-patient unit, or doctor's office.	Surgeon or urologist.	20–30 minutes.	Some soreness afterward.
Results Ready When	**Special Equipment**	**Risks/Complications**	**Average Cost**
Several days.	Surgical tools.	Possible bleeding and small risk of infection.	$$

Other names None.

Purpose

- To evaluate infertility.
- To rule out cancer.

How it works A tissue sample is removed and sent for laboratory analysis.

Preparation None.

Test procedure

- Local anesthetic is used.
- An incision is made in the scrotum to expose the testicles.
- A piece of testicular tissue—a little more than 1⁄16 of an inch in diameter—is removed.

After the test

- The incision is bandaged, and the patient is fitted with a protective scrotal support, after which the patient can go home.

- At home an ice pack may be used to ease soreness and reduce swelling.
- The patient can resume normal activities within a few days, but may be instructed to abstain from sexual activity for a few weeks.

Factors affecting results

- Illness.
- Previous vasectomy.
- Congenital abnormalities.
- Toxic exposures.
- Infections.

Interpretation The tissue is examined microscopically to check for any abnormal cells and for the absence or presence of normally maturing sperm.

Advantages The test may prevent or support further workup and treatment.

Disadvantages It's invasive.

The next step Proceed with treatment of diagnosed condition.

SCROTAL EXPLORATION

General information

Where It's Done	Who Does It	How Long It Takes	Discomfort/Pain
Surgical facility.	Urologist.	90 minutes.	Some soreness after procedure.
Results Ready When	**Special Equipment**	**Risks/Complications**	**Average Cost**
Immediately.	Surgical instruments and fluoroscope.	Bleeding and infection.	$$$

Other names Exploratory scrototomy.

Purpose To check for obstruction in the vas deferens or epididymis.

How it works The scrotum is surgically opened to examine the testicles for blockages.

Preparation If undergoing general anesthesia, you may have to fast the night before.

Test procedure

- Anesthesia may be local infiltration, epidural block, or general—the choice depending on the anticipated extent of surgery.
- The scrotum is opened and the testicles exposed to show blockage in the epididymis.
- A biopsy of testicular tissue is taken.

- If no blockage is evident, the scrotum is sutured closed.
- If the biopsy indicates a possible blockage, a vasogram (X-ray) may be performed by injecting contrast dye into the vas deferens.

After the test

- The area is bandaged.
- A scrotal support is applied.
- The patient may return home; if general anesthesia or spinal block was used, the patient should remain in recovery for two to three hours and then be accompanied home afterward.
- For at least seven days after the surgery, the scrotal area should remain dry and immobilized in the supportive structure.
- The patient may return to work after two to three days.

Factors affecting results

- Previous surgery or infection.
- Cystic fibrosis.

Interpretation Direct observation or X-rays may confirm blockage.

Advantages

- It's an effective method of confirming a testicular blockage.
- If the exact site of obstruction is determined, it may be correctable with additional surgery.

Disadvantages It's invasive.

The next step Surgical repair if indicated.

PROSTATIC BIOPSY

General information

Where It's Done	Who Does It	How Long It Takes	Discomfort/Pain
Surgical facility.	Urologist.	20 minutes.	Some, depending on anesthesia.
Results Ready When	**Special Equipment**	**Risks/Complications**	**Average Cost**
2–3 days.	For fine-needle aspiration, special needles and a needle guide; biopsy "gun" is often used.	From biopsy: bleeding and infection. Fine-needle aspiration may have fewer risks than core-needle biopsy but may provide less information.	$$–$$$

Other names Biopsy of the prostate.

Purpose To confirm or rule out prostate cancer.

How it works A sample of prostate tissue is removed and examined microscopically for cancerous cells.

Preparation

- You disrobe and don a surgical gown.
- You receive an injection of local anesthesia.
- You must remain still for the entire procedure.

Test procedure Ultrasound may be used to provide guidance for the test. For fine-needle aspiration:

- An anesthetic jelly may be used to numb the rectal area.
- A needle guide is inserted into the rectum.
- Once the prostate is reached, the long, thin aspiration needle is inserted, the sample taken, and the needle and guide removed.

For core-needle biopsy, tissue may be taken through the rectum or perineal area in front of the anus.

After the test

- You are free to leave and resume normal activities immediately.
- You may experience some soreness at the biopsy site for two to three days, for which you can take a nonprescription painkiller such as aspirin or acetaminophen.
- Any abnormal bleeding or fever should be reported to your doctor immediately.

Factors affecting results Failure to remain still during the procedure (under local anesthesia).

Interpretation A pathologist examines the biopsied tissue under a microscope for cancer.

Advantages The test provides a definitive diagnosis of prostate cancer.

Disadvantages It's invasive.

The next step If cancer is present, further tests, such as a CT and a bone scan, may be performed to check for its spread to other parts of the body. This will help determine the appropriate treatment. If no cancer is found, no further tests are immediately necessary, but follow-up PSA levels should be done every six months.

CAVERNOSOMETRY AND CAVERNOSONOGRAPHY

General information

Where It's Done	Who Does It	How Long It Takes	Discomfort/Pain
Urologist's office.	Urologist or radiologist.	1 hour.	Some, as the needles are inserted.

Results Ready When	Special Equipment	Risks/Complications	Average Cost
Immediately.	Arterial pressure monitor and perfusion pump.	Bruising; papaverine causes nausea in some patients.	$$

Other names None.

Purpose To determine whether erection disorders may be due to poor blood circulation.

How it works After injecting the drug papaverine (which dilates blood vessels) into the corpus cavernosa—the penile cavities that fill with blood during erection—local blood pressure is measured and recorded. Cavernosonography is an additional procedure, during which a contrast dye is injected and X-rays are taken.

Preparation None.

Test procedure

- You are given a gown to wear.
- You lie on an examination table.
- Two needles are inserted into the penis.
- A rubber band is placed at the base of the penis.
- Papaverine is injected, and an arterial pressure monitor measures blood pressure in the penis.
- The rubber band is removed after two minutes.
- A perfusion pump is used to increase the blood pressure in the penis.
- Pressures, are monitored and erectile activity of the penis observed until the pressure reaches a specific point.
- The pressure stabilizes at the maintenance rate—the rate necessary to maintain an erection. The infusion is then stopped and the dropping pressure is periodically recorded.
- If a blood leak is evidenced by rapidly dropping pressure, a contrast dye will be injected and X-rays taken.

After the test You may return immediately to normal activities.

Factors affecting results Venous leak (a leak in a vein).

Interpretation Any leak in the veins will be visible on the X-rays.

Advantages The test rapidly diagnoses blood leaks as the culprit in erectile disorders.

Disadvantages

- Some men are made dizzy and nauseated by the drug papaverine or the contrast dye.
- The procedure is uncomfortable.

The next step Treatment, either medical or surgical.

SEMEN ANALYSIS

General information

Where It's Done	Who Does It	How Long It Takes	Discomfort/Pain
Doctor's office, lab, or home.	You give a semen sample.	Varies—from 10–30 minutes.	None.
Results Ready When	**Special Equipment**	**Risks/Complications**	**Average Cost**
1–10 days, depending on the number and complexity of tests performed.	Urine specimen cup.	None.	$$

Other names Semen collection or sperm study.

Purpose To determine a man's fertility or infertility based on a variety of laboratory tests on the semen specimen.

How it works A semen specimen is submitted for laboratory analysis.

Preparation Some physicians recommend refraining from sexual activity for three days before the test.

Test procedure

- Either at home or in a doctor's office or laboratory, the man is required to masturbate to ejaculation and collect the semen in a sterile plastic container, usually the same kind used for a urine sample.

> **PATIENT TIP**
>
> When you masturbate for the test, do not use any lubricants, as these can kill sperm by attacking the sperm membranes.

- Obtaining the sample at the doctor's office or laboratory is more effective, ensuring a safe and fast delivery for analysis. Otherwise, the specimen must be delivered quickly to the doctor's office or laboratory and kept at room temperature and out of the light until delivery.

After the test You are free to leave and resume normal activities immediately.

Factors affecting results

- Improper collection procedure, especially affecting volume.
- Exposing semen to cold, heat, or strong light can destroy the sample.

Interpretation Various counts and analyses are done on the semen sample. These may include the following:

- *Volume:* Amount of semen in a single ejaculation.
- *Sperm concentration:* Number of sperm present in semen.
- *Viscosity:* The stickiness or resistance to flow of the semen.
- *Abnormal forms:* Percentage of sperm that are asymmetrical, unusually large, oddly shaped, or have double heads or tails.
- *Motility:* Percentage of sperm that are moving (variously interpreted as twitching in place, spinning in circles, or moving in one direction).
- *Migration:* Percentage of sperm showing forward progression.

A low sperm count or volume may be the reason for infertility. (Other infertility tests include the mixed erythrocyte-spermatozoa antiglobulin reaction [MAR test]—see table 10.4.)

Advantages

- It's noninvasive and inexpensive.
- It's a brief test that produces fast and reliable results.

Disadvantages You may be too embarrassed to masturbate and ejaculate in the doctor's office, and a sample from home may not be suitable for analysis because of exposure to heat or light.

The next step Treatment, depending on the diagnosis.

Peter E. Schwartz, MD ■ *David L. Olive, MD*

11 The Female Reproductive System

Tests Covered in This Chapter

The case of Michelle R., a 34-year-old mother of a 3-month-old son, Alex:

When my husband and I were married, we both wanted to have children right away, so I went off birth control pills, and we started trying to get pregnant. But after nine months of trying, we hadn't conceived, so I went to my physician for an evaluation. The physical examination revealed a cyst on one of my ovaries. Ultrasound confirmed the cyst, which had to be surgically removed. During the operation, the surgeon removed the cyst and part of the ovary, and he discovered that I had endometriosis, meaning that tissue normally found lining the uterus ends up elsewhere in the pelvic cavity. In my case, it caused scarring, which blocked my fallopian tubes and meant I probably was not going to be able to conceive on my own.

The Tests Because infertility may result from a combination of factors, Michelle's doctors started with the simplest tests. Her husband's sperm was tested and found to be normal. Michelle then had a postcoital test—a pelvic examination following intercourse. A sample of cervical mucus removed during the exam was then analyzed for the presence of sperm and to determine the quality of both the sperm and mucus. She also checked to be sure that she was ovulating by using a home ovulation detection kit that measures hormone levels in the urine.

The results of these tests were normal, leading Michelle's doctor to conclude that the scarring on her fallopian tubes was the major problem. He then ordered a hysterosalpingogram to evaluate the internal contour of her uterus and determine where the tubal blockage began.

The Outcome Because the hysterosalpingogram showed that Michelle's tubes were blocked at both ends, the couple decided to try in vitro fertilization. After two failed attempts, they were successful, and Michelle gave birth to a healthy baby boy.

INTRODUCTION

The femal reproductive system consists of a complex system of organs controlled by the monthly fluctuations of various hormones. Two ovaries, each about the size and shape of an almond, are located on either side of the uterus. The uterus, which has two parts, is a hollow, pear-shaped organ, located between the bladder and the rectum. The broad, upper portion, called the corpus, has two layers of tissue, the endometrium and the myometrium. The lower, narrow part is the cervix, which opens into the vagina.

Each month, in women of reproductive age, one ovary releases an egg, which travels through the fallopian tubes to the uterus. The ovaries also secrete the hormones estrogen and progesterone. These hormones regulate female body development, the menstrual cycle, and pregnancy. The monthly menstrual cycle begins when the endometrial tissue prepares to accept a fertilized egg by thickening and swelling. If the tissue is not used, it sheds and passes out of the vagina, causing menstruation. When a woman becomes pregnant, the fertilized egg attaches to the uterine wall and begins to grow, and the myometrium expands to hold the fetus. Eventually, all women experience menopause, when menstruation ceases and, with it, reproductive function. Menopause occurs when there are no more eggs left in the ovaries.

This chapter covers diagnosis and testing related to reproductive system disorders of women who are not pregnant. Chapter 25 focuses on pregnancy and related testing, while chapter 26 covers other diseases, including breast disease and osteoporosis, that affect primarily women.

REPRODUCTIVE SYSTEM DISORDERS

A wide range of disorders—including inflammation, tumors, infectious diseases, and infertility—can affect various parts of the female reproductive system. The most common disorders are described below.

Cancers. These include cervical, endometrial, ovarian, uterine, and vulvar cancer.

Endometriosis. A condition in which endometrial tissue grows in areas other than the uterus.

Fibroids. Noncancerous growths or tumors that occur, usually in multiples, in the uterus.

Hyperplasia. Extreme overgrowth of normal cells that line the uterus.

Infertility. The inability to conceive after a year or more of regular sexual activity without contraception.

Menopausal difficulties. Physical distress during menopause that can often be relieved with hormone therapy.

Sexually transmitted diseases (STDs). These diseases, which are spread by sexual intercourse or other genital contact, include AIDS, caused by a virus; the bacterial infections gonorrhea and syphilis; chlamydia, which is caused by cellular parasites; genital herpes and genital warts, which are caused by viruses; and pelvic inflammatory disease (PID), which is usually bacterial but may be caused by chlamydia. Diagnosis of these infectious diseases is discussed in chapter 22, with the exception of AIDS, which is discussed in chapter 21.

Vaginitis. A general term for inflammation of the vagina, often accompanied by itching and discharge. It may be caused by an overgrowth of yeast (also called fungus, *Monilia*, or *Candida*) normally found in the vagina; by an overgrowth of the bacteria (*Gardnerella*) that is normally found in the vagina or may be sexually transmitted; or by *Trichomonas*, a parasite that is sexually transmitted. It may also be a result of irritation from such diverse factors as excessive douching, laundry soap used to wash underpants, or the vaginal dryness and/or irritation that frequently occur after menopause.

REPRODUCTIVE SYSTEM SYMPTOMS

Many female reproductive disorders do not produce symptoms, which is why regular examinations and screening tests are necessary. However, the following is a list of possible indicators of the diseases listed for each symptom:

- *Abdominal or pelvic pain*. Pelvic inflammatory disease, fibroids, endometriosis, ectopic pregnancy, and cancers of the reproductive system.
- *Abnormal vaginal bleeding*. Pelvic inflammatory disease, fibroids, endometriosis, ectopic pregnancy, hormonal imbalance, and cancers of the reproductive system.
- *Abnormal vaginal discharge*. Pelvic inflammatory disease or vaginitis.
- *Amenorrhea (no menstrual bleeding)*. Ectopic pregnancy or hormonal abnormality.
- *Flulike symptoms, genital sores, and/or pain during urination*. Some sexually transmitted diseases.
- *Hot flashes and/or vaginal dryness*. May occur at menopause.
- *Itching or other irritation*. Menopausal difficulties, some sexually transmitted diseases, and vaginitis.
- *Pain during intercourse (dyspareunia)*. Ectopic pregnancy, menopausal difficulties, pelvic inflammatory disease, and endometriosis.

HOW YOUR DOCTOR DIAGNOSES REPRODUCTIVE SYSTEM DISORDERS

The first and most important element in any diagnosis is the history and physical exam, during which your doctor may ask you about your medical and family history and about any problems or changes you might have experienced since your last exam. These questions usually involve your reproductive history, menstrual cycle, and any symptoms you may experiencing, such as abnormal vaginal discharge.

The exam will include your height and weight, blood pressure, and possibly your temperature and pulse. Your breasts will be examined for any unusual lumps, tenderness, or discharge from the nipples.

The major part of the physical is the pelvic exam, during which the doctor looks for inflammation, discharge, masses, or tenderness that might indicate an infection or other disorder. If you have not had a recent Pap smear, your doctor will usually do one during the pelvic exam. The Pap smear is perhaps the most important tool in screening for cervical cancer because it shows cellular abnormalities that appear long before symptoms do and may indicate precancerous changes.

Depending on your symptoms and any findings from the exam, the doctor may perform additional tests or schedule you for more complicated diagnostic procedures at a later date. Over the past decade, development of more accurate and less invasive tests has made diagnosis of female reproductive system problems easier and more comfortable for women and has obviated the need for surgery in many cases. The disorders or circumstances described below require a more extensive workup.

Abnormal Vaginal Discharge

If you have any abnormal vaginal discharge or lesions, your doctor may examine a sample under a microscope (a procedure known as wet-mount) and/or may send it to a laboratory for a bacterial culture or a Gram stain test (see chapter 4) to find its origin. In some cases, antibiotic therapy will begin before the results of the culture are obtained.

Menstrual Irregularities

If your menstrual periods have been irregular or nonexistent (amenorrhea), the doctor will first try to ascertain whether the problem is the disorder itself or a result of another disorder. Also, your doctor will distinguish between primary amenorrhea, never having had any menses, and secondary amenorrhea, which develops after having experienced menses at some point.

Primary Amenorrhea. A physical examination is done to ascertain evidence of breast development and the presence or absence of a uterus. If a uterus is present and breast development is absent, puberty has been delayed. Measuring the level of the gonadotropin hormone follicle-stimulating hormone (FSH) in the blood determines if the disorder is a malfunctioning ovary or a central nervous system disorder. If the ovary is the culprit, a karyotype (mapping of genetic material) and blood tests may be performed to identify a possible genetic cause. If a central nervous system problem is noted, imaging studies of the skull are generally ordered.

If the uterus is absent and breast development is absent, the problem is usually a genetic blockade in making hormones. People with this problem have the genetic makeup of a male but appear as undeveloped females due to the inability to make hormones. Surgery to remove intra-abdominal testes is required.

If there is breast development but no uterus, the patient is a genetic male with androgen (male sex hormone) insensitivity syndrome, called testicular feminization; or the patient is a genetic female with a malfunction in uterine development. A blood test to measure testosterone level differentiates the two. If the woman has both uterus and breasts, the evaluation is identical to that of secondary amenorrhea.

Secondary Amenorrhea. First, a blood test for the level of the hormone prolactin is done. If it is elevated, the pituitary gland is evaluated by CT scan or magnetic resonance imaging (MRI). If the level is not elevated, the doctor prescribes a ten-day regimen of a progesterone-like hormone. If the woman bleeds after this treatment, the diagnosis is anovulation (lack of ovulation). If she does not bleed, she will take estrogen for a month, followed by ten days of a progesterone-like hormone. If she still does not bleed, a hysteroscopy is performed to search for an abnormal uterus. If she bleeds, a blood test to determine her level of follicle-stimulating hormone (FSH) will distinguish between premature ovarian failure and a central nervous system disorder. The latter requires imaging studies of the skull.

Suspected Ectopic Pregnancy

If the pregnancy is believed to be in the early stages, a blood sample is tested for human chorionic gonadotropin (hCG), a hormone secreted by the placenta. If the level is high, an ultrasound exam should show an intrauterine pregnancy. If it does not, an ectopic pregnancy is suspected. A dilation and curettage (D & C) is performed to remove the lining of the uterus. If no fetal tissue is found, laparoscopy is performed to locate the embryo.

If the level of hCG is low, the test is repeated after two days, by which time an increase of two-thirds is expected. If there is no change, a D & C, and possibly a laparoscopy, is done. If there is an increase, the level is monitored until it reaches a high level or until it stops climbing steadily, and then an ultrasound is done.

Abnormal Postmenopausal Bleeding

Abnormal bleeding in a postmenopausal woman requires prompt evaluation. The first step is a sampling of the inside lining of the uterus, which can often be performed in the office without anesthesia using aspiration biopsy equipment. If the biopsy reveals a cancer of the uterus, a total hysterectomy and removal of both fallopian tubes and ovaries is performed. If the biopsy reveals precancerous changes such as hyperplasia (abnormal increase of cells), a hysteroscopy may be necessary to further evaluate the lining of the uterus.

Abnormal Pap Smear

If Pap smear results are abnormal, a colposcopy exam is done to determine the site of the abnormal cells. The colposcope allows the examiner to observe abnormal blood vessel patterns often associated with precancerous or cancerous changes. Biopsies will be obtained from the worst-appearing sites as well as from the inside lining of the cervical canal. If the abnormality is limited to the outside surface of the cervix, the changes can be treated in the office. If it extends into the canal of the cervix, a large biopsy, called a cone biopsy, must be done to evaluate the extent and degree of the abnormality.

Rape

Following a rape, a woman is examined, in the presence of a witness, to document abrasions, bruising, or other evidence of trauma. Samples should be taken from under the fingernails, and the pubic hair should be combed for specimens. A complete search for semen stains should be done with a black light, which will make them show up as fluorescent. Pelvic and rectal exams should again look for evidence of trauma. The vagina should be swabbed for semen, and cultures for sexually transmitted diseases obtained.

Infertility

The first step in evaluating infertility is analysis of a semen sample from the male to determine the quality of the sperm (see chapter 10). In the female, a hysterosalpingogram is performed just after her menstrual period. Ovulation is monitored with a luteinizing hormone (LH) detection kit, ultrasound, and/or basal body temperature. At midcycle, a postcoital test is performed. An endometrial biopsy is performed ten to 12 days after ovulation. Finally, a laparoscopy completes the evaluation. If problems are identified in any of these screening tests, additional tests will be ordered to pinpoint the problem.

TESTS COMMONLY USED TO DIAGNOSE FEMALE REPRODUCTIVE SYSTEM DISORDERS

Tables 11.1 through 11.5 list and briefly describe a wide variety of tests used in the evaluation and diagnosis of disorders of the female reproductive system.

TABLE 11.1 Laboratory Tests Done on Blood Samples

All of the following tests are done on a sample of blood taken from a vein, usually in the arm. For more information about the venipuncture procedure, see chapter 4.

Test	Use
Human chorionic gonadotropin (hCG) (a hormone)	Can help identify ectopic pregnancy or threatened abortion. May also be used to monitor women with rare forms of ovarian cancer or those with cancerous changes in the placenta (gestational trophoblastic disease).
Complete blood count (CBC)	Routinely done to help identify cause of pelvic pain, such as ectopic pregnancy or vaginal bleeding. See chapter 4.
Erythrocyte sedimentation rate (ESR)	To help identify cause of pelvic pain and to rule out infection. See chapter 16.
Venereal Disease Research Laboratory (VDRL) test	To help identify cause of pelvic pain, especially when syphilis is suspected. Positive result indicates syphilis. Negative result rules it out or indicates that it has been adequately treated. Some false-positive results occur in people with other infectious diseases.
Follicle-stimulating hormone (FSH) and luteinizing hormone (LH)	To diagnose precocious puberty, menopausal problems, infertility, menstrual difficulties, and gonadal malfunctions, all of which cause excessive levels of these hormones. Low levels of these hormones indicate pituitary and hypothalamic disorders.
Estradiol (a hormone)	To identify causes of infertility, menstrual irregularity, or precocious puberty. Elevated levels indicate possible disorders. Oral contraceptives lower estradiol levels.
Thyroid function tests—thyroid-stimulating hormone (TSH), T_3, and T_4	To identify causes of infertility, abnormal bleeding, or galactorrhea. See chapter 9.
Prolactin (a hormone)	To diagnose galactorrhea (lactation at the wrong time), amenorrhea, or infertility. High levels occur normally during pregnancy, breast-feeding, and after a hysterectomy. Otherwise, high levels indicate a prolactin-secreting tumor. Many drugs, including estrogens and antihypertensives, can cause elevated levels.
Testosterone (a hormone)	Used to determine cause of hirsutism (excessive facial and body hair), lack of ovulation, or amenorrhea. Abnormally high levels in women may indicate a malfunction of the ovaries.
Dehydroepiandrosterone (DHEA) and DHEA-sulfate (DHEA-S)	To determine cause of hirsutism, amenorrhea, or infertility. Abnormally high levels may indicate an adrenal gland disorder. See chapter 9.

Lupus anticoagulant	To determine cause of recurrent miscarriage. High levels indicate an abnormal factor in the blood that causes clotting complications.
Chromosomal analysis	To identify precocious puberty, congenital anomalies, recurrent miscarriages, amenorrhea, or infertility. Chromosomal defects may explain the problems that prompted the test.
Rapid plasma reagin (RPR) test	To diagnose syphilis, which produces a positive test result.
Fluorescent treponemal antibody absorption (FTA-ABS) test	To confirm syphilis, especially in early stages. Determines whether positive result from nontreponemal antigen tests such as VDRL is false-positive or is indicative of syphilis.
Micromagglutination, treponema pallidum (MHA-TP)	To confirm syphilis.
CA 125	To diagnose, monitor progression of, and check for recurrence of ovarian cancer. Abnormally high level is commonly associated with ovarian cancer, but levels may be falsely elevated in many gynecological disorders such as endometriosis, benign ovarian cysts, first trimester of pregnancy, and pelvic inflammatory disease. It is also elevated in 70% of people with cirrhosis, 60% of people with pancreatic cancer, and 20% to 25% of all other malignancies.
Lipid-associated sialic acid (LSA, LASA-P) in plasma	To diagnose, monitor progression of, and check for recurrence of ovarian cancer. High levels are associated with malignancies and inflammatory conditions. This nonspecific test may be elevated in a variety of chronic, benign medical conditions.
NB/70K	To diagnose, monitor progression of, and check for recurrence of ovarian cancer.
CA 19–9	To diagnose, monitor progression of, and check for recurrence of pancreatic or ovarian cancers.
TAG 72.3	To diagnose, monitor progression of, and check for recurrence of colon or ovarian cancers. May be used along with other tumor markers to distinguish benign ovarian tumors from malignant ones.

TABLE 11.2 Imaging Tests

Test	Use
Barium enema	To detect endometriosis, cervical cancer, and ovarian cancer. See chapter 8.
Color-flow Doppler	See chapter 3.
CT scan	To detect pelvic masses, brain or pituitary lesions, and cervical cancer. See chapter 3.
Hysterosalpingography	See below for a full description.
Intravenous pyelogram	To detect or determine the cause of endometriosis, pelvic masses, cervical cancer, congenital anomalies, and postoperative complications. See chapter 12.
Magnetic resonance imaging (MRI)	See chapter 3.
Transabdominal ultrasound	To detect or determine the cause of ectopic pregnancy, pelvic inflammatory disease, or unexplained pelvic pain. See chapters 3 and 25.
Transvaginal ultrasound	See below for a full description.
Vaginogram	To detect fistulas, abnormal passages between two internal organs or between an internal organ and the body surface (such as an opening between the vagina and the rectum). The test involves injecting radiopaque dye into the vagina and taking X-rays of the area.
Voiding cystourethrogram	See chapter 12.

TABLE 11.3 Aspiration Tests

Test	Use
Culdocentesis	To detect causes of pelvic pain or intra-abdominal bleeding or to confirm suspected ectopic pregnancy. See below for a full description.
Dilation and curettage (D&C)	To confirm suspected ectopic pregnancy or determine cause of postmenopausal bleeding. See below for a full description.
Toluidine blue dye test	To evaluate abnormal changes in the vulva. Toluidine blue is a dye that is selectively taken up by tissue that exhibits precancerous changes.

TABLE 11.4 Other Laboratory Tests

Test	Use
Cervical/uterine/vaginal cultures	To detect or identify bacteria in cases of vaginitis or toxic shock syndrome. Fluid obtained with a swab or aspiration needle is sent to a laboratory to be grown in a culture medium. See chapter 4.
Urinalysis and culture	See chapter 12.
HPV subtyping	To screen for the human papillomavirus (HPV) and to determine the particular type if the test is positive. A tissue specimen is obtained during a biopsy or cervical swab (much like the Pap smear) and sent to a laboratory for analysis.
Dark-field examination	To diagnose syphilis. This is a microscopic technique that is useful when searching for the characteristic bacteria of syphilis. Serum is collected from the surface of a lesion (also called a chancre) and examined by dark-field microscopy. See chapter 17.

TABLE 11.5 Function Tests

Test	Use
Basal body temperature	To detect ovulation in infertility evaluation. See chapter 2.
Cystometry	To evaluate bladder function. See chapter 12.
GnRH (gonadotropin-releasing hormone) stimulation test	To differentiate hypothalamic from pituitary dysfunction in amenorrhea.
Postcoital test (Huhner test)	In cases of infertility, to determine the quality of cervical mucus and the penetrability of mucus by sperm, and to screen for anti-sperm antibodies. A day or two prior to ovulation, the couple has intercourse at a predesignated time, and the woman then goes to the doctor's office within two to eight hours. A pelvic examination is done, and a sample of cervical mucus (presumably containing sperm) is removed and examined under a microscope.

PELVIC EXAM AND PAP SMEAR

General information

Where It's Done	Who Does It	How Long It Takes	Discomfort/Pain
Doctor's office.	Physician or nurse practitioner.	About 10 minutes.	There may be minor discomfort when speculum is inserted.

Results Ready When	Special Equipment	Risks/Complications	Average Cost
Within a week for Pap smear.	Speculum and pelvic examination table with stirrups.	None.	$

Other names Pap test.

Purpose To diagnose any abnormalities that the doctor can feel or see without a microscope or that will show up on analysis of tissue from the cervix.

How it works The doctor inspects and palpates the reproductive organs and takes a sample of cervical tissue for microscopic examination in a laboratory.

Preparation You undress and don a hospital gown. If the exam does not include your breasts, you may only have to undress from the waist down.

Test procedure

- You lie on your back on an examining table with your feet in the stirrups while the doctor examines your vulva, the lips of your vagina (labia majora and labia minora), and your clitoris.
- The doctor then inserts a metal or plastic speculum into your vagina. This device, which will remain in place during the rest of the exam,

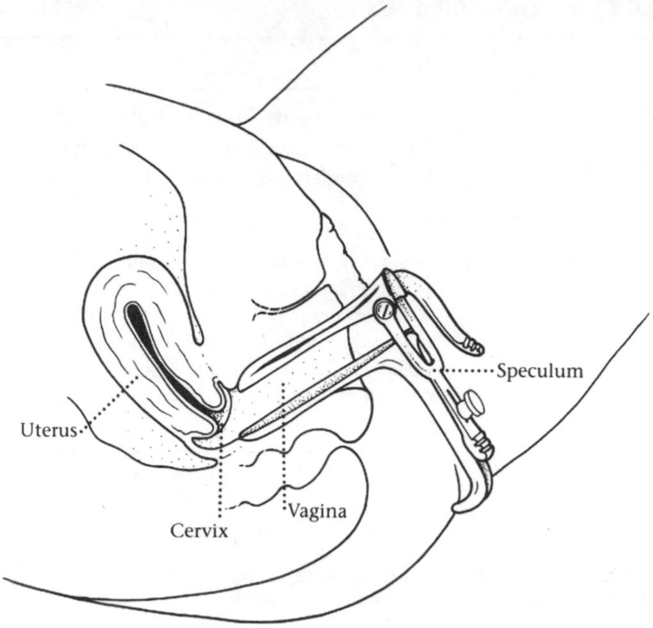

FIGURE 11.1 During a pelvic exam, an instrument called a speculum is inserted into the vagina to hold it open and allow the doctor to inspect the vaginal tissue and cervix. At this time, a swab can be inserted into the vagina to collect cells for a Pap smear.

has two adjustable paddles that spread the vaginal walls and hold them open, allowing a view of the upper vagina and cervix (see figure 11.1).

- A long cotton-tipped swab will be used to dab the cervix (a painless procedure) to take a sample of cells for a Pap smear.
- If you have vaginitis or the doctor suspects an infectious disease, a sample of vaginal discharge may also be taken.
- The doctor will insert one or two gloved, lubricated fingers into your vagina while pressing down on your abdomen with the other hand. The doctor will then insert one finger into your rectum and one into your vagina while continuing to press down on your abdomen. These steps help detect structural anomalies or abnormal growths.

After the test You get dressed and return immediately to normal activities.

Factors affecting results

- Full bladder.
- Obesity.

Interpretation The physician will determine if further tests are necessary in response to any abnormalities detected. A pathologist will examine the cervical tissue specimen for any changes in cells he or she may have seen, felt, or discovered from your reactions.

Advantages The test helps detect a variety of disorders at a minimum of discomfort and cost.

Disadvantages Further tests are usually required if an abnormality is found.

The next step

- If the Pap smear is normal, no further tests are necessary. The test will be repeated in one to three years, depending on your age and history (see chapter 2).
- If the Pap smear is abnormal, your doctor may recommend a procedure such as colposcopy (see below).
- Ultrasound, biopsy, or endoscopic procedures such as laparoscopy may be recommended, depending on the findings of the pelvic exam.

TRANSVAGINAL ULTRASOUND

General information

Where It's Done	Who Does It	How Long It Takes	Discomfort/Pain
Radiology section of hospital or doctor's office.	Radiology technician or physician.	Less than an hour.	There may be slight pressure when the ultrasound probe is inserted.
Results Ready When	**Special Equipment**	**Risks/Complications**	**Average Cost**
Immediately.	Ultrasonic imaging machine and handheld vaginal transducer.	None.	\$–\$\$ (depending on extent of test).

Other names Endovaginal ultrasound or ultrasonography.

Purpose

- To detect and delineate pelvic masses, ectopic pregnancy, ovarian cysts or tumors, pelvic inflammatory disease, and fibroid and bladder tumors.
- In an infertility workup, to assess ovulation.
- To confirm early pregnancy in the uterus.

How it works A transducer is used to transmit high-frequency sound waves, which bounce back to produce an image that can be recorded on X-ray film (see chapter 3).

Preparation
- You disrobe and don a hospital gown.
- Your bladder should be empty.

> **DID YOU KNOW?**
>
> Transvaginal ultrasound uses the same technology as abdominal ultrasound, but because the sound waves do not have to travel as far, there is less distortion and the test is more accurate. It may also be more comfortable because it does not require a full bladder.

Test procedure
- You lie on your back on an examining table with your feet in stirrups.
- A handheld transducer is inserted into your vagina. The transducer is shaped like and slightly smaller than a tampon.
- The images are seen on a video monitor and a hard copy may be made on film.

After the test You are free to return to normal activities.

Factors affecting results None.

Interpretation A radiologist or gynecologist examines the images for areas of abnormal tissue.

Advantages It's noninvasive and relatively inexpensive.

Disadvantages The image is not as high in resolution as a magnetic resonance image (MRI).

The next step
- If the test shows a fluid-filled ovarian cyst, the diagnosis is usually considered definitive and treatment can begin.
- If the test reveals a cyst that is solid, or liquid and solid, an X-ray or MRI may be recommended (see chapter 3).

COLPOSCOPY

General information

Where It's Done	Who Does It	How Long It Takes	Discomfort/Pain
Gynecologist's office or hospital outpatient department.	Doctor.	3–15 minutes depending on whether or not biopsies are taken.	The insertion of the speculum may cause some discomfort.

Results Ready When	Special Equipment	Risks/Complications	Average Cost
Colposcopic findings are immediately available. Biopsy reports take 2–5 days.	Colposcope and vaginal speculum.	None, unless a biopsy is performed at the same time (see below).	$$

Other names None.

Purpose

- To evaluate the cervical tissue following an abnormal Pap smear.
- Routinely to monitor women who are at increased risk of reproductive system cancers, such as women whose mothers took DES (diethylstilbestrol) during pregnancy.

How it works The colposcope, a specially lit microscope on a stand, allows the doctor to look directly at the abnormal tissue of the cervix. Sometimes a biopsy is done at the same time.

Preparation You remove all clothing from the waist down and don a hospital gown.

Test procedure

- You lie on your back on the examination table with your feet in the stirrups.
- The doctor will insert a speculum into your vagina (see the description of a pelvic exam) and may perform a Pap smear before using the colposcope, which is positioned about a foot from your body.
- If a biopsy is indicated, the doctor will remove a sample of cervical tissue (see the description of a cervical biopsy).

After the test The speculum is removed, and you are free to dress and return to normal activities, or follow the postbiopsy restrictions if you had a combined procedure.

Factors affecting results Creams or other obstructions in the vaginal area.

Interpretation Direct visualization may determine if there is abnormal tissue.

Advantages

- It's relatively noninvasive.
- It allows physician to view directly the tissue in question.

Disadvantages It does not allow for laboratory analysis of the tissue unless a biopsy is performed.

The next step

- If the results of the colposcopic exam are normal, the test is considered conclusive, but you may be scheduled for Pap tests at closer intervals than persons with normal Pap test results.
- If your doctor notices any abnormalities, a cervical biopsy may be done.

CERVICAL BIOPSY

General information

Where It's Done	Who Does It	How Long It Takes	Discomfort/Pain
Gynecologist's office or hospital outpatient department.	Doctor.	Less than 15 minutes.	Brief (a few seconds) but intensive pain when tissue is collected. Possible cramping afterward.

Results Ready When	Special Equipment	Risks/Complications	Average Cost
Within 1 week.	Vaginal speculum, colposcope, and punch for clipping tissue.	Small risk of excessive bleeding or infection.	$$

Other names Punch biopsy.

Purpose To evaluate abnormal cervical tissue found during a Pap smear or colposcopy.

How it works A sample of the tissue is removed for study in a pathology laboratory.

Preparation

- The physician will try to schedule you for the biopsy about one week after your menstrual period. (If you have your period at the time of the scheduled biopsy, you should reschedule.)
- Before the procedure, you undress from the waist down and don a surgical gown.

Test procedure

- Your doctor does a colposcopic exam (see above).
- The doctor then uses a small, scissors-like instrument called a punch to snip one or more tiny pieces of tissue (less than a ¼ of an inch in size) from your cervix.
- The specimen is sent to the pathology lab for analysis.

Variations

- *Loop electrical excision of the transformation zone (LETZ).* Rather than using a punch, in this procedure the doctor uses an electrocautery loop to remove a cervical tissue sample for biopsy.

- *Endocervical curettage.* Following a punch biopsy, your doctor may also take a sample of the tissue lining the endocervical canal, which is just past the opening of the cervix (cervical os) but not in the uterus itself. This is a precaution against missing any abnormal tissue in this area, which cannot be fully seen with the colposcope. A small, spoon-shaped instrument called a curette is inserted into the canal and briefly scraped against the lining. Although the procedure lasts only a few seconds, it may cause cramping.

After the test

- You dress and are free to leave.
- You may experience cramping after the procedure, so plan to take some time off to rest. (Ask if you can take a mild analgesic about half an hour before the procedure to lessen the cramps later.)
- Plan to wear a sanitary napkin for the first 24 hours or so after the biopsy.
- Avoid strenuous activity, douching, and sexual intercourse for at least 24 hours.
- You may experience bleeding or an unpleasant vaginal discharge for a day or so. This is usually not a cause for concern, but you should report any excessive bleeding immediately.

Factors affecting results Inadequate sample.

Interpretation A pathologist studies the tissue for abnormal cells and submits a report to your referring physician.

Advantages The test makes available the actual abnormal tissue for analysis.

Disadvantages It's invasive.

The next step

- If the tissue is normal, you may receive a clean bill of health or undergo further tests to determine the cause for the original referral. You may, however, be scheduled for Pap tests at closer intervals than persons with normal Pap test results.
- Abnormal tissue may indicate an infection or possible cancer. You may be referred for further tests to confirm the diagnosis, or treatment may be begun.

CULDOCENTESIS

General information

Where It's Done	Who Does It	How Long It Takes	Discomfort/Pain
Doctor's office or outpatient clinic.	Gynecologist.	About 10 minutes.	Possible mild discomfort from needle stick.

Results Ready When	Special Equipment	Risks/Complications	Average Cost
Immediately.	18-gauge spinal needle.	None.	$$

Other names None.

Purpose

- To identify the cause of pelvic inflammatory disease (PID).
- To diagnose ectopic pregnancy.

How it works Fluid withdrawn from the pelvic cavity is examined for abnormalities such as blood or infectious agents.

Preparation You undress and don a hospital gown.

Test procedure

- You lie on your back on an examination table with your feet in the stirrups as for a pelvic exam.
- The doctor inserts a needle through your vagina and into the cul-de-sac of Douglas, an area just behind the uterus that is defined by the membrane lining the abdomen and pelvic organs, and withdraws a sample of fluid from this cavity.

After the test You dress and are free to return to normal activities.

Factors affecting results Inadequate sample.

Interpretation If the fluid contains nonclotting blood, a ruptured ectopic pregnancy may be suspected. If PID is suspected, the fluid may be examined for infectious agents.

Advantages

- The test is quick and inexpensive.
- It provides immediate results.

Disadvantages It does not diagnose an ectopic pregnancy that has not already ruptured or produced nonclotting blood.

The next step

- If the results indicate a possible ectopic pregnancy, a laparoscopy may be performed to confirm the diagnosis and remove the fetus.
- If an infectious agent is identified as the cause of PID, treatment with antibiotics can begin.

HYSTEROSALPINGOGRAM

General information

Where It's Done	Who Does It	How Long It Takes	Discomfort/Pain
Hospital radiology suite.	Gynecologist and radiologist with nurse or technician.	15–30 minutes.	Cramping lasting several minutes when dye is instilled in uterus. May cause additional pain if fallopian tubes are blocked or go into spasm.

Results Ready When	Special Equipment	Risks/Complications	Average Cost
Preliminary results immediately; final report in 2–4 days.	Contrast dye, speculum, tenaculum, catheter, and X-ray machine.	Test should not be done on women who are pregnant or who have an infection. Slight risk of introducing or spreading pelvic infection. Rare risk of allergic reaction to iodine in dye.	$$

Other names Hysterogram, hysterosalpingography, uterography, uterotubography, and uterosalpingography.

Purpose

- To diagnose tubal obstruction as a cause of infertility.
- To detect suspected fibroids, polyps, or developmental abnormalities in the uterus and fallopian tubes.
- To evaluate the fallopian tubes before or after sterilization reversal surgery.
- To evaluate incompetent cervix in women with a history of miscarriage.

DID YOU KNOW?

Although hysterosalpingography is primarily a diagnostic technique, it sometimes acts as a treatment because the dye unblocks minor obstructions as it flows through the fallopian tubes. Some doctors think that oil-based dyes are more likely to do this than water-based dyes.

How it works Contrast dye is used to highlight the areas in question for the X-ray machine.

Preparation

- The test will be scheduled during the early part of your menstrual cycle (between menstruation and ovulation), when pregnancy is unlikely.
- You undress from the waist down and don a hospital gown.

Test procedure

- You lie on your back on an examination table with an X-ray machine suspended over your abdomen. Your legs will be placed in special stirrups that go behind your knees.
- A speculum is inserted into your vagina to hold open the vaginal walls. Then a thin, grasping instrument called a tenaculum is inserted to hold the cervix in place.
- A thin catheter is inserted through the cervix into the uterus. A small balloon inside the catheter is inflated to keep it in place, and radiopaque contrast dye is instilled through the catheter. This usually causes several minutes of cramping and may result in spasm.
- The gynecologist and radiologist watch the dye on a fluoroscope screen as it enters the uterus and spreads through the fallopian tubes, looking for abnormalities.
- Four to eight X-rays are taken at various intervals as the dye travels through your reproductive tract.

Special precautions

- If you suspect that you have a pelvic infection or may be pregnant, ask your doctor to reschedule the test.
- Tell your doctor if you are prone to pelvic infections. You may be given prophylactic antibiotics to take before the test is done. It may also affect the choice of dye since water-based dyes are believed less likely to spread infection.
- Be sure to take an analgesic such as ibuprofen about 30 minutes before the test to lessen the effect of the cramps.

Variations

Sonohysterogram, a test in which a catheter is inserted into the uterine cavity to instill fluid to distend the uterus, which is then examined via transvaginal ultrasound for space-occupying structures.

After the test

- You will remain on the examination table until any cramping subsides and to be sure that you do not experience any adverse effects from the dye.
- You may be asked to stay until the X-ray films are developed to be sure that no others are needed.
- Then you are free to dress and return to normal activities.
- If you experience severe cramping, you should not drive home.
- Wear a sanitary napkin for 24 hours after the procedure.
- Notify your doctor if you experience or notice excessive bleeding, fever, or unpleasant vaginal odor.

Factors affecting results

None.

Interpretation The radiologist will study the X-rays for a final report, but certain diagnoses can be made by watching the progress of the dye on the fluoroscope to see whether the shape of the uterine cavity appears normal or has apparent protrusions that might indicate a fibroid tumor or scar tissue; whether the dye leaks, indicating a tear in the uterine lining; and whether the dye flows through and out the fallopian tubes, indicating that they are patent (open).

Advantages

- It's relatively noninvasive.
- Negative results (showing that the fallopian tubes are open) are highly reliable.
- It shows the internal contours and patency of the fallopian tubes (ultrasound does not).
- The test itself may open small blockages.

Disadvantages It may produce false-positive results: what appears to be a tubal blockage close to the uterus may only be a spasm in that area.

The next step

- If the tubes appear to be open, and the uterine contour is normal, no further testing is necessary.
- If they appear to be closed, or the uterine cavity is irregular, additional tests (laparoscopy or hysteroscopy) or surgery may follow.

LAPAROSCOPY

General information

Where It's Done	Who Does It	How Long It Takes	Discomfort/Pain
Ambulatory or inpatient surgery department in hospital or surgical center.	Gynecologist.	30 minutes to 4 hours.	Minor discomfort from needle stick for the anesthesia; cramps and abdominal soreness afterwards. Possible referred pain in shoulder from carbon dioxide.
Results Ready When	**Special Equipment**	**Risks/Complications**	**Average Cost**
Laparoscopic findings, immediately; lab results, in 2–4 days.	Laparoscope, trocar, tenaculum, Veres needle, gas insufflator, and small surgical instruments (if a surgical procedure is combined with the examination).	There is a rare possibility of excessive bleeding or infection.	$$–$$$ (varies greatly according to the extent of the procedure).

Other names Peritoneoscopy, celioscopy, and pelvic endoscopy.

Purpose

- To determine the cause of chronic pelvic pain.
- To identify tumors, ovarian cysts, and endometrial growths, and possibly to drain or remove them.
- To determine the cause of fertility problems.
- To perform a tubal ligation—cutting and tying off the fallopian tubes—for purposes of sterilization.

How it works

A laparoscope—a narrow tube with a fiber-optic light on the end—introduced through the abdominal wall allows the doctor a direct view of the pelvic organs.

Preparation

- Because you are undergoing general anesthesia, you must not have anything to eat or drink for eight hours before the procedure.
- You remove all clothing and don a hospital gown.
- In some cases, a local anesthetic will be administered with the general anesthesia.

Test procedure

- Once the anesthesia takes effect, the doctor makes a 1-inch incision just below your navel.
- A gas insufflator is used to fill your abdominal cavity with carbon dioxide or nitrous oxide. This elevates the abdominal wall and allows a better view of your organs.
- The laparoscope is then introduced into the cavity through the incision. The physician looks at the reproductive organs, notes any abnormalities, and takes biopsy specimens if necessary. Surgical procedures may also be performed at this time using tiny instruments that fit into small sheaths inserted elsewhere in the abdomen.
- When the procedure is over, the gas is allowed to escape, and the incision is closed with a few stitches and dressed. Any tissue specimens will be sent to the laboratory for analysis.

Variations

In *hysteroscopy,* a hysteroscope—an endoscopic instrument similar to a laparoscope—is inserted through the vagina and cervix into the uterine cavity in order to examine the endometrium, the tissue that lines the uterus. A small electrified loop can be used to take biopsy samples of the endometrium for laboratory analysis.

After the test

- You will remain in the recovery room for two to three hours while the anesthesia wears off and your vital signs are monitored. You will be encouraged to walk around as soon as possible.
- Unless this is an inpatient procedure, you will be allowed to leave and resume a normal diet.
- You may experience some cramping, and you may experience referred pain in one or both shoulders as a result of the gas. These effects can be treated with nonprescription painkillers and should last no more than a day or two.

- You can shower as usual if you keep the dressing dry, but you should restrict your activity and avoid sexual intercourse for two or three days.
- Call your doctor if you have any severe pain, bleeding from your incision, or fever.

Factors affecting results Obesity.

Interpretation The physician may be able to report some results immediately. Any laboratory specimens will be examined by a pathologist, who will submit a report to your doctor. Abnormalities may include fallopian tube malfunctions, ectopic pregnancy, endometriosis, uterine fibroid tumors, ovarian cysts, or evidence of pelvic inflammatory disease (PID).

Advantages

- It provides direct view of female reproductive organs.
- In many cases, it eliminates the need for more invasive surgical procedures.

Disadvantages It's a surgical procedure with some risk attached.

The next step

- If laparoscopy is performed for tubal ligation or to terminate an ectopic pregnancy, or if the procedure allows complete removal of a cyst, a tumor, or endometrial tissue, no further procedures are necessary.
- If endometrial tissue or fibroid tumors are extensive, more invasive surgery may be necessary.

DILATION AND CURETTAGE (D & C)

General Information

Where It's Done	Who Does It	How Long It Takes	Discomfort/Pain
Hospital operating room or ambulatory surgery clinic.	Gynecologist.	Less than 30 minutes for scraping, but entire procedure will take most of a day.	None if general anesthesia is used; possible cramping if local anesthesia.

Results Ready When	Special Equipment	Risks/Complications	Average Cost
1–3 days.	Speculum, tenaculum, metal sound, metal rods of increasing thickness, and curette.	Small risk of excessive bleeding or uterine perforation and infection. Rarely, damage to bowel or bladder. Repeat D & Cs or overscraping may lead to scar tissue, which may cause infertility or menstrual problems.	$$

Other names None.

Purpose

- To help diagnose the cause of abnormal menstrual bleeding or infertility when an endometrial biopsy cannot be done.
- As treatment, to stop heavy bleeding or remove residual tissue following miscarriage, abortion, or occasionally, childbirth.

PATIENT TIP

If your doctor recommends a D & C, ask if a suction endometrial biopsy can be done instead. It carries a lesser risk of complications, but cannot be substituted in all cases.

How it works The cervical opening is dilated, and a tissue sample from the lining of the uterus is scraped out.

Preparation

- You may have to go to the hospital or doctor's office one or two days before the D & C for blood and urine tests and to rule out pregnancy if the procedure is diagnostic.
- You must have nothing to eat or drink for eight hours before surgery if you are having general anesthesia.
- You undress and don a hospital gown.
- You will be given general anesthesia intravenously.
- If the procedure is to be performed under local anesthetic, you may be given an oral sedative about 30 minutes before the procedure. You lie on a table with your feet in stirrups as for a pelvic exam. Once you are sedated, a local anesthetic is injected into the cervix.

Test procedure

- The doctor inserts a speculum into your vagina and then uses a special clamp called a tenaculum to grip the cervix.
- A thin metal rod called a sound is then inserted to determine the angle of the cervical canal and the depth of your uterus.
- Your cervix is slowly dilated, using metal rods of increasing diameter up to about ½ inch (see figure 11.2).
- A spoon-shaped curette is used to scrape tissue from the uterine lining. (In a therapeutic D & C, polyps or other unwanted tissue are removed as well.)
- The tenaculum and speculum are then removed.

After the test

- A tissue sample is sent to the lab for examination.
- If you have had general anesthesia, you will remain in a recovery room, and your vital signs will be monitored for about one hour until the anesthesia wears off.
- Once you are up and moving around, you are free to dress and leave, but you should arrange to have a friend or family member drive you home.

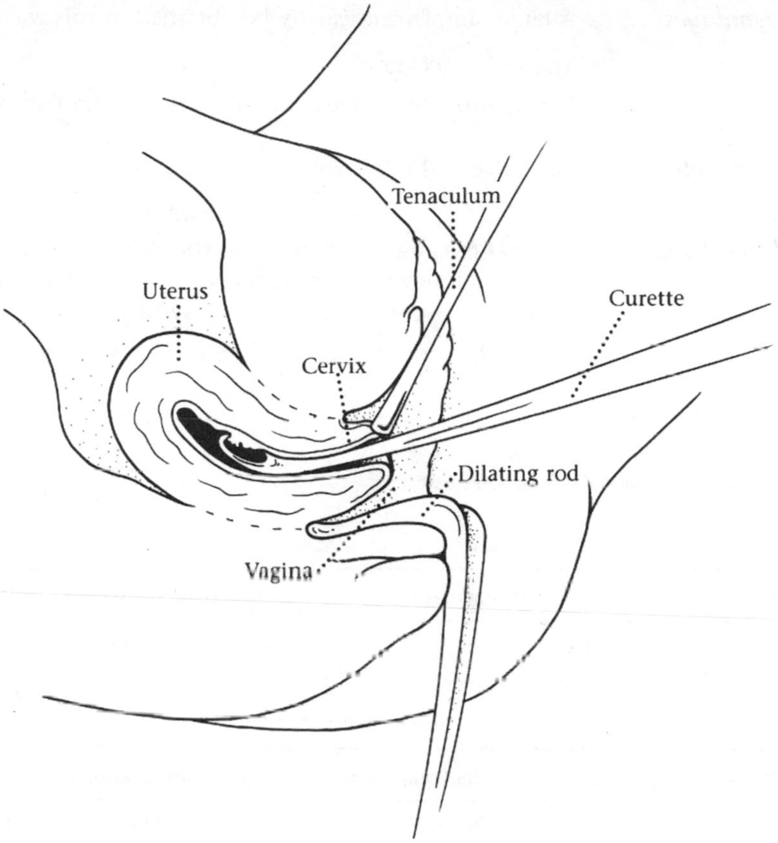

FIGURE 11.2 During dilation and curettage, or a D & C, the cervix is opened, or dilated, by using metal rods of increasing size. A spoon-shaped curette is then used to scrape tissue from the uterine lining.

- You may experience mild to moderate cramping over the next 24 hours or so, and you may be given a prescription for a painkiller.
- You can return to work or other usual activities as soon as you feel able, within hours or one or two days.
- You may have bleeding requiring you to wear sanitary napkins for two weeks or more.
- You should avoid sexual intercourse, tampons, and douching for at least two weeks to prevent infection.
- If you experience heavy bleeding, strong cramping, unusual vaginal discharge, or fever, notify your doctor immediately.

Factors affecting results Inadequate sample.

Interpretation A pathologist will examine the tissue sample for any abnormalities.

Advantages

- A large sample can usually be obtained in this way.
- The test is accurate.
- It may provide the cure if abnormal cells are removed.

Disadvantages It's invasive and relatively expensive.

The next step

- If the D & C was performed to stop heavy bleeding or remove residual tissue following a miscarriage or abortion, or to remove polyps, no further testing or treatment may be necessary.
- If the laboratory results indicate cancer, surgery may be scheduled.

ENDOMETRIAL BIOPSY

General information

Where It's Done	Who Does It	How Long It Takes	Discomfort/Pain
Doctor's office or outpatient clinic.	Gynecologist.	About 10 minutes.	Possible moderate to strong cramping, which can be minimized with a local anesthetic.
Results Ready When	**Special Equipment**	**Risks/Complications**	**Average Cost**
3–5 days.	Curette, or catheter attached to a vacuum.	Slight risk of heavy bleeding and rare risk of perforation and infection of the uterus.	$$

Other names: Uterine biopsy.

Purpose

- To diagnose the cause of vaginal bleeding, especially in women over 35 who have a family history of endometrial cancer.
- To help determine the cause of the infertility.
- To check for any cancerous or precancerous changes in women who are taking estrogen replacement therapy without progesterone.

DID YOU KNOW?

The endometrial lining provides information about ovulation and hormone activity, which can be useful in determining the cause of infertility.

How it works A sample of endometrial tissue is removed for examination by a pathologist.

Preparation

- You undress from the waist down and cover your lap with a sheet.
- If a local anesthetic is not being used, you may be given a mild painkiller such as ibuprofen 30 minutes before the procedure.
- You lie on your back on an examination table with your feet in the stirrups as for a pelvic exam.
- A local anesthetic will then be injected into the cervix.

Test procedure A narrow, flexible tube (catheter) is inserted into the uterus. The other end of the tube is attached to a vacuum. Suction is then used to remove a sample of endometrial tissue.

After the test

- You are free to leave and return to normal activities.
- You may experience some bleeding for a day or so, for which you should wear a sanitary napkin (avoid tampons).
- You may experience some cramping, for which you can take an over-the-counter pain reliever such as ibuprofen.
- If you experience heavy bleeding, notify your doctor immediately.

Factors affecting results Inadequate sample.

Interpretation The sample will be analyzed by a pathologist for any cancerous or precancerous changes and possibly tested for the presence of hormones.

Advantages It's quick, accurate, and inexpensive.

Disadvantages

- It's invasive.
- As with any biopsy, there is some risk of serious complications.

The next step

- If the test was done to monitor a woman taking estrogen replacement therapy without progesterone, it may be rescheduled periodically, even if results are normal.
- If tissue changes are noted, a D & C or other surgical procedure may be scheduled.

CONE BIOPSY

General information

Where It's Done	Who Does It	How Long It Takes	Discomfort/Pain
Hospital outpatient surgical unit.	Gynecological surgeon and nurse.	Less than 30 minutes for biopsy, but entire procedure will take most of a day.	Minor from needle stick for IV anesthesia; some bleeding and cramps.

Results Ready When	Special Equipment	Risks/Complications	Average Cost
3–5 days.	Scalpel.	Possible heavy bleeding; rarely, perforation or infection of the uterus. Possible miscarriage from incompetent cervix; possible infertility; scar tissue may interfere with vaginal childbirth or menstrual flow (rare).	$$

Other names Cervical biopsy or conization.

Purpose

- To check cervical cells for cancer, especially when colposcopy and cervical biopsy do not provide adequate evidence to confirm or rule out the diagnosis.
- As treatment, to remove abnormal cells.

How it works A sample of cells is removed from the cervix for direct examination in the laboratory.

> **PATIENT TIP**
>
> Complications from cone biopsy can be significant. If your doctor recommends this procedure, ask if colposcopy or cervical biopsy can be done instead.

Preparation

- You will go to the hospital for blood and urine tests one or two days before the surgery.
- You must have nothing to eat or drink for eight hours before surgery if you are having general anesthesia.
- You undress and don a hospital gown.
- You will be given general anesthesia intravenously.
- The procedure is sometimes modified so that local anesthesia is adequate. In this case, you will be given an oral sedative, and once you are sedated (about 30 minutes), the anesthesia will be injected into your cervix.

Test procedure

- The surgeon uses a scalpel to remove a cone-shaped tissue sample from the center of the cylindrical cervix. The base of the cone is

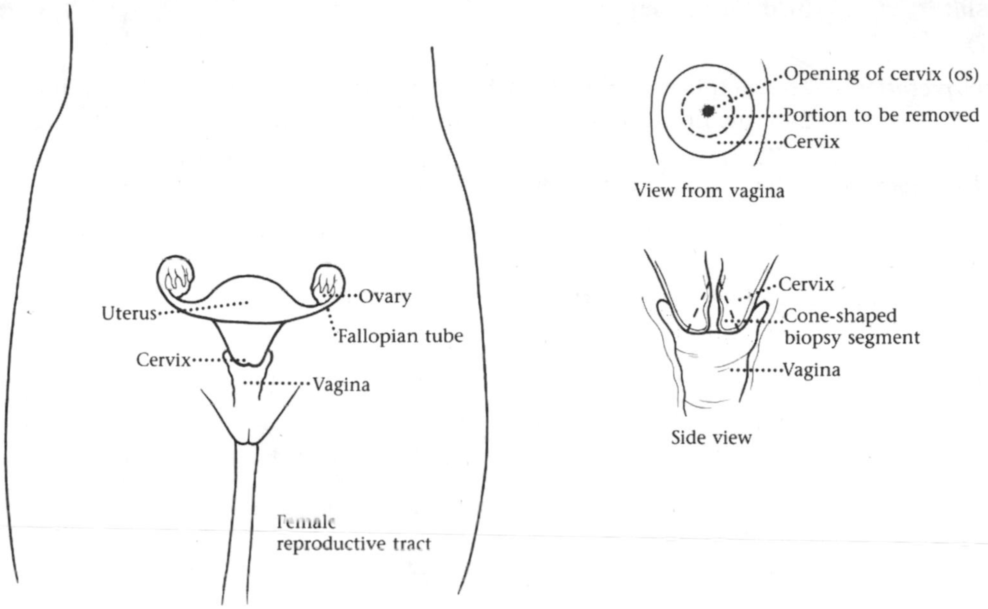

FIGURE 11.3 A cone biopsy entails removal of a wedge- or cone-shaped segment from the central portion of the cervix.

taken from the opening of the cervix (cervical os); the middle and tip of the cone, from the cervical canal (see figure 11.3).

- The cut edges of the cervix are then sutured or cauterized.
- If the procedure is being done as treatment, laser or electrocautery techniques may be used instead and will not require sutures.

After the test

- The sample is sent to the lab for examination.
- You will remain in a recovery room, and your vital signs will be monitored for about one hour until the anesthesia wears off.
- Once you are up and moving around, you are free to dress and leave, but you should arrange to have someone drive you home.
- You may experience mild to moderate cramping over the next 24 hours or so, and you may be given a prescription for a painkiller.
- You can return to work or other usual activities within two or three days.
- You may have bleeding requiring you to wear sanitary napkins for several days. Lighter bleeding can occur for a week or more as the stitches are absorbed.
- You should avoid sexual intercourse, tampons, and douching until your incision completely heals, which may take five to six weeks.
- If you experience heavy bleeding, notify your physician immediately.

Factors affecting results Inadequate sample.

Interpretation The sample is examined in the laboratory for abnormal cells that may indicate a precancerous or cancerous condition.

Advantages

- It provides a large sample.
- It may remove any cancerous tissue in the process.

Disadvantages It's a major surgery that carries the potential for severe complications.

The next step

- If biopsied tissue is not cancerous, no other testing is necessary.
- If biopsied tissue is cancerous, additional surgery may be scheduled, or if tissue has been completely removed, radiation may be scheduled.

Margaret J. Bia, MD

12 The Renal System

Tests Covered in This Chapter

The case of Deborah O., a 38-year-old attorney and mother of one:

One day during my freshman year in college I went to the bathroom and discovered blood in my urine. I was in the middle of finals so I ignored it, thinking it was just an unusual period. When it didn't recur, I assumed everything was fine, until a year or so later when I had a routine blood test and ended up being diagnosed with high blood pressure and chronic glomerulonephritis, a progressive inflammation of the renal filtering units.

I started taking medication for my blood pressure and led a pretty normal life for the next ten years, even though my kidneys were functioning at only about half of normal capacity. Then my creatinine began rising steadily. A kidney biopsy revealed interstitial nephritis, an inflammation of another area of the kidney. My doctors explained that my kidneys were so damaged, it was only a matter of time before they would stop working altogether. Eventually, I went on dialysis and was placed on transplant waiting lists, hoping for a new kidney.

The Tests Deborah's blood test showed high levels of creatinine, a by-product of muscle metabolism that accurately reflects a kidney problem but can't identify its cause. For that, she needed a kidney biopsy (in which a tiny piece of renal tissue is obtained surgically or with a needle for laboratory examination). Later, in preparation for transplant, she underwent various tests to be sure she was a good candidate. These included an X-ray scan of the gallbladder (cholecystography), which revealed a suspicious spot on one of her kidneys. It was too small to identify, even with CT and MRI scans, so doctors removed the kidney as a safeguard. It turned out to be a malignant tumor, but fortunately, the cancer had not spread and required no further treatment.

The Outcome A year or so after she started dialysis, Deborah received her transplant. Her recuperation was rapid, and although her body tried to reject the new kidney, she weathered the episode with immunosuppressant drugs. She has monthly urine and blood tests, including creatinine tests to monitor her kidney function. Every few months her blood is tested for cholesterol and calcium, and the proteins in her urine are measured with a 24-hour urine collection. Her doctor says she couldn't be doing better, and she now looks forward to returning to work.

INTRODUCTION

The renal system—the kidneys and the urinary tract—performs many vital functions necessary for survival. The kidneys remove waste products from the body and regulate the body's fluid and acid-base balance. The renal system releases hormones to regulate blood pressure, synthesizes vitamins that control growth, and regulates red blood cell production.

The kidneys, each about 4 inches long, are located on either side of the spine near the bottom of the rib cage. To perform their tasks, they require more blood than any other organ—about 2 pints every minute—and a complex circulation system to control the flow of this massive blood volume.

Here's how the system works: Blood reaches the kidneys through the renal arteries and passes through a set of filtering systems called nephrons. Both kidneys contain about 1 million of these microscopic nephrons, each resembling a tiny funnel (glomerulus) with a long stem and two twisted tubes (tubules) attached. The glomerulus allows blood cells, protein, other large particles, and some of the water to remain in the bloodstream, but filters out everything else and passes the blood on to the tubules. The tubules reclaim about 99% of the water, nutrients, and salts and return them to the bloodstream. Although this might seem like double work, it allows the nephrons to make an enormous number of intricate adjustments in order to keep the body in balance and compensate for daily fluctuations in fluid and salt intake. In the meantime, the mix of waste chemicals and water left behind is excreted as urine. It flows first into the center of the kidneys and then into the ureters, the tubes that connect the kidneys to the bladder. From the bladder, the urine is expelled from the body through a small tube called the urethra.

The kidneys are instrumental in regulating blood pressure by controlling the release of a hormone called renin. The amount of renin circulating in the blood ultimately causes the muscles in the blood vessel walls to contract (constricting the walls and raising blood pressure) if the blood pressure is too low, or to relax (dilating the vessels and lowering blood pressure) if the blood pressure is too high. Renin also affects blood pressure through the endocrine (glandular) system by signaling the adrenal glands at the top of the kidneys to secrete the hormone aldosterone into the blood. Aldosterone tells the kidneys to retrieve more water and salt from the urine, which increases blood volume and thus causes blood pressure on the vessel walls to rise.

HOW YOUR DOCTOR DIAGNOSES RENAL DISEASE

Kidney and urinary tract diseases range from mild infections treatable with antibiotics to total renal failure, which requires a kidney transplant or treatment on an artificial kidney (dialysis) machine. You may experience symptoms (see the accompanying box) or you may be

Common Symptoms of Kidney and Urinary Tract Disorders

Recognizing the earliest warning signs and getting prompt treatment can sometimes prevent chronic renal failure. Many kidney disorders share the same initial symptoms. The most common symptoms are the following:

- *Fluid retention (edema),* causing swelling and puffiness, especially in the hands, ankles, face, and eyelids.
- *Flank pain,* felt in the small of the back below the ribs.
- *Burning and increased frequency of urination (dysuria).*
- *Red, rusty, smoky, coffee-colored, or cola-colored urine,* indicating the presence of blood (hematuria).
- *A decrease in the amount of urine.*

Blood Tests: Markers for Renal Disease

A simple blood test (see chapter 4) can be analyzed for a number of elements that indicate problems with kidney function. These include the following:

- *Blood urea nitrogen (BUN) and creatinine.* These chemicals are formed in the body by normal metabolism and removed by the kidneys. Measuring the level of these chemicals is one way to assess filtration function: The higher the level in the blood, the poorer the filtration.
- *Calcium and phosphate.* These elements are excreted by the kidney. In kidney disease, the level of calcium may be low and that of phosphate high. Abnormal levels in the blood may also indicate bone disease.
- *Potassium.* Potassium is retained and the level increases during renal failure.
- *Bicarbonate.* The level of bicarbonate reflects blood acid content. The level decreases when renal disease is present and acids build up.
- *Hematocrit.* Hematocrit is a measure of blood count. It decreases when renal failure is present, causing anemia.

unaware of a problem even though your kidneys are functioning at only 10% to 15% of normal capacity. Whatever the reason for your visit, your doctor will start with your medical and family history. If kidney disease is suspected, he or she will want to know about any kidney disease, high blood pressure, or diabetes in your family (certain types of renal disease run in families, and diabetes and high blood pressure are common causes of kidney failure).

The doctor will usually order a series of routine blood tests (see the accompanying box). A test of your blood sugar level, for example, can confirm or rule out diabetes. Because the kidneys maintain normal blood levels of many elements, such as potassium, sodium, calcium, phosphate, and acid, abnormalities in routine blood tests are often the first indications of defects in renal system function. In addition, because the kidneys produce a hormone that is critical for normal blood production, anemia can also be a sign of kidney failure. Tests of these minerals and hormones in the blood are used not only to diagnose kidney disorders, but also, if disease is found, to monitor its course and its response to therapy.

Analyzing your urine for such elements as protein, blood, bacteria, and calcium provides your doctor with another key to kidney disease. Since protein is usually returned to the bloodstream during the filtering process, excess protein in the urine (proteinuria) is the hallmark of a defect in the kidneys' filtration units that is associated with many kidney diseases, especially diabetes, hypertension, and glomerulonephritis. If protein is present on the initial screen, you may be asked to collect urine over a 24-hour period (see the accompanying

24-Hour Urine Collection

Test Procedure: A 24-hour urine collection measures the amount of substances, such as protein, creatinine, and calcium, excreted in the urine in 24 hours. You will be given a container for the collection. For the results to be valid, you must adhere to the following procedure:

- Begin the collection upon arising in the morning.
- Discard the first voided urine.
- Each time you void for the rest of the day and during the night, put the urine into the collection jug.
- Put the next morning's first voided urine into the jug to end the collection.

Special Considerations:

- The urine should be kept in a refrigerator or other cool place to prevent bacterial growth and odor.
- If you go out during the day of the collection, you can collect urine samples in a small jar and empty them into the jug when you get home.
- If you forget to add some of your urine, the collection is inaccurate and not worth analyzing. If this happens, notify your nurse or doctor to schedule a new collection rather than submit an inaccurate one.

Interpretation: From the collection, the amount of protein you are excreting can be measured. In addition, the amount of blood serum you are filtering (known as creatinine clearance) can be estimated and compared to normal values to see how well your kidneys are working. Other substances can also be measured when indicated. For instance, your doctor can determine the amount of stone-forming elements excreted by your kidneys each day to assess your risk factors for kidney stones.

box). Since the presence of protein may indicate serious disease, your doctor may also want to do a kidney biopsy (see below).

Blood in the urine (hematuria) can be caused by injury, kidney stones, inflammation, cancer, bleeding cysts, infection, blood-clotting disorders, or renal damage from sickle-cell anemia. A kidney biopsy is sometimes necessary to distinguish among these possibilities in order to determine the appropriate therapy.

If a physical exam and test results suggest infection or impaired renal function, other tests and procedures may be ordered. Kidney X-rays and scanning and ultrasound techniques provide images of the kidneys' internal structure and are instrumental in locating obstructions, tumors, and other malformations.

If these procedures do not confirm that your problem is caused by kidney or urinary tract impairment, your physician may refer you for tests of other organ systems. For instance, heart disease frequently causes impaired kidney function, and assessment by a cardiologist may confirm this diagnosis (see chapter 5).

COMMON KIDNEY AND URINARY TRACT DISORDERS

Some of the more common diseases and disorders of the kidneys and urinary tract are described below.

Diabetic kidney disease (diabetic glomerulosclerosis) is a scarring of the kidneys as a result of damage to the glomeruli, the kidneys' filtering units. The leading cause of chronic renal failure, it ultimately affects about 40% of all individuals who develop diabetes in childhood (Type 1 diabetes).

Hypertensive renal disease, the result of severe, uncontrolled hypertension, destroys kidney tissue and impairs the kidneys' filtering ability, ultimately leading to chronic renal failure. Conversely, kidney disease can *cause* hypertension by disrupting the mechanisms through which the kidneys help regulate blood pressure.

Kidney stones, usually made of calcium or some other crystal, can develop in the kidneys or anywhere along the urinary tract. If the stones block the flow of urine, they can cause infection or even permanent kidney damage, but this is usually a treatable condition.

Urinary tract infections are the second most common infections after respiratory infections. More common in women than in men, they are usually confined to the bladder and are referred to as *cystitis*. If untreated, the infection can spread up into the kidneys, where it becomes *pyelonephritis*, causing chills, fever, and pain that must be treated with antibiotics.

Glomerulonephritis is an inflammation of the glomeruli, the part of the kidneys that filters the blood. It may be chronic and severe, leading to rapid or slowly progressive loss of kidney function. It may also be acute, in which case it may require drug treatment or short-term dialysis, or it may clear up on its own.

Urinary tract obstruction is the term for a blockage anywhere along the urinary tract. It may be caused by kidney stones, a cancerous mass, or, in men, enlargement of the prostate gland that lies at the base of the bladder. Blockages should be treated promptly to prevent permanent kidney damage and kidney failure.

Hereditary kidney disorders are transmitted genetically. The most common of these is *polycystic kidney disease (PKD)*, in which large cysts develop in the kidneys, distorting the nephrons and rendering them increasingly ineffective. It leads to renal failure later in life in about half of all cases.

KIDNEY-URETER-BLADDER (KUB) RADIOGRAPHY

General information

Where It's Done	Who Does It	How Long It Takes	Discomfort/Pain
Hospital radiology suite or office of radiologist.	X-ray technician.	About 5 minutes.	None.

Results Ready When	Special Equipment	Risks/Complications	Average Cost
In a few minutes (interpretation and reporting may take longer).	X-ray table and machine.	Minimal radiation risk.	$$

Other names Abdominal X-rays or flat plate of the abdomen.

Purpose

- To very roughly evaluate the structure, size, and position of the kidneys.
- To detect abnormalities such as kidney stones, tumors, or other obstructions.

How it works This test uses standard X-ray technology (see chapter 3) to obtain pictures of internal organs.

Preparation

- You disrobe and don a hospital gown.
- You may be given a lead shield to protect your ovaries or testicles from unnecessary radiation.

Test procedure

- You lie on your stomach on a table with the X-ray equipment positioned above you.
- You must remain still in a specific position while the X-rays are taken.

After the test You can return to normal activities immediately.

Factors affecting results

- Bowel gas, obesity, feces, fluid, ovarian lesions, or calcified uterine fibromas in the intestine.
- Dye or barium remaining from previous tests.

Interpretation A radiologist reads the X-rays for kidney anomalies or obstructions.

Advantages No contrast dye is used when the KUB is done alone. Usually, however, it is done in conjunction with an intravenous pyelography (see below).

Disadvantages The image quality may not be sufficient to show details of the kidney's structures.

The next step If the test shows a mass, blockage, or other kidney abnormality, additional tests, such as renal ultrasound or intravenous pyelography, may be ordered to pinpoint the problem.

RENAL ULTRASOUND

General information

Where It's Done	Who Does It	How Long It Takes	Discomfort/Pain
Hospital radiology suite.	Radiology technician.	30–45 minutes.	Positioning may cause some minor discomfort, as may coolness of room or equipment.

When Results Ready	Special Equipment	Risks/Complications	Average Cost
A few minutes to a few days.	Imaging equipment, ultrasound transducer, oscilloscope, cathode-ray tube and amplifier, water-soluble gel, and instant camera.	None.	$$

Other names Doppler ultrasound.

Purpose

- To detect a mass, cyst, kidney stone, or other obstruction in the kidney.
- To determine kidney size and shape.
- To locate the kidney during a kidney biopsy.
- To determine circulation in the renal arteries and veins by the use of a Doppler monitor (see chapter 3). This variation does not alter the test from the patient's standpoint but yields additional information.

How it works A transducer passed over your kidneys emits sound waves that, like sonar, bounce off your kidney, transmitting a picture of the organ that can be displayed on a video screen.

Preparation

- You disrobe and don a hospital gown.
- A water-soluble gel is applied to the skin on your torso as a medium for the transducer (see below).

Test procedure

- You lie on an examining table while a transducer, a handheld unit that emits sound waves, is passed over the skin above your kidneys.
- A video screen shows the images, which are assessed or photographed for later assessment.

After the test You dress and return to normal activities.

Factors affecting results In very obese people, the outline of the kidneys may be obscured by fatty tissue.

Interpretation A radiologist studies the ultrasound images for abnormal masses or blockages. Kidneys that appear too small may explain chronic renal malfunctioning.

Advantages

- It's painless and noninvasive.
- It does not involve exposure to radiation.
- It requires little preparation.

Disadvantages The images produced are not as exact as those of more direct visualization techniques, such as intravenous pyelography.

The next step If an abnormal mass or obstruction is found, additional tests, such as a biopsy or pyelography will be performed to detect the exact cause.

INTRAVENOUS PYELOGRAPHY (IVP)

General information

Where It's Done	Who Does It	How Long It Takes	Discomfort/Pain
Hospital radiology suite or office of radiologist.	Technician.	About 1 hour.	Minor discomfort of injection; possible flushing or light-headedness during dye injection. Positioning and coolness of room and equipment may cause some minor discomfort.

Results Ready Wen	Special Equipment	Risks/Complications	Average Cost
A few minutes to a few days.	X-ray table and machine, contrast dye, and tomographic equipment.	Possible allergic reaction to the contrast dye (see chapter 3). Some radiation risk if the procedure is repeated several times. People with diabetes and renal system impairment are at risk of acute renal failure.	$$

Other names Excretory urography or intravenous urography (IVU).

Purpose

- To pinpoint tumors and anatomical abnormalities of the kidneys, ureters, and bladder.

- To detect kidney stones.
- To assess renal blood flow.
- Can detect outlet obstruction.

How it works Contrast dye, injected intravenously, allows visualization of some structures that are not normally seen on regular X-rays (see chapter 3).

Preparation

- The procedure may be done on an outpatient or inpatient basis.
- You may be asked to fast for eight hours before the procedure.
- On the day before the test, you may be given an oral laxative, and on the morning of the test, a laxative suppository.
- You disrobe and don a hospital gown.

Test procedure

- Your reproductive organs are covered by a lead shield, and you lie face up on an X-ray table while an initial X-ray is taken.
- Contrast dye is injected into a vein, usually in your arm, and X-rays are taken at timed intervals as the dye travels through the kidneys and urinary tract.
- A band, something like a blood pressure cuff, is wrapped around your waist at one point to compress internal structures, making it easier to see collecting systems within the kidneys clearly.
- You go to a bathroom to urinate, or are given a bedpan, after which a final X-ray is taken to look at the amount of the contrast agent remaining in the bladder.

PATIENT TIP

You may feel a warm flush when the dye is injected. Some patients have the sensation of tasting the liquid; others feel momentarily nauseated. However, these effects rarely last more than 30 seconds.

After the test

- Your fluid intake and urinary output are monitored over the next 24 hours.
- Blood in your urine may indicate a complication that would require further follow-up. Otherwise, you can return to normal activities.

Factors affecting results

- Bowel gas.
- Obesity.
- Poor kidney function that prevents the kidneys from concentrating the dye from the bloodstream and "lighting up."
- Failure to fast before the test.

Interpretation A radiologist studies the X-ray images for indications of abnormal renal function.

Advantages The test allows direct visualization of the kidneys.

Disadvantages

- It requires some patient preparation.
- There is some danger of temporarily damaging the kidneys with the contrast dye.

The next step If a kidney stone is identified, it will be followed until it has passed. If a mass is suggested, a follow-up CT scan or angiography may be required. Certain anatomic abnormalities (eg, papillary necrosis or medullary sponge kidney) can be definitively detected with IVP. With recurrent kidney stone disease, you may need to repeat the IVP at intervals.

VOIDING CYSTOURETHROGRAPHY (VCUG)

General information

Where It's Done	Who Does It	How Long It Takes	Discomfort/Pain
Hospital radiology suite or office of radiologist.	Technician and radiologist.	About 1–2 hours.	Some discomfort when catheter is inserted.
Results Ready When	**Special Equipment**	**Risks/Complications**	**Average Cost**
A few minutes to a few days.	X-ray machine, foley catheter, fluoroscope and screen, and dye.	Minimal radiation risk. Because of foley catheter placement, there is a risk of bladder infection.	$$

Other names None.

Purpose

- To determine whether the bladder empties completely when you urinate.
- To diagnose reflux (in which urine backs up to the kidneys instead of flowing out through the urethra).
- To detect abnormalities of the urethra (used for this purpose more often in children than in adults).

How it works The use of a radiopaque contrast dye to highlight internal structures and a fluoroscope (moving X-ray) allows the radiologist to actually see what happens internally when you urinate.

Preparation You must disrobe and put on a hospital gown.

Test procedure

- The technician will take a series of X-rays while you assume different positions.
- A catheter is then inserted into your bladder in order to drain urine and inject the contrast dye.
- When your bladder is full, the catheter is removed and you are asked to urinate.
- More X-rays are taken.

After the test

- You may be asked to wait until the X-rays are developed, after which you may resume normal activities.
- You should drink plenty of fluids after the test to help flush out the dye from your bladder and reduce burning during urination.
- Notify your doctor if you see blood in your urine or experience lower-abdominal pain or fever.

Factors affecting results

- Feces or gas in the bowels.
- Inability to urinate in a steady stream without muscle spasms.

Interpretation A radiologist examines the flow of urine on the moving X-rays for signs of reflux.

Advantages

- It is the only test that can diagnose reflux.
- It's a good way to determine how well the bladder empties.

Disadvantages

- It requires insertion of a foley catheter.
- Some patients are embarrassed about having to urinate in front of a radiology screen.

The next step

- If there is a diagnosis of reflux, surgical correction may be recommended, especially for young children and kidney transplant patients.
- If the test indicates a problem with bladder contraction, further urologic testing may be recommended, or drugs such as urocholine may be prescribed to improve bladder function.
- In patients preparing for renal transplant, the presence of severe reflux may be an indication that the diseased kidney should be removed before the transplant.

RENAL COMPUTED TOMOGRAPHY

General information

Where It's Done	Who Does It	How Long It Takes	Discomfort/Pain
Hospital radiology suite or office of radiologist.	A technician.	About 1 hour.	Minor, from injection. Possible flush or light-headedness, metallic taste in mouth, or slight nausea during dye injection. Machinery is loud; some feel claustrophobic in scanner.

Results Ready When	Special Equipment	Risks/Complications	Average Cost
In a few minutes (interpretation and reporting may take longer).	X-ray table, CT scanner, contrast dye, IV infusion kit, oscilloscope screen, and camera.	Dye may cause allergic reaction or, rarely, impaired kidney function. For known allergy to dye, a nonionic contrast solution, along with pretreatment with steroids and antihistamines, can lessen this problem.	$$$

Other names CT scan of the kidneys.

Purpose

- To evaluate the structure, size, and position of the kidneys.
- To detect abnormalities such as kidney stones, tumors, or other obstructions.

How it works CT scan technology (see chapter 3) allows visualization of the kidneys that is more sensitive than conventional X-rays.

Preparation

- You fast for about 12 hours before the test.
- If you are claustrophobic, ask for a tranquilizer before the test begins.
- Since the noise level inside the scanner is quite high, you may want to ask about bringing headphones and a radio or tape player to drown it out and take your mind off the test.
- You disrobe and don a hospital gown.

Test procedure

- You may or may not receive an injection of a contrast dye as you lie on a narrow table that slides into a large tube, called the CT scanner. You must remain motionless during the scan.
- The scanner revolves around your body and takes multiple X-rays, which are then analyzed by a computer to provide a cross-sectional view of your kidneys.

After the test You are monitored for about 30 minutes for any ill effects from the dye, after which you can resume normal activities.

Factors affecting results

- Failure to fast before the procedure.
- Failure to lie motionless during the scan.
- Recent tests involving dye or other foreign substances may affect the accuracy of the test images.

Interpretation The radiologist reads the series of cross-sectional views of the kidney to see exactly where abnormalities lie.

Advantages It provides a high-resolution image of kidney structure and anatomy.

Disadvantages

- The test involves some, although relatively minimal, radiation as well as the injection of radiopaque contrast dye.
- Some people find the scanner tube claustrophobic.

The next step Some blockages or other kidney abnormalities can be explained or diagnosed on the basis of the scan. Other visible masses may require additional tests, such as a biopsy or angiography, to determine their cause.

RENAL SCAN

Other names Renal scintigram or captopril renal scan.

For a full description of this test, see chapter 20.

RENAL ANGIOGRAPHY

General information

Where It's Done	Who Does It	How Long It Takes	Discomfort/Pain
Hospital radiology suite or office of radiologist.	A doctor known as a vascular angiographer.	About 3–5 hours.	Minor discomfort from injection, line insertion, or remaining still in a cool room for a prolonged period. Possible abdominal pressure/ fullness during endoscopy. Possible flush, burning sensation, or slight nausea during dye injection.

Results Ready When	Special Equipment	Risks/Complications	Average Cost
A few minutes to a few days.	X-ray machines, fluoroscope with video monitor, catheters, flexible guide wire, dye, and pressure-injection device.	Bleeding and clotting at the line-insertion site, possible internal bleeding outside the renal artery, blood clots, kidney failure, or loss of kidney function. Cholesterol plaques can be dislodged from the walls of blood vessels, possibly causing a blockage.	$$$

Other names Renal arteriography.

Purpose

- To examine the renal blood vessels (which supply blood to the kidneys) for signs of blockage or abnormality, which may be causing bleeding.
- To repair a bleeding renal vessel.
- To determine whether a mass in the kidney is a tumor or vascular tissue.

How it works A contrast dye injected via a catheter threaded into the blood vessels of the kidneys makes them visible on a fluoroscope, allowing detection of any abnormalities affecting the blood supply to the kidneys.

Preparation

- You fast for 12 hours before the procedure.
- You disrobe and don a hospital gown.

Test procedure

- Local anesthesia is injected into your skin near an artery in your arm or leg.
- When the site is numbed, a catheter is inserted into the artery and threaded up through the aorta and into the renal artery.
- Dye is injected through the catheter, and a series of X-rays is taken. During the X-rays, you must remain absolutely still.

After the test

- The catheter is removed, and you may be asked to wait while the X-ray films are developed.
- Pressure is applied to the catether site (usually with a sandbag) to stop any bleeding.
- You will go to a recovery room for a short while so your vital signs can be checked. You may receive pain medication if the catheter insertion site is sore.
- You should restrict your activities and remain relatively quiet during the next 24 hours, after which you can resume normal activities.
- You must check the incision and report any excessive bleeding, soreness, or swelling to your doctor.

Factors affecting results

- Moving during the X-rays.
- Failure to fast overnight.
- Feces or gas in your intestinal tract or remnants of other tests such as a barium enema.

Interpretation After studying the X-rays, the physician may be able to detect abnormalities such as a clogged renal artery, or a tumor or cyst.

Advantages It provides the highest-resolution image of the renal blood vessels of any test available.

Disadvantages

- It's invasive.
- It involves a radiopaque contrast material and radiation.
- It may dislodge plaque lining the arteries of patients with atherosclerosis; the plaque can travel in the bloodstream and cause a blockage (embolus) elsewhere.

The next step

- If a tumor or cyst is found, a renal biopsy may be ordered to determine its nature.
- If there is a rupture in a renal blood vessel, it will be repaired immediately.
- If the angiography reveals a blocked artery, balloon angioplasty may be necessary to open up the artery. The angioplasty may be performed at the same time or at a later date.

CYSTOSCOPY

General information

Where It's Done	Who Does It	How Long It Takes	Discomfort/Pain
Urologist's office or hospital urology suite.	Urologist.	About 30 minutes.	If local rather than general anesthesia is used, there may be some discomfort or burning sensation when endoscopes are inserted and bladder is filled.

Results Ready When	Special Equipment	Risks/Complications	Average Cost
Immediately.	Endoscopes (cystoscope and urethroscope), sheath, and light source.	In rare cases, damage to internal structures may occur. Should not be done if patient has an infection of the urethra, bladder, or prostate gland.	$$

Other names Cystourethroscopy.

Purpose To detect structural abnormalities or obstructions, such as tumors or stones, inside the bladder and along the urinary tract.

How it works Fiber-optic technology allows a doctor to actually see inside internal organs through a scope, an instrument with a flexible tube and a viewing device inserted into the urinary tract through the urethra.

Preparation

- If general anesthesia is used, you will be asked to fast for eight to 12 hours before the procedure.
- Your urine will be tested for signs of urinary tract infection; if found, the test will be postponed.

Test procedure

- You disrobe and don a hospital gown.
- As you lie on your back with your knees bent, your legs spread apart, and your feet in stirrups, anesthetic jelly is injected into your urethra to numb the pain.
- The physician inserts an instrument containing two separate tubes, the cystoscope and the urethroscope, into your urethra (through the penis in males) and then into the bladder. If you are unable to withstand the catheter insertion, local anesthesia with IV sedation or general anesthesia will be administered.
- In order to get a better image, the physician may expand the bladder by filling it with fluid through the tube inserted into it.
- During the procedure, a biopsy sample may be taken using tiny tools threaded through the catether. Urine may also be collected through the catheter.

PATIENT TIP

Ask your doctor to use a flexible scope, which most patients find more comfortable than a rigid scope.

After the test

- Your vital signs are checked, and you receive pain medication if desired.
- You may be given antibiotics to prevent infection.
- You should drink plenty of fluids—but no alcoholic beverages—to lessen the burning sensation you will feel when you first urinate.
- Report any severe abdominal, back, or side pain; chills; fever; problems urinating; or excessive bleeding to your physician.

Factors affecting results Failure to fast before the procedure.

Interpretation Because the physician views the area directly through the scope, abnormalities are immediately apparent. Biopsy and urine specimens taken during the procedure are used to confirm a diagnosis.

Advantages This is the best test for immediate detection of lesions (changes in tissue structure as a result of disease or injury) along the lower urinary tract.

Disadvantages

- It involves some pain on catheter insertion.
- There is an increased risk of urinary tract infection because of the trauma caused by the scope.
- It requires general anesthesia.
- Some patients find the procedure embarrassing.

The next step Treatment can begin.

PERCUTANEOUS KIDNEY BIOPSY

General information

Where It's Done	Who Does It	How Long It Takes	Discomfort/Pain
Hospital radiology suite.	Nephrologist with the help of a radiologist or radiology technician.	1–2 hours; more if kidney is deep or small.	Possible deep pain when the biopsy is obtained, but this is often minimized by the use of an anesthetic. Possible dull ache in the back for several days.
Results Ready When	**Special Equipment**	**Risks/Complications**	**Average Cost**
2–3 days for preliminary results; a week for final results.	Biopsy needle and diagnostic imaging equipment.	The major risk is bleeding (usually not significant). In less than 5% of cases, bleeding is severe enough to require further treatment (and possibly a blood transfusion). In less than 0.1% of cases, the kidney has to be removed because of uncontrollable bleeding.	$$ (may be higher when the the radiologic guidance is added).

Other names Kidney biopsy.

Purpose

- To determine the cause of protein or blood in the urine (proteinuria and hematuria).
- To monitor the effectiveness of treatment.

How it works A tiny sample of kidney tissue is obtained with a long needle and examined by a pathologist under the microscope for damage or abnormalities.

Preparation

- You discontinue any nonsteroidal anti-inflammatory drugs, including aspirin and ibuprofen, ten to 14 days before the test, as these drugs impair the blood's clotting ability.
- You have initial blood tests to screen for bleeding abnormalities. If you have clotting problems, you may be admitted to the hospital the evening before the biopsy for treatment to diminish this, or the biopsy may be canceled.
- You fast on the day of the biopsy to avoid any potential stomach upset that sometimes accompanies anxiety about the procedure.

PATIENT TIP

If you tend to be anxious about medical tests, ask for a sedative before you are taken to the radiology department.

Test procedure

- You lie facedown on a bed or stretcher while your kidneys are visualized using an X-ray, ultrasound, or CT scan to guide the nephrologist in inserting the needle.
- The area just under your ribs is then anesthetized with novocaine.
- A thin, 4- to 6-inch biopsy needle is passed through your skin down to your kidney.
- You hold your breath while a tiny piece (about ¼ of an inch long) of kidney tissue is obtained. Sometimes this procedure must be repeated a few times until an adequate specimen is obtained.
- No incision is made and no stitches are required.

DID YOU KNOW?

Because the kidneys sit below the diaphragm, they move up and down when you breathe. This is why you must hold your breath each time the needle is moved.

After the test

- You will be kept in bed for several hours after the biopsy to prevent excessive internal bleeding, or you may be admitted to the hospital to monitor possible bleeding.
- Your blood pressure is monitored frequently because a drop can indicate abnormal bleeding.
- One out of three patients experiences red urine in the first 24 hours or so (this is not a sign of excessive bleeding).
- Your blood count and blood pressure are checked 12 to 24 hours after the biopsy. If they are stable, you will be discharged.
- You must avoid any "bouncing activity" (eg, aerobic exercise, jogging, tennis, or bouncing when coming down stairs) for two weeks so that the small blood clot that temporarily forms over the biopsy site does not become dislodged.

- Report to your doctor any abdominal pain, or pain that radiates down into the groin. However, mild aching and discomfort in the loin area (due to irritation of the back muscles) is typical and not cause for concern.

Factors affecting results Occasionally the kidney tissue sample obtained is not adequate for diagnosis, and the biopsy must be repeated.

Interpretation The biopsy sample will be examined by a pathologist and reviewed by your nephrologist.

Advantages It provides the most accurate assessment of abnormalities in kidney tissue.

Disadvantages It's an invasive procedure accompanied by a risk of moderate to severe kidney damage.

The next step If your kidney biopsy shows a treatable problem, you may be offered therapy with specific drugs. Otherwise, you may receive treatment for risk factors, such as high blood pressure or high blood cholesterol, that may have an impact on your kidneys.

Leo M. Cooney Jr, MD

13 Rheumatoid and Musculoskeletal Disorders

Tests Covered in This Chapter

The case of Enid J., a 65-year-old grandmother and retired nurse's aide:

More than 20 years ago the fingers in my right hand became so numb that it affected my work. I was diagnosed with carpal tunnel syndrome and had to have surgery on my wrist. Later I developed it in the other hand and had surgery again. But by that time, I had such pain and numbness traveling up both arms and into my shoulders that I was referred to an arthritis specialist.

I was diagnosed with rheumatoid arthritis and put on prednisone and other drugs. But one day the pain became so bad, I ended up in the emergency room. I saw an arthritis specialist who kept me on the prednisone but prescribed a new drug, sulfasalazine, plus ibuprofen for controlling pain.

The Tests The primary test to confirm rheumatoid arthritis measures rheumatoid factor, an antibody found in high concentrations in the blood of people with severe arthritis. Although this test is generally reliable, it tends to produce both false-negative and false-positive results. That is, it may produce negative results in people who have the disease, and positive results in people who don't. For this reason, the results must be correlated with a patient's symptoms and other conditions. In Enid's case, the carpal tunnel syndrome was one clue to diagnosis. Although most people with carpal tunnel syndrome do not develop rheumatoid arthritis, many people who have rheumatoid arthritis tend to have carpal tunnel syndrome.

The Outcome Enid continues to take her drugs. Although she has flare-ups, especially pain and itchiness in her hands when the weather turns damp or rainy, she finds that the medications work well. She suffers from morning stiffness, but by afternoon is able to take regular walks, an important key to maintaining mobility.

INTRODUCTION

The musculoskeletal system consists of the skeleton and the muscles attached to its bones, called skeletal muscles. The skeleton provides a strong framework for the body that enables it to move, and provides support and protection to various organs. The skeletal muscles, also referred to as voluntary muscles because they are under conscious control, open and close joints and move various parts of the body.

The adult body contains 206 bones. The bone has several layers: a thin outer membrane (periosteum) containing blood vessels and nerves; a hard, dense shell that gives the bone its strength; and an internal layer that is spongy or porous. Contrary to a common misconception, bone tissue—which is made up of a supporting matrix impregnated with minerals, particularly calcium salts—is far from inert: Its cells are continuously dissolved and replaced, playing an important role in regulating calcium in the body. Many bones are hollow inside and contain soft fatty tissue called bone marrow, which produces red and white blood cells and other blood components.

Areas where two bones come into contact are known as joints. They are held together by ligaments and tendons, which keep the joint stable while allowing movement. The ends of the bones are covered with cartilage, which allows them to move smoothly against each other. The joint is lined with a thin layer of tissue called synovium or synovial membrane, which further reduces friction between bone surfaces. Adjacent to many joints is a small saclike structure (the bursa) that is lined with the same synovial tissue as the joint and acts as a buffer between tendon and bone, also serving to reduce friction.

Skeletal muscles, which account for 40% to 45% of body weight, consist of fibers that can relax or contract when they receive appropriate nerve impulses from the brain. The muscles remain in a constant state of slight contraction, which is referred to as muscle tone. The activity of the muscle depends on the proper functioning of the nerves and on the condition of muscle tissue itself. It is also affected by enzymes, minerals, and other chemicals present in fluids surrounding muscle cells.

HOW YOUR DOCTOR DIAGNOSES MUSCULOSKELETAL PROBLEMS

Disorders of the musculoskeletal system are very common: about one in six visits to a doctor is prompted by musculoskeletal complaints. Although they can occur at any age, they are particularly common in the elderly, who often have more than one musculoskeletal disease (see the accompanying box, which lists some different types of musculoskeletal disorders).

Types of Musculoskeletal Disorders

Musculoskeletal disorders fall into the following major categories:

- *Inflammatory disorders,* characterized by inflammation of joints or other tissues. The main types include the following:

  Rheumatic disorders: rheumatoid arthritis, systemic lupus erythematosus, ankylosing spondylitis, Reiter's syndrome, psoriatic arthritis, gout, and pseudogout.

  Connective tissue disorders: scleroderma, vasculitis, polymyositis, and sarcoidosis.

  Infectious arthritis: Lyme disease, gonococcal arthritis, other bacterial arthritis, and viral arthritis.
- *Mechanical disorders,* characterized by injury to bones, ligaments, tendons, cartilage, or other structures in or around joints. Common examples include bone fractures, ruptures or tears of ligaments, meniscal tears, tendinitis, bursitis, disc degeneration, and herniated discs.
- *Osteoarthritis,* which is the disintegration of cartilage in the joints.
- *Metabolic bone diseases,* in which the normal functioning of the cells in the bones is disrupted. These include osteoporosis, osteomalacia, and Paget's disease of the bone.
- *Bone cancer,* in which the proliferation of cancer cells interferes with cell functioning.

Signs and Symptoms of Musculoskeletal Disorders

- Joint pain (sometimes only during movement or with certain movements).
- Joint swelling.
- Pain in bones.
- Loss of motion.
- Morning stiffness.
- Weight loss.
- Fatigue.
- Muscle weakness.
- Loss of function of body parts.

Because many symptoms of musculoskeletal problems (see the accompanying box) resolve themselves with time and appropriate rest, your doctor will take a careful history and examine you thoroughly before deciding whether you have a problem that requires immediate testing and treatment. If, for example, you have joint pain, which is one of the most common reasons people see doctors, the physician will ask you questions about the nature of the pain. These may include the following:

- How often does the pain appear?
- What alleviates it, and what makes it worse?
- Is the pain intermittent, or has it been gradually getting worse?

Pain that is intermittent and occurs after exercise is less likely to be a sign of a serious disorder; it may indicate a mechanical problem inside a joint, such as irritation of a tendon or cartilage. On the other hand, pain that is persistent and severe may be a cause for more immediate concern.

The doctor will try to establish whether the abnormality is located in or near the joint. Swelling of the joint usually indicates that the space inside the joint is affected. The swelling results from excess secretion of fluids that lubricate the joint in response to irritation, inflammation, or mechanical problems. To determine the cause of swelling, the fluid may be drained and analyzed in a procedure called arthrocentesis.

If you have lost motion in the joint, the doctor will try to determine whether the loss is due to a mechanical problem, such as a torn cartilage of the knee, or chronic inflammation that leads to scarring of the synovium. If you notice gradual loss of movement in the joint, you should consult a doctor. In most cases it can be treated; without treatment, however, it may develop into a major problem that will restrict your movements or affect your gait.

The presence of other symptoms helps narrow down the diagnosis. For example, fatigue is likely to occur in people with inflammatory diseases but not in those with osteoarthritis or bursitis. Weight loss is common in people with infectious diseases or tumors but not in those with mechanical injuries.

During the physical examination, the doctor first evaluates the part of the body affected by symptoms. However, disease may not originate in the area where you experience pain. For example, tendinitis of the shoulder may also cause pain in the upper arm, while hip disease often causes symptoms in the thigh, knee, and lower back. Therefore, the examination usually includes all the major muscles, bones, and joints of the body.

The doctor may ask you to bend or extend your limbs at different angles or to lift your shoulders or flex your elbows against resistance. You may be asked to stand, sit, turn, and walk so the doctor can observe your gait and movements. If a mechanical injury is suspected, the exam is the most important diagnostic tool. Mechanical problems usually produce pain on certain maneuvers—for example, people with a disease of the rotator cuff tendon (the tendon that reinforces the shoulder joint) often have pain when lifting the shoulder against resistance.

Diagnostic tests should be ordered only after the doctor has determined the general nature of your musculoskeletal problem. If tests are ordered sooner, their results can be misinterpreted, because many tests may produce results that are unrelated to your problem. For example, the majority of people over 55 have abnormalities in the upper spine that are detected by X-rays but often cause no symptoms. After a certain age, having abnormal X-rays may be quite normal, making a diagnosis based on these results alone erroneous.

While tests can now provide excellent views of the bones and muscles, they may be overused. Even if a test is likely to reveal the cause of symptoms, it should only be performed if the results will affect treatment or provide important information about the prognosis, or likely outcome, of a condition. For example, if you have a slight pain in the knee that would not warrant surgery regardless of test results, there is no need for extensive testing. Another example is acute back pain, which usually resolves itself. If an infection or tumor is suspected, tests are crucial, but if the pain is likely due to a mechanical problem and there is little need for drugs or surgery, tests may be unnecessary. In some cases, predicting the progress of a disease is a valid reason for testing. For example, some lab tests can help predict the severity and future course of arthritis. But the costs, risks, discomfort, and inconvenience associated with tests should always be carefully weighed against their potential benefits.

There is no standard battery of tests for musculoskeletal problems. If there is fluid in the joint, the most informative test is arthrocentesis. Most other tests involve obtaining images of the joints, bones, and soft tissues and vary with the suspected problem. If you have shoulder pain, for example, the doctor may order an X-ray to check for abnormal calcium deposits or changes in the joint space. But if your symptoms suggest a tendon rupture, the test of choice is magnetic resonance imaging (MRI), which provides excellent images of soft tissues such as tendons, ligaments, and cartilage. If surgery is considered, arthroscopy allows the doctor to view the joint directly and to perform minor surgery if necessary.

Depending on your most likely diagnosis, any of the tests described below may be performed.

For an inflammatory disorder, the doctor may order such blood tests as erythrocyte sedimentation rate (ESR), which detects inflammation but doesn't identify its cause; autoimmune antibody tests to diagnose autoimmune disorders (see chapter 15); rheumatoid factor for rheumatoid arthritis; and Lyme disease antibody test for Lyme disease.

For a mechanical injury, tests may be performed if a fracture or tumor is suspected. Apart from arthrocentesis, a standard X-ray is the most common test. Magnetic resonance imaging, or MRI, is very helpful for such mechanical problems as tears of the ligaments or cartilage in the knee, or rupture of shoulder tendons.

For muscle disease, the doctor will try to determine whether your symptoms originate in the muscle or other tissues: general muscle weakness may be caused by neurological disorders such as stroke or multiple sclerosis, while weakness in individual muscles may result from tendon tears. Disease of the muscle itself, which is a relatively uncommon cause of muscle problems, usually causes symmetrical weakness in the muscles of the arms and legs and generally involves inflammation. When muscle disease is suspected, tests usually include creatine kinase (CK), which signals muscle damage; electromyography (see chapter 23), which evaluates the function of nerves that supply muscles as well as the function of the muscles themselves; and muscle biopsy, which allows the doctor to examine muscle tissue under a microscope.

For bone disease, tests may include standard X-rays; a CT scan, MRI, or bone scan; and occasionally, bone biopsy. Osteonecrosis (bone destruction) is usually diagnosed by MRI, and osteoporosis by bone densitometry (see chapter 26). Blood tests may be performed to measure various substances, including calcium, levels of which help evaluate bone metabolism, and alkaline phosphatase. Vitamin D levels may be measured if a deficiency is suspected as a cause of a bone disorder called osteomalacia. Since bone may be affected by disorders of other organs, including the kidneys and parathyroid glands, hormones and other substances in the blood may be measured to diagnose these disorders (for more information, see chapter 9).

ARTHROCENTESIS

General information

Where It's Done	Who Does It	How Long It Takes	Discomfort/Pain
Hospital or doctor's office.	Doctor.	3–5 minutes.	Minor discomfort associated with needle insertion.

Results Ready When	Special Equipment	Risks/Complications	Average Cost
3–4 hours.	Syringe and needle, collecting tubes, and elastic wrap.	Infection (extremely rare if sterile conditions are strictly applied), bleeding or accumulation of blood, and joint pain.	$$

Other names Joint tap, synovial fluid analysis, and closed joint aspiration.

Purpose

- To establish the cause of joint swelling.
- To distinguish between different types of arthritis.
- To monitor the effects of antibiotic treatment on septic arthritis.
- As treatment, to drain excess fluid from a joint or to inject corticosteroids or other medications into the joint to relieve pain.

How it works Synovial fluid (which helps lubricate the surface of bones and cartilage inside the joints) is withdrawn and analyzed in a laboratory for substances that may help establish the cause of joint swelling.

Preparation You remove clothing as necessary to expose the joint.

Test procedure

- The doctor examines your joint for excess fluid.
- The doctor marks the spot at which arthrocentesis will be performed, cleans the skin with an antiseptic liquid, and applies to the skin or injects a local anesthetic.
- A needle is inserted into the marked spot and guided into the joint space. You may feel a "pop" when it penetrates the joint capsule.
- After excess synovial fluid is removed, the needle is withdrawn and the fluid is sent to a lab for analysis.

PATIENT TIP

Insertion of the needle is normally painless, although you may feel temporary pain when the joint capsule is penetrated. Let the doctor know if you experience persistent pain during arthrocentesis as this may mean that the cartilage or the membrane covering the bone is irritated. In this case, the doctor will usually withdraw the needle and insert it at a different angle.

After the test

- You will receive special instructions on joint care following arthrocentesis.
- In some cases, you may resume regular use of the joint immediately after the procedure, or you may be instructed to avoid excessive use of the joint.
- You may apply an ice pack to the joint if it is painful and swollen.

Factors affecting results None.

Interpretation Synovial fluid that is opaque and turbid (instead of clear and viscous) may indicate inflammatory diseases, while the presence of pus may signal septic arthritis. Blood in the fluid may indicate a fracture or blood disorder, while crystals may signal gout or pseudogout. A high white blood cell count may indicate an inflammatory disorder. Various other tests, such as Gram stains for certain bacteria, cultures for infectious organisms, and glucose measurement, may be done if other problems are suspected.

Advantages

- The test is indispensable for diagnosing septic arthritis and joint diseases associated with crystals.
- There is a low risk of complications.

Disadvantages None.

The next step

- If blood is present, trauma or fracture may be diagnosed and an X-ray may be performed.
- If no blood is present, a culture and other tests may be performed.

ARTHROSCOPY

General information

Where It's Done	Who Does It	How Long It Takes	Discomfort/Pain
Doctor's office or hospital.	Orthopedic surgeon, assisted by anesthesiologist and nurses.	30–40 minutes for diagnosis; additional hour for repair.	Minor.
Results Ready When	**Special Equipment**	**Risks/Complications**	**Average Cost**
Immediately.	2 mm arthroscope, micro TV equipment, and special tables.	Pain and possibility of infection or joint damage.	$$–$$$ (Cost varies depending on joint examined and whether therapy is added.)

Other names Office arthroscopy, or knee endoscopy (if performed on the knee).

Purpose

- To observe the interior of a joint (primarily the knee, but also the shoulder, ankle, or elbow).
- To irrigate the joint with salt water if the fluid in the joint is causing irritation or discomfort.
- To obtain a biopsy to aid in diagnosing infections, gout, rheumatoid arthritis, or collagen disorders (those that affect the connective tissue).
- To surgically repair the menisci (knee cartilage), ligaments, or tendons.
- To remove loose growths in the elbow (osteophytes) or in the ankle (osteochondral lesions).

DID YOU KNOW?

The name "office arthroscopy" is something of a misnomer because the procedure usually takes place in what is called a special procedures room, actually a type of operating room. When it's performed in an office, the doctor must take special care to maintain the same meticulous levels of cleanliness and sterility as in a hospital operating room.

How it works A thin fiber-optic tube is inserted directly into the joint (see figure 13.1).

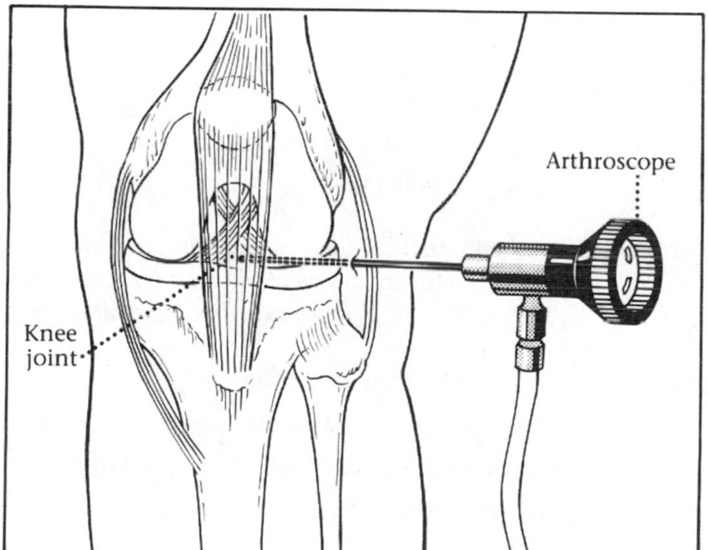

FIGURE 13.1 Arthroscopy

A fiber-optic viewing tube is inserted directly into the joint, allowing a doctor to examine its interior by using special magnifying devices. During arthroscopy, other procedures, including collection of tissue samples and surgical repair, can be carried out.

Preparation

- You may be asked to fast the morning of the test.
- You undress and don a surgical gown.
- You lie down on a special table, and the area to be examined is cleaned, prepped, and locally anesthetized. For some procedures, you may receive general anesthesia.
- You may receive a sedative before the procedure to help you relax.

Test procedure

- The doctor inserts a fiber-optic tube directly into the joint.
- The doctor inspects the entire joint through direct visualization and with a microscopic camera.

After the test

- You rest and recover from the anesthesia and any additional sedation.
- Your joint may be wrapped in elastic bandages or, for a shoulder or elbow, your arm placed in a sling.
- You must be driven home if you had general anesthesia.
- Your activity is restricted for at least one to two days, longer if surgery was involved.
- You will probably experience some pain and swelling for the next week.
- You should notify your doctor if you see significant swelling (indicating internal bleeding) or signs of infection, such as fever, or redness or pus at the incision site.

Factors affecting results

- If you are unable to relax and lie still, the physician will have trouble seeing the structures of the joint.
- Heavy bleeding can obstruct the view.

Interpretation

A specially trained doctor compares your joint to a normal joint and makes recommendations for further diagnostic testing or treatment such as reconstructive ligament surgery or cartilage repair or removal.

Advantages

- It's an outpatient procedure.
- It provides immediate diagnostic information.
- It makes it possible to obtain biopsy samples.
- It's less invasive than open surgery.

Disadvantages

- It's invasive.
- It's more expensive than some noninvasive tests, such as MRI.
- It does not always allow for treatment (which may require more arthroscopy).
- There is a risk of infection and joint damage.
- It can't detect problems in surrounding bones and ligaments as MRI can.

The next step Additional diagnostic tests, such as arthrography with CT scan, or treatment, such as reconstructive ligament surgery or cartilage repair or removal.

RHEUMATOID FACTOR (RF)

General information

Where It's Done	Who Does It	How Long It Takes	Discomfort/Pain
Doctor's office, hospital, or commercial laboratory.	Doctor, nurse, or lab technician.	Less than 5 minutes.	Minor discomfort associated with drawing blood.

Results Ready When	Special Equipment	Risks/Complications	Average Cost
1–2 days.	Needle, syringe, and collecting tubes.	Negligible.	$

Other names Rheumatoid arthritis factor.

Purpose

- To help distinguish rheumatoid arthritis from other disorders.
- To predict the course of rheumatoid arthritis.

How it works Rheumatoid factor (RF) is an antibody found in the blood of many people with rheumatoid arthritis and is believed to play a role in tissue destruction associated with this disease.

Preparation None.

Test procedure A sample of your blood is drawn from a vein in your arm and sent to the laboratory for analysis.

After the test You follow procedures for venipuncture (see chapter 4) and are free to leave.

Factors affecting results

- RF is found in the blood of up to 5% of healthy elderly people, and sometimes although much less frequently in the blood of healthy young people.
- Several infectious disorders, chronic inflammation, and other diseases may trigger production of RF.

Interpretation

- Since the blood does not normally contain RF, its presence, along with other characteristic symptoms, helps confirm rheumatoid arthritis and helps distinguish it from rheumatic disorders, such as osteoarthritis, ankylosing spondylitis, psoriatic arthritis, and gout, which are not associated with RF production.

- High RF levels are generally found in people with more severe and active disease and may be associated with a worse prognosis.
- The presence of RF in a blood sample, particularly in low concentrations, does not provide definitive diagnosis of rheumatoid arthritis because it may also be found in many other diseases, including bacterial endocarditis, malaria, syphilis, tuberculosis, cirrhosis of the liver, hepatitis, and infectious mononucleosis. Moreover, some people produce RF in the absence of any disease, particularly in old age.
- Conversely, failure to find RF does not rule out rheumatoid arthritis because up to 20% of people with this disorder produce no RF or have it at very low levels. In particular, young people with juvenile rheumatoid arthritis often have no RF in their blood.

Advantages

- There's no risk to the patient.
- It may help confirm or rule out the diagnosis of rheumatoid arthritis when interpreted together with signs and symptoms.

Disadvantages False-negative and false-positive results are common.

The next step The presence or absence of RF in a person's blood does not definitively establish or rule out a diagnosis of rheumatoid arthritis. Taken together with symptoms and the doctor's observations, however, the result may be sufficient to begin treatment.

LYME DISEASE ANTIBODY

General information

Where It's Done	Who Does It	How Long It Takes	Discomfort/Pain
Hospital, doctor's office, or commercial laboratory.	Doctor, nurse, or lab technician.	Time required to draw blood or cerebrospinal fluid.	Minor discomfort associated with needle insertion.
Results Ready When	**Special Equipment**	**Risks/Complications**	**Average Cost**
3–7 days.	Syringe and needle; collecting tubes.	Negligible for blood testing; for risks of CSF drawing, see Lumbar Puncture, chapter 23.	$

Other names Lyme arthritis serology or Lyme titer.

Purpose To confirm the diagnosis of Lyme disease, a disorder that causes skin rash and arthritislike symptoms in the joints, among other symptoms.

How it works Since Lyme disease is caused by an organism that is difficult to detect in body fluids, tests for Lyme disease look for antibodies produced in response to the organism and found in the blood or cerebrospinal fluid (CSF). Antigens from spirochetes that cause Lyme disease are added to the blood or fluid sample. If antibodies are present, they bind with the antigens and can be detected and counted with the help of immunofluorescence or enzyme-linked immunosorbent assay (ELISA) technology (see chapter 4 for more information on this technique).

Preparation None.

Test procedure Blood is drawn from a vein in your arm, or a sample of CSF is obtained and sent to a laboratory for analysis. (For a full description of a cerebrospinal tap, see Lumbar Puncture, chapter 23.) If initial testing produces ambiguous results, the test may be repeated with the help of Western blot technology (see chapter 4).

After the test You follow procedures for venipuncture (see chapter 4) and are free to leave. For care after drawing of CSF, see Lumbar Puncture, chapter 23.

Factors affecting results

- False-negative results are common three to five weeks after infection, when the antibodies are present in small amounts.
- Antibody levels tend to rise after the initial infection, peak after six to eight weeks of illness, and decline after four to six months, although in some people they remain elevated indefinitely.
- False-positive results may be caused by a variety of disorders, including infectious mononucleosis, rheumatoid arthritis, lupus, periodontal disease, and other diseases caused by spirochetes.
- Tests performed in various laboratories differ in their reliability. Identical blood or CSF samples sent to different laboratories may produce different results.

Interpretation

- Because of the high rate of false-positives and false-negatives, test results are helpful in establishing a diagnosis only when closely correlated with the person's symptoms.
- When the doctor considers Lyme disease unlikely, negative test results may help rule it out.
- Some people harbor antibodies to the spirochete but have no symptoms; when another illness develops, its symptoms may be attributed to Lyme disease on the basis of a positive test for Lyme disease antibodies.

Advantages It provides the most practical way of confirming the diagnosis of Lyme disease.

Disadvantages

- False-negative and false-positive results are common.
- False-positive results may lead to inappropriate and ineffective treatment.

The next step Together with the presence of symptoms and the doctor's observations, a positive test is often sufficient to begin treatment.

ALKALINE PHOSPHATASE (ALP)

General information

Where It's Done	Who Does It	How Long It Takes	Discomfort/Pain
Hospital, doctor's office, or commercial laboratory.	Doctor, nurse, or lab technician.	Less than 5 minutes.	Minor discomfort associated with blood drawing.
Results Ready When	**Special Equipment**	**Risks/Complications**	**Average Cost**
2–4 hours.	Syringe and needle; collecting tubes.	Negligible.	$

Other names None.

Purpose

- To diagnose bone disorders in which the activity of bone cells is decreased or increased.
- The test may also be performed to diagnose liver disease (see Liver Function Tests, chapter 8).

How it works Alkaline phosphatase (ALP) is an enzyme produced in several organs, including the bones, liver, and intestines, and found in the blood of healthy people. Blood concentrations of ALP may rise whenever there is increased activity of bone cells (eg, during childhood growth periods or after a bone fracture) or as a result of bone disorders, including osteomalacia, bone cancer, and Paget's disease of bone.

Preparation You must avoid ingesting food and drink for several hours before the test.

Test procedure Blood is drawn from a vein in your arm (see chapter 4) and sent to a laboratory for analysis.

After the test You follow procedures for venipuncture (see chapter 4) and are free to leave.

Factors affecting results

- Certain drugs.
- Pregnancy.

- Chronic alcoholism.
- Excessive consumption of vitamin D.
- Occasionally, lung and breast cancer.
- Failure to fast prior to the test, particularly if a fatty meal was consumed.

Interpretation ALP levels vary depending on the person's age and sex and can be influenced by a number of other factors ranging from an underactive thyroid gland to pernicious anemia. Results must be correlated with the patient's history and symptoms.

Advantages It's minimally invasive.

Disadvantages It detects an abnormality but not its cause.

The next step If ALP levels are abnormally high or low, further tests must be performed to detect the underlying abnormality. To determine whether increased ALP is due to bone or liver disease, a test may be ordered in which ALP is exposed to heat. This may not require a second venipuncture if there is sufficient serum stored from the first blood sample.

CREATINE KINASE (CK)

General information

Where It's Done	Who Does It	How Long It Takes	Discomfort/Pain
Hospital, doctor's office, or commercial laboratory.	Doctor, nurse, or lab technician.	Less than 5 minutes.	Minor discomfort associated with drawing blood.
Results Ready When	**Special Equipment**	**Risks/Complications**	**Average Cost**
2–4 hours.	Syringe and needle; collecting tubes.	Negligible.	$

Other names Creatine phosphokinase (CPK).

Purpose

- To diagnose muscle disorders and monitor their course.
- To help verify a suspected heart attack (see chapter 5).
- To identify female carriers of Duchenne muscular dystrophy, although more accurate genetic tests are now available for detecting this disorder.

How it works Creatine kinase (CK) is an enzyme present in skeletal muscle, heart muscle, and the brain. When muscle is damaged or diseased, CK flows into the bloodstream, where it can be measured.

Preparation Avoid exercise and strenuous physical activity for three or four hours before the test.

Test procedure Blood is drawn from a vein in your arm (see chapter 4) and sent to a laboratory for analysis.

After the test You follow standard procedures for venipuncture (see chapter 4) and are free to leave.

Factors affecting results

- Exercise or strenuous physical activity within the previous 24 hours.
- Surgery that involved incision through muscle.
- Intramuscular injections.

Interpretation Decreased CK concentrations in the blood may indicate metastatic cancer, alcoholic liver disease, and connective tissue diseases. Increased levels may signal muscular dystrophy, polymyositis, dermatomyositis, and sometimes myositis, as well as heart attack. CK may also be elevated after surgery, or in some people with underactive thyroid gland or malignant hyperthermia, an abnormally high fever that develops in response to certain anesthetics.

Advantages It's noninvasive.

Disadvantages It detects an abnormality but not its cause.

The next step An abnormal CK level in itself cannot diagnose a muscle disorder. Therefore, additional tests must be ordered, depending on the patient's history and symptoms. These might include an electromyogram and a muscle biopsy.

BONE X-RAYS

General information

Where It's Done	Who Does It	How Long It Takes	Discomfort/Pain
Hospital, doctor's office, or commercial X-ray facility.	Radiologist or X-ray technician.	5–10 minutes.	You may have to assume uncomfortable positions, such as flexing and extending your neck for skull X-rays.

Results Ready When	Special Equipment	Risks/Complications	Average Cost
Immediately.	X-ray machine (portable or stationary).	Risks associated with exposure to radiation, particularly during pregnancy.	\$–\$\$

Other names Plain X-rays of bones, scoliosis series (if spine curvature is evaluated), and skeletal survey.

Purpose

- To detect bone fractures.
- To detect bone cancer and cancer metastases to the bone.
- To diagnose infectious diseases of the bones.
- To diagnose different types of arthritis.
- To determine bone age in children.
- To evaluate intervertebral disc spaces in the lower spine.
- To evaluate abnormal curvature of the spine or other deformities.
- To detect congenital skull deformities.
- To detect injuries in a battered child.

How it works X-rays (electromagnetic energy emitted by an X-ray tube) are absorbed by the body tissue. When the tissue is exposed to special photographic film, various types of tissue show up as shadows, as dark gray areas, or as white opaque areas.

Preparation

- You remove all clothing and jewelry and don a hospital gown.
- For skull X-rays, you will have to remove hairpins, glass eyes, contact lenses, glasses, and dentures.

Test procedure

- The technician places you against the X-ray machine in a position dependent on which bones are to be examined. For example, for an X-ray of the upper spine in the absence of injury, you will stand with your side to the X-ray machine while dropping your shoulders as much as possible. You may have to hold heavy weights in your arms to help you lower the shoulders.
- You must remain perfectly still during the X-ray picture, which takes only a few seconds.
- The X-ray picture may be taken from different angles or of different parts of your skeleton. The number of views depends on the purpose of the test. A single X-ray is sufficient to determine bone age.

After the test

- You get dressed and are free to leave.
- The film is processed in a developing machine and X-ray pictures are produced.

Factors affecting results

- Metal jewelry.
- Movement during the test.

Interpretation

- The X-ray films are analyzed for abnormalities. In arthritis, the loss of cartilage produces a narrowed space between bones. The pattern of joint space narrowing can help distinguish among types of arthritis. Bone spurs and erosions (characteristic indentations of the bone) also help diagnose arthritis.
- Infectious diseases, such as osteomyelitis and septic arthritis, produce bone changes that appear on X-rays within several weeks, but a bone scan is a better test for picking up early signs of bone and joint infection.
- The age of the bones, which can be determined by comparing an X-ray of the hand and wrist with a standard X-ray from a child of the same age and gender, helps assess the physical development of the child. A bone that is too mature for a child's age may signal precocious puberty, while immature bones may be due to delayed development. The doctor can also assess the mineral content of the child's bones and scars resulting from interrupted growth that may have been caused by past illnesses or other mishaps.

Advantages

- It's simple, quick, and noninvasive.
- It's also inexpensive and widely available.

Disadvantages

- It involves exposure to radiation (although minimal).
- It's less sensitive than a bone scan in detecting bone destruction.

MUSCULOSKELETAL MAGNETIC RESONANCE IMAGING (MRI)

Other names Magnetic resonance scan of the shoulder, knee, spine, hip, or neck.

For a full description of this test, see chapter 3.

Purpose

- While X-rays are used to evaluate dense tissues, such as bones, MRI is most useful in detecting problems in soft tissues, such as tendons, ligaments, cartilage, and structures inside the bone, including bone marrow.
- In musculoskeletal medicine, MRI is used most often to detect disc abnormalities (especially herniated discs) in the lower spine; tears in tendons; abnormalities in the ligaments, cartilage, and muscle; and the presence of cysts, tumors, and infection in the shoulder, lower spine, and knee; less commonly, it is used to diagnose these problems in the neck and hip.

Interpretation The doctor studies for abnormalities the pictures obtained with MRI on a video screen or on film.

MUSCULOSKELETAL COMPUTED TOMOGRAPHY (CT) SCAN

Other names Computed axial tomography.

For a full description of this test, see chapter 3.

Purpose

- To diagnose problems in the upper and lower spine, including herniated discs and spinal stenosis (narrowing of the spinal canal).
- To diagnose disorders of the hip joint.
- To identify abnormalities of various nerves in the spine.
- To detect tumors in bones or surrounding tissues.
- To establish the location of an abscess.
- To examine skeletal changes in osteoporosis and other metabolic bone diseases.

Interpretation The doctor studies the images, looking for abnormalities that may signal disease of the musculoskeletal system.

MUSCULOSKELETAL ULTRASOUND

Other names Extremity ultrasound (if the arms or legs are examined) or soft-tissue mass ultrasound.

For a full description of this test, see chapter 3.

Purpose

- To detect cysts, abnormal blood vessels, abscesses, and tumors.
- To assist in guiding the needle for a needle biopsy, or when a cyst, abscess, or excess fluid in a joint or cyst needs to be drained.
- To evaluate the size of tumors and distinguish solid tumors from fluid-filled cysts.
- To help identify blood vessel abnormalities, such as popliteal aneurysm, an abnormal bulging of the artery under the knee.

Interpretation The doctor studies the image, called an ultrasonogram, and assesses the size, shape, and composition of different structures.

BONE SCAN

Other names Radionuclide bone scan or bone scintigraphy.

For a full description of this test, see chapter 3.

Purpose

- To detect or rule out bone cancer when X-rays reveal no abnormalities but a malignancy is suspected.
- To detect bone infection.
- To determine the location of an abnormality before bone biopsy or surgery is performed.
- To diagnose stress fractures that do not always appear on X-rays.

Factors affecting results

- Injury resulting from trauma may be missed within the first 24 hours.
- In people with poor kidney function, the bone may not absorb sufficient radionuclide to perform the scan.

Interpretation The distribution of the radioactive material (radionuclide) helps evaluate the structure of the bone and the processes inside bone tissue (see figure 13.2). When bone tissue is healthy, the radionuclide is spread in a uniform fashion. An increased concentration of the material is usually found in diseased areas. Such areas may correspond to infection, inflammation, fracture, a cancerous tumor in which the cells are dividing rapidly, or another abnormality. The scan can pick up these abnormalities in early stages when X-ray findings are completely normal (X-rays detect them only after they produce structural deformities).

BONE BIOPSY

General information

Where It's Done	Who Does It	How Long It Takes	Discomfort/Pain
Hospital, doctor's office, or commercial surgical facility.	Doctor.	20–30 minutes.	Minor discomfort associated with needle insertion.
Results Ready When	**Special Equipment**	**Risks/Complications**	**Average Cost**
2–8 weeks.	Biopsy needle, collecting tube, adhesive bandage, and fluoroscope or CT scanner.	Bleeding from biopsy site (rare); infection (extremely rare if sterile conditions are strictly applied).	$$$

Other names None.

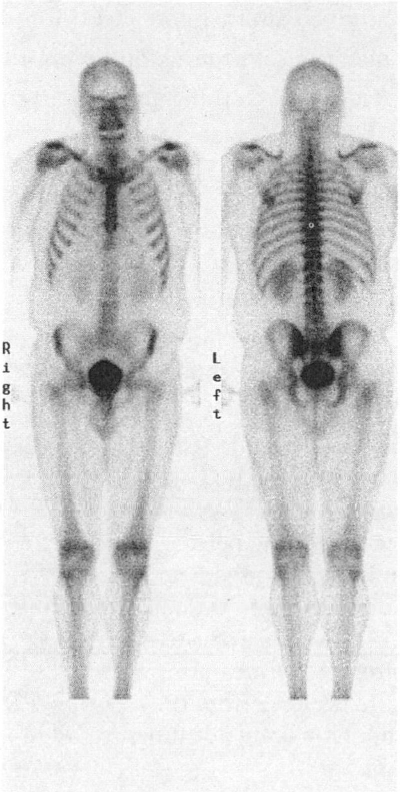

FIGURE 13.2 This is an example of a normal bone scan with the front view at the left and back view at the right.

Purpose

- To diagnose bone diseases such as osteoporosis, osteomalacia, and osteopenia when less invasive tests fail to provide definitive results.
- To distinguish between benign bone tumors and bone cancer.
- To determine which organism may be causing osteomyelitis.

How it works

A sample of the bone is removed and sent to a laboratory for analysis.

Preparation

- For diagnosing suspected cases of osteoporosis, osteomalacia, and osteopenia, you will be given oral

DID YOU KNOW?

Calcium in the body is in a constant state of flux, being absorbed and stored in the bones, then resorbed into the bloodstream. Because tetracycline attaches to the calcium in your blood it can be used to "label" bone. By comparing the tetracycline in the bone from the initial dose to the dose given at the time of the biopsy, a pathologist can evaluate the rate at which calcium is absorbed by the bones.

tetracycline (an antibiotic) three weeks prior to the procedure. You will be given another dose just before the biopsy.

- You may not eat or drink on the morning of the procedure.
- You remove all clothing and don a hospital gown.

Test procedure

- Local anesthesia is administered at the biopsy site. (Occasionally general anesthesia may be used.) The anesthetic is injected into the skin and sometimes into the portion of the bone itself where the nerve fibers run.
- A sedative is given intravenously.
- A hollow needle is introduced into your body and guided to the area of suspected bone abnormality with the help of a fluoroscope or CT scanner.
- In cases of systemic (affecting the entire body) bone disease, such as osteoporosis, the pelvic bone is usually used because it is close to the surface of the skin. The site is determined by measuring a specific distance from the hip bone, making a scanner unnecessary.

PATIENT TIP

The only pain you should feel as the bone sample is taken is in the periosteum that lines the bone, not the bone itself. Let your doctor know if you experience radiating pain during the procedure. In this case, the biopsy needle may be positioned differently.

- A tiny core of bone (a bit more than ⅙ of an inch in diameter) is removed with the help of a ratchetlike device on the needle. A sample of the synovium, the lining covering bone cartilage, may also be removed.
- Bone tissue obtained during the biopsy is sent to a laboratory for analysis.

After the test

- A pressure bandage is applied to the biopsy site, and you may be asked to lie on the site to apply additional pressure.
- If the biopsy was performed on the spine, you may have to spend 24 hours in the hospital. Otherwise you may leave in about an hour, assuming there is no bleeding (a rare complication) and that your pulse, blood pressure, breathing, and temperature are found to be normal.
- You should have someone drive you home, as you may experience some discomfort at the biopsy site.
- You must keep the biopsy site covered and dry (showers are okay, baths are not) for 48 hours.
- If you experience pain or discomfort, take acetaminophen (Tylenol, etc) or acetaminophen with codeine.

- Let your doctor know immediately if you experience bleeding through the bandage or signs of infection such as fever, pain on movement, or redness near the biopsy site.

Factors affecting results The site at which the biopsy is performed: If the site is not carefully chosen, cancer cells or other cells affected by disease may be missed; if bone density is measured, the density may vary depending on the part of the bone examined.

Interpretation The shape and appearance of bone cells are analyzed under a microscope in order to distinguish benign tumors from cancer. The presence of cells that play a role in inflammation may signal an inflammatory disorder, such as osteomyelitis. The sample may be stained with special dyes to detect other abnormalities, and certain chemicals in the tissue may be labeled so that they can be detected and measured. For example, low levels of certain minerals may lead to a diagnosis of osteomalacia, a disorder characterized by bone softening in adults.

Advantages It may establish definitive diagnosis without surgery.

Disadvantages It's invasive.

The next step A positive test indicates that treatment may begin.

MUSCLE BIOPSY

Other names Skeletal muscle biopsy.

For a full description of this test, see chapter 23.

Purpose

- To diagnose muscle disorders, including muscular dystrophies, polymyositis, myositis, and generalized vasculitis.
- To identify muscle inflammation that may be due to infection or immune abnormalities.
- To diagnose muscle disorders associated with hormone disruption.

Interpretation

- Analysis of muscle tissue under a microscope makes it possible to determine which muscle fibers are involved in disease. The presence of certain abnormal cells may signal inflammation of the muscle.
- Excess fat in the sample may signal a disease caused by abnormal accumulation of fats in the muscle.
- The activity of various enzymes will be assessed. Enzymes (particularly aldolase, which helps convert sugars to energy) are responsible for producing energy in the muscle and performing important tasks in metabolism. Several muscle diseases are caused by enzyme abnormalities.

14

Fred S. Kantor, MD

Allergies

Tests Covered in This Chapter

The case of Margaret S., 37, a home care nurse and mother of two:

> *I've had allergies ever since I was a child. Summers used to leave me miserable with hay fever, but I always refused to have allergy shots. When I moved from New York City to the country, the allergies grew unbearable. Along with constant sneezing and difficulty breathing, I'd get these terrible sinus headaches and have to lie down for hours. Finally I went to see an allergist. He took a detailed history, including information about illnesses that run in my family. But he was most interested in my symptoms and how they were limiting my life.*

The Tests To pinpoint the allergies, the allergist injected a number of allergens into Margaret's arm and observed the sites for rashlike reactions. Large, itchy wheals appeared at most of the test sites. It turned out that she was severely allergic to virtually all the substances tested, including dust, mites, mold, mildews, feathers, animal hair, grass, trees, and various flowers and weeds. Ironically, she wasn't allergic to ragweed, which she'd always assumed to be the cause of her allergy problems.

The Outcome Because Margaret's allergies were so severe, her allergist recommended shots (extracts made up from the allergens themselves) to desensitize her, which Margaret found to be quite tolerable after all. It took almost a year before she felt relief, but her symptoms, such as occasional earaches, have become so mild that most of the time she's unaware of them. She was able to taper down from weekly to monthly shots, and at one point, knowing that some people find they can live without the shots, she tried discontinuing them. But within a year the symptoms returned and she resumed taking the shots. She must still take other precautions, such as frequently dusting and vacuuming her home.

INTRODUCTION

Allergies occur when the body's immune system works *too* well. Normally, the task of the immune system is to recognize antigens—bacteria, viruses, and other invading agents—and destroy them. In some people, however, the system is overly sensitive. It mistakenly attacks otherwise harmless substances, such as house dust or certain foods, causing an allergic reaction.

Allergic reactions usually work like this: An allergen—say, ragweed pollen—enters the body where blood cells called lymphocytes recognize it. Within days to weeks, they form antibodies, or immunoglobulins, a type of protein. The antibodies attach themselves to tissue cells called mast cells, found in the airways, skin, and digestive tract. Later, when pollen is inhaled again, the antibodies react with it, causing the mast cells to release chemicals responsible for inflammation, irritation, and other symptoms of an allergic response. The best known of these is histamine, which can cause sneezing, a runny nose, swelling of the airways, and a skin rash.

Every antibody produced by the immune system is programmed to respond to a specific allergen. For example, an antibody made against cat dander will trigger an allergic reaction only to a cat, not to a dog.

Although the antibody IgE is responsible for the majority of allergic reactions, some reactions may involve a type of white blood cell called a T cell, which attacks the allergen directly. The most common allergic reaction that is due to this so-called cell-mediated immunity is contact dermatitis.

Allergic diseases can be acute or chronic, and can range from mild conditions that produce a minor inconvenience to severe disorders that can be life-threatening. Many symptoms of allergy can result from other causes, but when they are triggered by an allergic reaction, they tend to be more severe and chronic.

Allergies usually appear first in childhood and tend to diminish or disappear completely with age. Doctors don't know why people develop them, but the tendency often runs in families. Types of allergies include those described below.

Respiratory allergies. These are the most common allergies, affecting millions of people. Best known is *hay fever*, or allergic rhinitis, which is characterized by runny nose and eyes, sneezing, and nasal congestion. Although hay fever is the common name, it is not caused by hay, nor does it produce fever. The most common allergens that trigger allergic rhinitis include grass, tree, and weed pollens (particularly ragweed), spores from molds, household dust mites, and animal dander.

In contrast to allergic rhinitis, which mostly affects the nose and upper respiratory airways, *asthma* is a reaction that occurs in the lungs. In most children and many adults with asthma, symptoms of the disease can be triggered by common respiratory allergens.

Skin allergies. Allergic skin reactions can take different forms. *Contact urticaria* (hives) develops on direct contact with an allergen, as for example when a person allergic to cat dander strokes a cat. *Contact dermatitis* is a rash that develops after contact with a substance containing chemicals that are not allergens themselves but can turn into allergens in the body. Common triggers include poison ivy, poison oak, poison sumac, cosmetics, perfumes, metals, dyes, and various chemicals. *Atopic dermatitis* (eczema) is an allergic response that is not dependent on contact and that manifests itself as an extremely itchy rash.

Food allergies. These are the most controversial and the least understood of all allergies. They are often confused with food intolerance, which is an inability to digest a particular substance, such as lactose in milk or gluten in wheat. A bad reaction to food or food intolerance produces mainly digestive symptoms, while a true food allergy usually causes other allergic symptoms, such as eczema, swelling of the eyes, lips, face, and tongue, and occasionally hay fever–like reactions. Common food allergens include dairy products, nuts, eggs, fish and shellfish, chocolate, wheat, corn, berries, peas, and beans.

Drug allergies. Nearly every drug can cause an allergic reaction, but some of the most common ones are penicillin and several other antibiotics, horse serum, insulin, barbiturates, local anesthetics, and certain hormones. Most often, drugs cause a mild allergic response consisting of fever or itching and hives, but in rare cases they may lead to a severe reaction and shock.

Insect allergies. In allergic individuals, bites of certain insects can trigger hives, itching, dry cough, constriction in the throat, and often abdominal pain, nausea, and vomiting. Biting flies, mosquitoes, ticks, and a few spiders generally cause mild reactions, but several stinging insects, including honeybees, bumblebees, wasps, hornets, yellow jackets, and fire ants, can cause a severe, life-threatening response.

Anaphylactic shock. Anaphylactic shock, although rare, is the most severe allergic reaction. It may develop within seconds or minutes of exposure to insect venom, drugs, and certain foods, and it requires immediate medical help. The symptoms may include itching all over, difficulty breathing, dizziness, rapid pulse, fainting, tightness in the chest, wheezing, and a sudden drop in blood pressure that can cause shock.

HOW YOUR DOCTOR DIAGNOSES AN ALLERGY

The doctor starts the diagnostic workup by taking a thorough medical history, examining you (paying special attention to the organ system involved, such as the lungs or skin), and discussing your symptoms. In order to better understand your symptoms, your doctor may ask the following questions:

- *When do your symptoms appear, and what makes them worse? Can you identify any foods or circumstances that seem to cause them?* Since allergies often come and go, the examination is likely to yield the most information if it is conducted while the symptoms are most severe.
- *Do any of your family members have allergies?* The tendency toward allergy may be a more important predictor than the specific allergy.
- *Do you suffer from any chronic diseases?* These may affect your immune system and produce allergylike responses or affect the results of diagnostic tests.
- *Where do you live and work?* For example, factory workers may be exposed to more chemicals than office workers, and allergens common in cities may differ from those prevalent in rural areas.
- *What drugs are you taking?* If a drug is suspected of causing the allergy, your doctor may ask you to bring it with you to the office. Some people take many medications for various conditions, and the precise composition of these drugs may be important in establishing the cause of the allergy.

In about 90% of cases, a presumptive diagnosis can be made on the basis of your medical history and an examination, but the doctor may order tests to confirm this. The tests are to evaluate physical impairment, such as a decrease in lung function in asthmatics, and to pinpoint the specific cause of the allergy. In the latter case, results must always be correlated with your history and clinical exam, because it is not unusual for people to test positive for substances to which they are not actually allergic. For example, pollen may stimulate your blood to produce antibodies but cause no allergic reaction.

Skin tests generally correspond more closely to actual allergies than blood tests, although some people's skin is so sensitive that a test may cause irritation even in the absence of an allergic reaction. Conversely, a skin test may occasionally be negative while in fact there is an allergy present, but this is relatively rare.

When a food allergy is suspected, your doctor may suggest an approach known as "avoidance and challenge." First, you will be asked to eliminate the suspected food from your diet for a few days or several weeks. Then you'll be instructed to eat the food in large amounts for three days to see if symptoms appear. To pinpoint the foods linked with symptoms, you may be asked to keep a food diary.

If symptoms occur too often to suspect a particular food, you may be placed on an elimination diet, in which you will eliminate everything except a food such as rice, which rarely produces allergic reactions. Then you will reintroduce food items one by one until a reaction occurs.

If these tests do not lead to a diagnosis, your doctor may perform a food challenge test, in which you will be given concentrations of the suspected allergenic food in capsule form.

SKIN TESTS

General information

Where It's Done	Who Does It	How Long It Takes	Discomfort/Pain
Doctor's office or clinic.	Doctor, lab technician, or nurse; doctor must be present in the area.	About 15 minutes.	Minor discomfort associated with the needle scratch, prick, or puncture.
Results Ready When	**Special Equipment**	**Risks/Complications**	**Average Cost**
15 minutes.	Commercially prepared extracts of allergens in a saline solution, plus a separate needle and/or syringe for each allergen.	Itching, arm swelling, fatigue, and a small risk (less than 1%) of a severe allergic reaction.	$

Other names Skin allergy testing: scratch test, prick test, puncture test, and intradermal test; immediate hypersensitivity skin tests; and intracutaneous (intradermal) or percutaneous allergy testing.

Purpose To demonstrate or rule out an allergic reaction to a particular substance, such as pollens, grasses, animal dander, or stinging-insect venom.

How it works If an allergy is present, application of a small amount of the suspected allergen will produce an allergic reaction—a red, raised spot, called a wheal, at the test site.

Preparation You may be asked to avoid taking certain drugs, particularly antihistamines, for several days prior to the test. Long-acting antihistamines may have to be avoided for two to three weeks.

Test procedure

- A normal-looking patch of skin on your forearm or back is cleaned with alcohol.
- A drop of a solution containing an allergen is placed on the skin. Depending on the method, the skin is lightly scratched with the tip of a needle (scratch test), pricked with the tip of a needle to pick up the superficial layer of the skin (prick test), or punctured with a needle (puncture test).
- In the intradermal test, a lower concentration of the allergen solution is injected under the skin.
- Several dozen allergen solutions (or up to 15 in the intradermal test) may be tested in one session, their drops placed in parallel rows about an inch apart.
- Test sites are examined after about 15 minutes for the presence of a red, raised wheal.
- The different test methods may be used separately or during one session. Sometimes, the scratch, prick, or puncture test is performed first, followed by the intradermal tests if the first test yields no positive results but an allergy is strongly suspected.

After the test

- You will be asked to wait 20 to 30 minutes to be sure there is no severe allergic reaction.
- You may experience two to three hours of itching in the test area. Highly allergic individuals may experience arm swelling, particularly after intradermal testing. People who react to several allergens may experience fatigue during the rest of the day.
- Notify your doctor immediately if you experience wheezing, lightheadedness, severe itching, or shortness of breath later in the day.
- Be sure to keep the test area clean until it completely heals.

Factors affecting results

- Poor circulation under the skin may blunt the results in the scratch, prick, and puncture tests.
- Antihistamines, tricyclic antidepressants, phenothiazines, and other drugs may block allergic reactions.
- Location: Reactions on the back, particularly the upper back, may be stronger than those on the arm.
- Overall health: Dialysis or widespread cancer may blunt the allergic response.
- Redness and wheals can also be caused by skin irritation, not allergy.

Interpretation The presence of a red, raised wheal larger than 5 millimeters (a little less than ¼ of an inch) in diameter indicates that you have antibodies against the tested allergen. The larger the red area and wheal, the greater the severity of the allergy. The response is measured and graded on a scale of 0 to 4+.

Advantages

- It's simple, relatively painless, and inexpensive.
- It provides immediate results.
- It's generally safe, although the intradermal test has slightly higher risk of a severe reaction than others.
- It allows several allergens to be tested simultaneously.

Disadvantages

- False-negative results are possible, particularly with the scratch, prick, and puncture tests.
- More elaborate tests may be required for a definitive diagnosis or to prescribe immunotherapy.
- Only a limited number of allergen extracts is available for testing.

The next step

- If the response is strong (grade 3 to 4+), allergy can be assumed. The allergist may advise avoidance of the allergen (such as animal dander), use of antihistmine, or allergy shots to build up tolerance.
- If a prick or RAST test is negative, an intradermal test may be recommended. A RAST test (see below) may be recommended, or a skin test may be repeated at a later date.

PENICILLIN SKIN TESTS

General information

Where It's Done	Who Does It	How Long It Takes	Discomfort/Pain
Doctor's office, commercial laboratory, or hospital.	Doctor, nurse, or lab technician; doctor must be present in testing area.	15–20 minutes.	Minor discomfort from needle stick.
Results Ready When	**Special Equipment**	**Risks/Complications**	**Average Cost**
Immediately.	Extracts of penicillin in a saline solution; needle and syringe.	Minor bleeding under the skin, itching, skin irritation, and slight risk of a widespread allergic reaction (less than 1% of cases). Should not be performed in people who have prevously had a severe reaction to penicillin.	\$–\$\$ (depending on number of tests).

Other names Skin tests for penicillin allergy.

Purpose

- To identify people at risk of a severe allergic reaction to penicillin.
- To determine the safety of penicillin and its derivatives for those who have had allergies to antibiotics.

How it works If an allergy is present, a small amount of penicillin will produce a red, raised spot, called a wheal, at the test site.

Preparation For several days before the test, avoid taking antihistamines, hydroxyzine (Atarax), tricyclic antidepressants, phenothiazines, and other medications that may block an allergic response.

Test procedure Reaction to penicillin is assessed first by a prick test, then by an intradermal test (see above).

After the test

- You will be asked to wait 20 to 30 minutes to be sure there is no severe allergic reaction.
- Do not cover the injection site, but keep it clean until it completely heals.
- Notify the doctor immediately if you experience light-headedness, wheezing, severe itching, or shortness of breath later in the day.

Factors affecting results

- Poor circulation under the skin may blunt the results in the scratch, prick, and puncture tests.
- Antihistamines, tricyclic antidepressants, phenothiazines, and other drugs may block allergic reactions.
- Overall health: Dialysis or widespread cancer may blunt the allergic response.

Interpretation The presence of a red, raised wheal larger than 5 millimeters (a little less than ¼ of an inch) in diameter indicates allergy to penicillin. The larger the wheal, the greater the severity of the allergy.

Advantages If you have no history of penicillin allergy, a negative test virtually rules out the risk of a life-threatening reaction to penicillin-type antibiotics.

Disadvantages

- Minor reactions, such as rash and itching, may occur during penicillin therapy, even if a penicillin allergy test was negative.
- Test results do not apply to other classes of antibiotics.
- The test assesses only allergic reactions caused by IgE antibodies (see above).
- Such adverse effects as serum sickness (most commonly, hives, pain, and swelling) and drug fever (a high temperature due to a drug reaction) may still occur, even if penicillin skin test is negative.

The next step

- A negative result in the absence of symptoms is sufficient to rule out penicillin allergy; no further testing is required.
- If the test is positive, you should not be treated with penicillin if possible. If penicillin must be given, you can be desensitized in the hospital.

DELAYED-TYPE HYPERSENSITIVITY TEST (DTH)

General information

Where It's Done	Who Does It	How Long It Takes	Discomfort/Pain
Doctor's office, commercial lab, or hospital.	Doctor, nurse, or lab technician; a doctor should always be present in testing area.	1–2 minutes.	Minor discomfort associated with injection.
Results Ready When	**Special Equipment**	**Risks/Complications**	**Average Cost**
3 days.	Syringe, needle, and concentrated tuberculin.	Fever, pain, redness, swelling, or possibly ulcers at the site of injection.	$ (per allergen)

Other names Tuberculin-type skin testing, Mantoux test, and anergy battery test.

Purpose

- To detect a type of allergic response referred to as delayed or delayed-type hypersensitivity because it takes 24 to 72 hours to appear.
- To detect tuberculosis (see chapter 7).

How it works Extracts of various suspected allergens are injected under the skin, which is watched for the development of symptoms (soreness or redness). By isolating a suspected allergen at a particular site, it is possible to determine the cause of delayed hypersensitivity, which can otherwise be difficult to diagnose because of the time lag and possibility of intervening allergic responses.

Preparation None.

Test procedure

- A small amount of a solution containing a suspected allergen, or an extract of tubercle bacteria known as tuberculin, is injected under your skin, usually in the forearm.
- A variant of this test is the anergy battery, in which you are exposed to a series of substances that commonly produce delayed hypersensitivity reactions.

After the test

- You are free to leave within several minutes of injection if no adverse reaction occurs.

- You should keep the test site clean for 72 hours. Let your doctor know immediately if you develop a severe reaction at the site of injection, fever, or difficulty breathing.
- You will be asked to return to the test center in two or three days to be examined by a nurse or physician.

Factors affecting results

- Age: Responses are diminished in infants and older people, giving false-negative results.
- Recent viral infection or vaccination, particularly against measles, or a weakened immune system may also produce a false-negative result.

Interpretation

- If you are allergic to the tested substance, redness and swelling will appear within 24 to 72 hours at the site of the injection.
- If you have no response to any of the substances used in the anergy battery test ("anergy" means lack of a reaction), your immune system may be suppressed by an inflammatory disease, cancer, or an infectious agent such as the human immunodeficiency virus.

Advantages

- It's inexpensive.
- It's easy to perform.

Disadvantages Discomfort at the site of the test.

The next step

- A positive response indicates the presence of an allergy or tuberculosis; and avoidance, desensitizing injections, or treatment (for tuberculosis) can begin.
- A negative test requires no further action unless it is suspected that your immune system is suppressed by a systemic disease such as cancer or AIDS.

RADIOALLERGOSORBENT TEST (RAST)

General information

Where It's Done	Who Does It	How Long It Takes	Discomfort/Pain
Doctor's office, hospital, or commercial laboratory.	Doctor, nurse, or lab technician.	Less than 5 minutes.	Minor discomfort associated with drawing blood.
Results Ready When	**Special Equipment**	**Risks/Complications**	**Average Cost**
7–14 days.	Supplies for drawing blood.	Negligible.	$ (per allergen)

Other names Allergen profile and IgE allergen specific.

Purpose

- To detect an allergy to a substance in the environment, such as animal dander, grasses, house mites, or insects, particularly if a skin test cannot be performed or has produced ambiguous results.
- To confirm an allergy to a particular substance prior to allergy shots (immunotherapy).

How it works

A sample of your blood serum is exposed to a small disk to which the test allergen has been attached. If you are allergic, your IgE antibodies will attach to the allergen in the disk. A radioactive reagent is used to quantitate the attached antibodies.

Preparation

- No procedures involving radioactive substances in your blood should be done prior to this test.
- You may be asked to avoid ingesting certain foods and medications in the days preceding the test.

Test procedure

Blood is drawn from a vein in your arm and sent to a laboratory for analysis.

Variations

Variations on the RAST test differ in the material to which the allergen is attached and the method by which antibodies are counted. The most popular one, known as FAST (fluorescence allergosorbent test), uses cellulose film in place of paper discs and a fluorescent chemical to tag the antibodies, which are then counted with the help of ultraviolet light.

After the test

Follow procedures for venous blood drawing (see chapter 4).

Factors affecting results

- Presence of radioactive substances in your blood (from other procedures in the previous few days).
- Presence of diseases such as atopic dermatitis and parasitic infections, which cause increased Ig E antibody levels even if there is no allergic reaction to the substance being tested.

Interpretation

Test results show the amount of antibodies in a milliliter of serum. If you are not allergic to the tested substance, the amount may be very low or nonexistent. If you are allergic, it may be elevated.

Advantages

It can be used in people with extensive eczema or dermatitis who cannot undergo skin testing.

Disadvantages

- Results must be interpreted in the light of your symptoms and history: A positive response to an allergen indicates only a potential allergic reaction that may not be the cause of your symptoms.
- It's at least twice as expensive as skin testing.
- Results are not immediately available.

- It may produce negative results for drugs or insect venom when in fact an allergy exists.
- Only a limited number of allergen extracts is available for this test.

The next step

- If results are equivocal, a skin test or provocation test may be done.
- If the test is positive, especially if it follows a positive skin test, immunotherapy may be begun if indicated.
- Test results must be correlated with symptoms for a positive diagnosis.

PAPER RADIOIMMUNOSORBENT TEST (PRIST)

General information

Where It's Done	Who Does It	How Long It Takes	Discomfort/Pain
Doctor's office, hospital, or commercial laboratory.	Doctor, nurse, or lab technician.	Less than 5 minutes.	Minor discomfort associated with drawing blood.

Results Ready When	Special Equipment	Risks/Complications	Average Cost
7–14 days.	Supplies for drawing blood.	Negligible.	$

Other names Total IgE levels.

Purpose

- To monitor the effectiveness of treatment and to predict recurrence in patients with allergic bronchopulmonary aspergillosis, a fungal infestation of the airways.
- Occasionally used to measure total levels of IgE antibodies in the blood. This helps interpret results of RAST in people with diseases such as atopic dermatitis that result in high IgE levels.
- May predict allergic disorders in infants when performed on blood taken from the umbilical cord.

How it works IgE is the most common antibody produced in allergic reactions. A high concentration in the blood usually indicates that an allergy (or allergies) is present but does not identify specific allergens.

Preparation No procedures involving radioactive substances in your blood should be done in the days prior to this test.

Test procedure Blood is drawn from a vein in your arm and sent to a laboratory for analysis using a method similar to that of RAST (see above).

After the test Follow procedures for venous blood drawing (see chapter 4).

Factors affecting results

- Injection of radioactive substances into your blood (from other tests) prior to testing.
- IgE levels can be elevated by parasitic or viral infections, immune abnormalities and other diseases, tobacco smoking, and certain other environmental factors.

Interpretation The results show the total amount of IgE antibodies in a milliliter of serum. Their interpretation depends on the reason for ordering the test. For example, if a RAST is to be performed on a person with atopic dermatitis, a PRIST might be done first to establish total IgE level. Since IgE levels tend to be extremely high in people with this skin disorder, the RAST results will only be meaningful if the total IgE levels are known.

Advantages The risk to the patient is negligible.

Disadvantages

- Results correspond poorly with the individual's predisposition to allergy.
- It's at least twice as expensive as skin testing.
- Results are not immediately available.

The next step Usually, no further testing is necessary; however, determining the levels of other antibodies, such as IgA, IgG, and IgM (see below), may be helpful in interpreting results.

ENZYME-LINKED IMMUNOSORBENT ASSAY (ELISA)

General information

Where It's Done	Who Does It	How Long It Takes	Discomfort/Pain
Hospital or commercial laboratory.	Doctor, nurse, or lab technician.	Less than 5 minutes.	Minor discomfort associated with drawing blood.
Results Ready When	**Special Equipment**	**Risks/Complications**	**Average Cost**
7–14 days.	Supplies for drawing blood.	Negligible.	$ per antibody.

Other names IgA, IgG, or IgM antibody testing.

Purpose

- To monitor treatment for an insect allergy.
- To measure antibodies that develop in certain infectious diseases, such as aspergillosis, a fungal lung infection, or AIDS.

- To measure the levels of antibodies other than IgE in the blood.
- Rarely used for diagnosis of an allergy.

How it works A sample of blood serum is applied to a plastic disk to which the test antigen or allergen is attached. An enzyme-linked marker is added, which causes a color change if your serum contains antibodies to the antigen tested.

Preparation None.

Test procedure Blood is drawn from your vein and sent to a laboratory for analysis.

After the test Follow procedures for venous blood drawing (see chapter 4).

Factors affecting results High levels of one type of antibody may prevent low levels of another antibody against the same substance from being detected.

Interpretation The test demonstrates the amount of IgA, IgG, and IgM antibodies in a milliliter of serum. Interpretation varies with the reason for the test. Since treatment of insect allergies leads to production of IgG, a high level can mean that the treatment is successful. Similarly, since IgG is produced in response to an aspergillosis infection, a high level indicates a recent infection.

Advantages

- It's relatively inexpensive.
- No radioactive materials are involved.

Disadvantages It does not detect IgE, the antibody most commonly involved in allergic reactions.

The next step

- No further testing is necessary, except for monitoring purposes.
- If immunodeficiency is suspected and levels of IgAs are normal, you will be vaccinated and the response to the vaccine will be monitored.

PRECIPITATING ANTIBODIES

General information

Where It's Done	Who Does It	How Long It Takes	Discomfort/Pain
Doctor's office, commercial laboratory, or hospital.	Doctor, nurse, or lab technician.	Less than 5 minutes.	Discomfort associated with drawing blood.

Results Ready When	Special Equipment	Risks/Complications	Average Cost
1–2 weeks.	Supplies for drawing blood.	Negligible.	$

Other names Allergic lung serology.

Purpose To diagnose farmer's lung disease and other lung disorders caused by an allergic reaction to inhaled fungi, molds, or other organic substances.

How it works If an allergy is present, antibodies will be found in the serum part of the blood. When the serum is placed in a clear gel containing the suspected allergen, the antibodies will bind with the allergen and form a precipitate that clouds the gel.

Preparation None.

Test procedure Blood is drawn from your vein and sent to a laboratory for analysis.

After the test Follow procedures for venous blood drawing (see chapter 4).

Factors affecting results The levels of precipitating antibodies may vary with fluctuations in the disease.

Interpretation A cloudy, whitish band in the clear gel after the serum is added indicates that you may be allergic to the tested antigen. The test detects the antibodies only if they are present in large amounts.

Advantages It entails no risk.

Disadvantages There is a possibility of false-negatives and false-positives if test results aren't carefully correlated with history of disease.

The next step

- A positive test in the presence of symptoms is considered definitive for diagnosis, and no further tests are necessary. However, your environment must be surveyed for sources of the allergen, eg, moldy hay.
- A negative test, if there is a history of symptoms, may be false, and the test may be repeated.

BLOOD AND URINE HISTAMINE

General information

Where It's Done	Who Does It	How Long It Takes	Discomfort/Pain
Commercial lab or hospital (test is available in a limited number of labs).	Doctor, nurse, or lab technician.	Less than 5 minutes.	Minor discomfort associated with drawing blood.

Results Ready When	Special Equipment	Risks/Complications	Average Cost
1–2 weeks.	Supplies for drawing blood, and container for collecting urine.	Negligible for drawing blood; none for testing urine.	$$

Other names None.

Purpose

- To confirm or rule out the presence of an allergy (but the test doesn't identify its cause).
- To help diagnose the nonallergic disorder mastocytosis (a proliferation of tissue cells that produce histamine).

How it works Histamine is a chemical responsible for numerous symptoms of allergic reaction. The amount present in the blood or urine can help confirm or rule out the presence of an allergy.

Preparation For three days prior to the test, avoid ingesting foods that increase histamine levels (particularly cheeses and sauerkraut).

Test procedure

- Blood will be drawn from your vein, or you will urinate into a cup.
- The sample will be sent to a laboratory for analysis.

After the test You are free to leave. If blood was drawn, follow procedures for blood drawing (see chapter 4).

Factors affecting results

- Urinary tract infections may lead to false-positive results.
- Some cancerous tumors, particularly in the digestive tract, produce excessive amounts of histamine, while other cancers may decrease histamine levels in the body.

Interpretation Histamine levels that are slightly elevated suggest that symptoms may be due to an allergic reaction, while extremely high levels suggest mastocytosis.

Advantages It's noninvasive.

Disadvantages

- False-positive and false-negative results are possible.

- There may be no close correlation between histamine levels measured by the test and the role of histamine in the disease process.

The next step

- Depending on symptoms, additional tests (such as skin tests, RAST, or challenge tests) will be necessary to determine the cause of elevated histamine levels.
- An extremely high level may indicate mastocytosis, or possibly cancer. To diagnose or rule out mastocytosis, a biopsy and CT scan may be necessary.

NASAL CHALLENGE TEST

General information

Where It's Done	Who Does It	How Long It Takes	Discomfort/Pain
Doctor's office or hospital lab.	Doctor, nurse, or lab technician.	2 hours.	Discomfort associated with spraying inside the nose.

Results Ready When	Special Equipment	Risks/Complications	Average Cost
Immediately.	Allergen spray, powder, or paper disc, and rhinomanometer.	Can cause all the usual symptoms of the allergy or a severe allergic reaction all over the body.	$$

Other names Nasal provocation test or rhinomanometry.

Purpose

- To confirm an allergic reaction, particularly when there is a discrepancy between skin and blood tests or in preparation for immunotherapy. (However, it is not used widely or often for this.)
- To test reaction to allergens present in the workplace.

How it works Histamine released during an allergic reaction causes inflammation of the tissue lining the nasal passages, which impedes airflow. A rhinomanometer measures airflow and air pressure in the nose.

Preparation Avoid taking antihistamines and other medications that may block an allergic response for several days prior to the test.

Test procedure

- A control test is performed with a neutral spray containing no potential allergens, and the passage of air through the airways is assessed with a rhinomanometer.
- One to two hours later, the suspected allergen is sprayed into the nose or introduced as a powder or on a paper disc.
- Airway resistance is measured again. Symptoms produced by the challenge, such as sneezing, runny nose, and nasal blockage, are recorded.

After the test Once your breathing returns to normal, you are free to leave.

Factors affecting results

- Medications that block an allergic reaction.
- The presence of viral infections and other disorders.
- Pollen in the air, if you have a pollen allergy.

Interpretation An increase in pressure and a decrease in airflow in the nasal passages after exposure to an allergen may indicate the presence of an allergy.

Advantages Negative results mean it is unlikely that the allergic reaction is due to the tested allergen.

Disadvantages

- It's time-consuming, unpleasant, and expensive.
- It may not correspond to real-life conditions because the amount of allergen in the spray is greater than that in natural surroundings.
- Test results vary, depending on how much of the offending allergen is in the air on a given day.

The next step

- A negative result is usually definitive, and no further testing is necessary.
- A positive test that confirms a positive skin or blood test is usually definitive; immunotherapy can be started.
- A positive result, if this is an initial allergy test, may not be indicative of an allergy to the substance tested, but rather the reaction may be caused by another allergen present in the environment. Caution must be used in initiating treatment based on this single test.

BRONCHIAL CHALLENGE TEST

General information

Where It's Done	Who Does It	How Long It Takes	Discomfort/Pain
Doctor's office, commercial laboratory, or hospital.	Doctor or lab technician; a doctor must always be present in the test area.	4–9 hours.	Some discomfort in breathing.

Results Ready When	Special Equipment	Risks/Complications	Average Cost
The same day.	Spirometer, mouthpiece, nose clip, nebulizers, dosimeter, and various doses of suspected allergen extracts.	Severe constriction of the airways and difficulty breathing. Should be avoided when breathing is disrupted by severe lung disease.	$$

Other names Bronchial provocation test.

Purpose

- To detect allergic asthma at times when no symptoms are present.
- To diagnose occupational asthma when the allergen is unknown; can evaluate response to workplace allergens such as industrial gas, vapor, and fumes in factories or flour in bakeries.

PATIENT TIP

Keep careful note of any prior illnesses or asthma symptoms. The test will not be conducted if you have had a viral infection within the past month or worsening of asthma in the past week.

How it works If allergic asthma is present, exposure to the allergen will cause constriction of the bronchial tubes. The resulting decrease in lung function can be measured with a spirometer.

Preparation Before the test, avoid smoking (for 12 hours); caffeine, eg, coffee, tea, cola, or chocolate (for six hours); significant exercise (for two hours); exposure to cold air (for two hours); and inhalers used to facilitate breathing and certain other medications (for six hours).

Test procedure

- Your lung function is measured using spirometry (for more information, see chapter 7).
- You inhale vapors of a neutral (saline) solution through the mouthpiece, and spirometry is repeated. If no decrease in lung function is observed, the testing continues.
- Vapors of an allergen extract are introduced into the air of the spirometer, and airflow through your lungs is evaluated again. If the flow drops too sharply, testing is discontinued. The test may be repeated with different allergens.

After the test After your breathing returns to normal, you are free to leave.

Factors affecting results

- Failure to follow instructions on avoiding drugs and other exposures prior to the test.
- Failure to follow instructions on breathing during the test.
- The presence of viral infections or obstruction in the lungs.
- Exposure to pollutants.

Interpretation Lung function before and after exposure to the allergen are compared. A drop in function signals an allergic reaction and possibly allergic asthma.

Advantages It allows testing with vapors and fumes in the same form as that encountered in workplace settings.

Disadvantages

- You are exposed to a single high dose of an allergen corresponding to months or years of natural exposure.
- False-negative results may occur.

The next step

- A positive test usually indicates an allergic reaction and requires monitoring and possible repeat testing.
- A negative test, if you have symptoms, may be a false-negative result, and you may need to repeat the test.

FOOD ALLERGY TEST

General information

Where It's Done	Who Does It	How Long It Takes	Discomfort/Pain
Doctor's office or patient's home.	Doctor or patient.	5 minutes to 7 days.	None.

Results Ready When	Special Equipment	Risks/Complications	Average Cost
5 minutes to 7 days.	Gelatin capsules that contain an extract of the food. Capsules containing a neutral substance may also be used.	Risk of a serious, possibly life-threatening reaction. Performing the test without the presence of a doctor can be risky. A previous severe reaction to a particular food or drug is reason to avoid testing with this substance. Less serious complications include nausea, diarrhea, runny nose, and hives.	$$

Other names Food (oral) provocation test, food (oral) challenge test, and ingestion challenge test.

Purpose Used infrequently and usually as a last resort to confirm an allergy to a food or food additive that has been suggested by medical history, physical exam, and the avoidance-and-challenge approach.

How it works The suspected allergen is injected or ingested in capsule form. If an allergy is present, the allergen will produce typical symptoms, such as angioedema or respiratory problems.

Preparation

- Avoid ingesting all foods suspected of causing an allergy for one to two weeks before the test.
- Do not take antihistamines or other drugs that might block an allergic response prior to the test.

Test procedure

- You receive an injection or swallow a test capsule and are observed for symptoms that may appear within minutes or take up to several days.
- To ensure objective results, the test may be repeated with a neutral capsule or injection (placebo). The substances should be coded by a third party, and neither the doctor nor the patient should know which is which (this approach is known as a double-blind food allergy test).

PATIENT TIPS

- Be sure to tell your doctor if you are taking astemizole (Hismanal), an antihistamine known to remain in the body for three weeks.
- If you are suffering from a severe cold or dehydration from severe diarrhea, postpone the test until you are feeling better.

After the test

You will be asked to remain in the doctor's office for 20 minutes to check for severe reactions. If symptoms appear, they may persist for several days. If you develop symptoms several hours after leaving the testing area, inform your doctor immediately.

Factors affecting results

- Diarrhea or other digestive problems.
- Certain medications.
- Psychological factors—anticipation of symptoms if the content of the capsule is known.

Interpretation

If typical symptoms of allergy appear shortly after swallowing a food capsule (but not the placebo), you may be allergic to the tested substance.

Advantages

It's more reliable than skin testing for a food allergy because the food is digested in the same way as when it is eaten.

Disadvantages

- It's time-consuming and expensive.
- Adequate extracts for many foods are not available.

The next step

- Positive results, if the double-blind test is used, are considered conclusive; no further tests are necessary. The food being tested should be avoided.
- Negative results are usually conclusive; no further tests are needed.

NASAL SMEAR FOR EOSINOPHILS

General information

Where It's Done	Who Does It	How Long It Takes	Discomfort/Pain
Doctor's office, commercial lab, or hospital.	Doctor, nurse, or lab technician.	Less than 1 minute.	None.

Results Ready When	Special Equipment	Risks/Complications	Average Cost
4 hours.	Sterile cotton swabs; glass or plastic slides.	None.	$

Other names Eosinophil smear.

Purpose The nasal smear is used to determine whether symptoms are caused by allergy or infection.

How it works Mucus is examined for the presence of eosinophil cells, which indicate an allergic reaction.

Preparation Avoid taking or using nasal sprays (particularly corticosteroids), oral steroids, and antihistamines for 24 hours prior to the test.

Test procedure A sample of secretions from your nose is removed with a cotton swab and sent to a laboratory for analysis.

After the test You are free to leave.

Factors affecting results

- Nasal sprays, particularly corticosteroid sprays.
- Oral steroids or antihistamines.

Interpretation The presence of eosinophils, especially in high concentrations, indicates an allergic reaction.

Advantages

- It's noninvasive.
- It's simple and inexpensive.

Disadvantages False-negative and false-positive results are common.

The next step

- Since false-negative and false-positive results are common, the test results must be interpreted in the light of other symptoms.
- A positive test may be repeated in a few weeks to be sure it was not caused by infection, or skin testing may be ordered, depending on symptoms. A culture may also be done of the nasal discharge and your sinuses may be X-rayed.

TRANSILLUMINATION OF THE SINUSES

General information

Where It's Done	Who Does It	How Long It Takes	Discomfort/Pain
Doctor's office.	Doctor.	1 minute.	None.
Results Ready When	**Special Equipment**	**Risks/Complications**	**Average Cost**
Immediately.	A fine-tipped light source.	None.	Part of doctor's fee.

Other names None.

Purpose To detect obstruction of the sinuses or openings to the sinuses that may result from an allergic reaction.

How it works Since light is able to pass through the delicate skin covering the hollow sinus cavities, a light source held against the upper cheek will produce a red dot on the palate if the sinuses are normal (filled with air rather than obstructed).

Preparation None.

Test procedure The doctor presses the light source against your upper cheek, close to the nose, asks you to open your mouth widely, and looks at your palate to see if the light passes through.

After the test You close your mouth, and the test is over.

Factors affecting results The presence of fluids, pus, or other debris in the sinus cavities.

Interpretation If the sinus cavities are obstructed (by a tumor, infection, or inflammation due to an allergic reaction), no red dot will be seen. X-rays or other tests must be performed to establish the cause.

Advantages

- It's simple, quick, and noninvasive.
- It's inexpensive.

Disadvantages It detects obstruction of the sinuses but not its cause.

The next step

- If test result is negative, no further testing is required.
- If test result is positive, X-rays of the sinuses may be taken.

Joseph E. Craft, MD ■ Fred Kantor, MD

15 The Immune System

Tests Covered in This Chapter

The case of Aubré B., a 23-year-old senior bank teller:

I was diagnosed with systemic lupus, an autoimmune disease, in March. But looking back, I realize I'd actually been ill since the previous fall, though I ignored the symptoms. Wrist pain came on first. Then pain started building in both ankles. Gradually it spread to my knees, elbows, wrists, and my jaw. I also suffered hot and cold flashes, which made me think it might be some kind of flu virus, but nothing serious.

One night my whole body was aching so much I couldn't move. I was taken to the emergency room. Because my joints were warm and swollen, this made them suspect acute arthritis. So they ordered tests and admitted me to the hospital. The next day, when I looked in the mirror I saw a blotchy butterfly-shaped rash covering my face.

The Tests The body's immune system manufactures special protein antibodies that travel in the bloodstream and attack such invaders as viruses and bacteria. Patients with systemic lupus erythematosus—lupus for short—produce excessive amounts of *auto*antibodies, abnormal proteins that attack the body's own tissue as if it were a foreign invader, causing inflammation. Although lupus primarily affects the skin, joints, and kidneys, it can inflame virtually any organ. When Aubré's tests showed a high level of creatinine in his blood as well as proteins and white and red blood cells in his urine—all signs of kidney trouble—a kidney biopsy was done to judge the extent of damage.

Lupus itself can usually be diagnosed by analyzing the blood for evidence of antinuclear antibodies (ANAs), which are present in almost all lupus patients. But ANAs are also associated with other autoimmune diseases, so doctors also check for anti-DNA antibody, a type of ANA unique to lupus.

The Outcome Aubré received two anti-inflammatory drugs: one to treat the lupus itself and kidney inflammation, and the other to control inflammation of the skin and joints. His spirits improved, the stiffness in his knees lessened, and he was able to return to work.

Lupus frequently goes into remission for a few years, and in a few people, it never comes back. By taking medication, most patients are able to lead normal lives and feel well. Aubré was encouraged to eat a good diet, exercise sensibly, and stay out of the sun, because too much exposure to ultraviolet rays can trigger flare-ups.

INTRODUCTION

Our immune systems shield our bodies from assault by harmful agents. While the most common attackers are pollutants in the air we breathe and infectious organisms—foreign invaders such as viruses, parasites, and bacteria—the immune system also keeps watch against internal attackers, such as normal cells that have changed (mutated) into cancerous forms (see figures 15.1 and 15.2).

Disease affecting the immune system may be the result of a malfunction in one of the interactions that make up the body's immune response. Of the two major types of immune abnormalities, autoimmune disorders, in which the body mistakenly attacks its own tissues, account for the majority of immune system problems. Immunodefi-

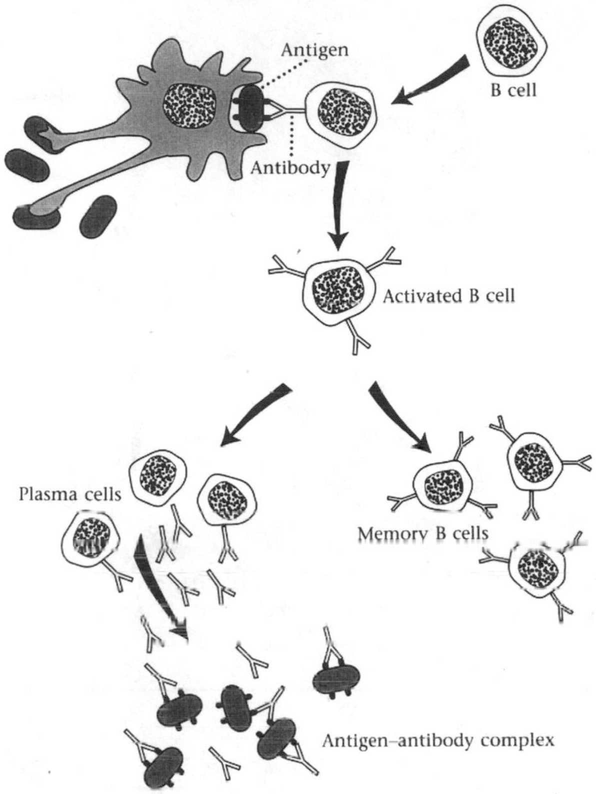

FIGURE 15.1 Humoral immunity

The body's immune system is activated when a foreign protein (antigen) enters the body, prompting white blood cells (macrophages) to produce antibodies and special memory B cells that are programmed to recognize the antigen. When these B cells are activated, they call into action plasma cells that destroy the antigen by forming antigen–antibody complexes.

ciency disorders, in which the body lacks the resources to fight off disease, are, with the exception of AIDS, much less common.

Autoimmune Disorders

The precise cause of autoimmune diseases is unknown, but scientists believe that heredity plays a part in predisposing people to them. Because they are much more common in females, the female hormone estrogen is thought to play a role in spurring their development.

Autoimmune breakdowns may play a part in diseases affecting organs such as the liver, the pancreas (in juvenile diabetes), and the nervous system (in multiple sclerosis and myasthenia gravis). Major

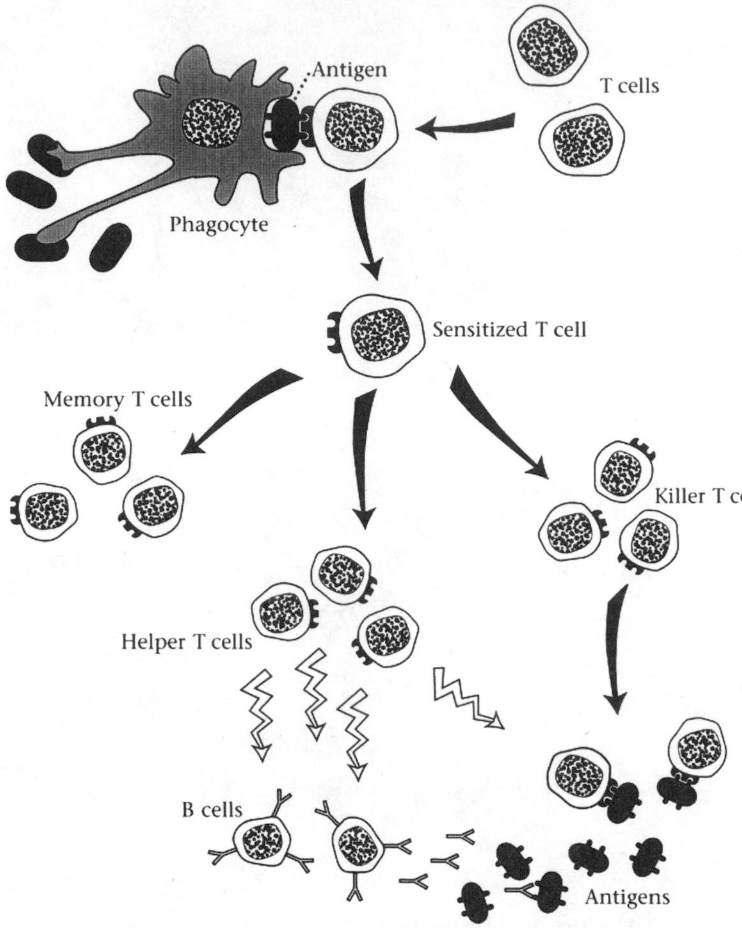

FIGURE 15.2 Cellular immunity

Another line of defense involves T cells, which attack both outside invaders and internal threats, such as cancer cells. They also help B cells destroy the invading antigens.

disorders in which autoimmunity is central to the disease process include the following:

- *Systemic lupus erythematosus,* a chronic inflammatory disease of connective tissues, joints, muscles, skin, and blood vessels. Tests used to diagnose lupus include complete blood count (CBC), erythrocyte sedimentation rate (ESR), autoimmune hemolytic anemia (AHA), antiphospholipid antibody tests, complement assay, and tests to evaluate damage to individual organs (see chapters 4 and 16).
- *Scleroderma,* a rare disease that affects many tissues and organs and may cause such symptoms as extreme sensitivity to cold in the fingers, tightening and thickening of the skin, heartburn, difficulty breathing, and sometimes constipation and diarrhea.

Scleroderma is often diagnosed using such tests as CBC, ANA, ESR, and tests to evaluate organ damage, particularly pulmonary function tests, barium swallow, and kidney function tests.

- *Sjögren's syndrome,* a disorder affecting mostly women and characterized by excessive dryness of the eyes, mouth, and vagina. Tests such as CBC, Schirmer's test, and a lower lip biopsy are used to diagnose it.
- *Polymyositis,* a disorder that causes the muscles, primarily those of the upper arms and thighs, to weaken and become inflamed. (When the skin is affected, the disorder is called *dermatomyositis.*) It is diagnosed with the help of such tests as creatinine phosphokinase, electromyography, and muscle biopsy.
- *Vasculitis,* a condition in which the blood vessels become inflamed, which may lead to bruiselike patches caused by bleeding into the skin, and in some elderly patients, headaches, difficulty chewing, and vision changes.
- *Polyarteritis,* a disorder caused by inflammation of blood vessels that lead to organs such as the lungs, kidneys, or organs of the digestive tract. It is diagnosed with the aid of ESR tests, X-rays, tissue biopsy, and arteriograms.

Immunodeficiency Disorders

A deficiency in any type of immune cell or immune protein can lead to disease. Immunodeficiencies hamper your ability to fight off infections and tumors and increase susceptibility to infectious disorders and certain forms of cancer. Immunodeficiencies that may be inherited or acquired include the following:

- *Severe combined immunodeficiency (SCID).* Babies born with SCID possess almost no immune defenses. Without treatment, these infants rarely survive beyond one year.
- *Acquired immunodeficiency syndrome (AIDS).* Perhaps the best known acquired immunodeficiency, this condition is caused by a virus that destroys the immune system (see chapter 21).
- *Immune system suppression.* The immune system may be suppressed by drugs, such as those taken for cancer chemotherapy, or by cancer itself. Severe malnutrition may also deplete the immune system, leading to a deficiency.

HOW YOUR DOCTOR DIAGNOSES IMMUNE DISORDERS AND DEFICIENCIES

Your doctor will start by taking a careful history of your disease, noting not only your symptoms (see the accompanying box) but also their pattern: Do they appear and then abate? Do certain conditions, such as stress, cause them to return or worsen? The doctor will do a thorough physical exam and then order tests that provide general

Symptoms of Autoimmune Disorders and Immunodeficiencies

- *Joint pain and stiffness* that tend to be severe in the morning.
- *Muscle weakness*, which may affect one particular muscle group or the entire body.
- *Fingers sensitive to cold (Raynaud's phenomenon)*. Sensitivity may also be linked to stress, result from trauma associated with operating a vibrating machine like a jackhammer, or, rarely, be caused by blood clots in the arm.
- *Skin rash*, including a butterfly-shaped rash over the bridge of the nose and cheeks in lupus and *livido*, a red, lacelike rash on the legs or, less often, the arms, which may also occur in healthy infants and adults.
- *Taut skin*, which, when accompanied by swelling of the fingers, may be an early sign of scleroderma. It may also occur during normal pregnancies.
- *Chronic fatigue*, which strikes nearly all those with autoimmune disorders at some time during their illness, but which also occurs in otherwise healthy people.
- *Hair loss*, which may occur during periods of stress or disease.

information about your health and immune status. (See the accompanying box, which lists and describes some techniques commonly used in these tests.)

Autoimmune Disorders

When your doctor suspects an autoimmune disorder, laboratory tests alone can seldom diagnose the problem. In fact, the tests that rule out autoimmune disorders may be easier to interpret than those that confirm them. Most often these include a complete blood count (see chapter 4), which may show anemia or white blood cell abnormalities. Next the doctor will order blood tests, such as sedimentation rate, rheumatoid factor, and antinuclear antibodies tests, that provide some information about autoimmune disorders. No single test definitively establishes or rules out any autoimmune disorder. Some tests produce false-positive or false-negative results, while others show abnormal results no matter what the autoimmune disease and cannot be used to specify the problem. Test results by themselves are often difficult to interpret because immune function varies widely even in people with normal health, and also changes with age.

After these general tests, the decision to conduct further tests depends on your symptoms. When all the test results are in, your doctor will interpret the results in light of your history of the disease and his or her observations during the physical exam.

Immunodeficiencies

Diagnosis of immunodeficiency disorders, like autoimmune disorders, depends on a thorough history and physical examination as well as laboratory tests. If your doctor suspects that your illness may be due to

Common Techniques Used in Immunologic Tests

These methods can also be used to detect other substances, such as hormones.

- *Enzyme-linked immunosorbent assay (ELISA).* Usually performed to detect antibodies, the test tags antibodies with enzymes that combine with other chemicals and change color. From these color changes, a machine called a spectrophotometer measures the antibody level. ELISA can also be used to detect antigens.
- *Radioimmunoassay.* Measures antigens or antibodies by tagging them with radioactive isotopes and counting them with a gamma counter.
- *Immunoelectrophoresis.* Most commonly used to measure proteins in blood or urine, particularly antibodies. Blood or urine is placed on specially treated film and then electrical current is run through it. The electric field causes different antibodies to move at various speeds in different directions. This movement forms dark bands that reveal the types of antibodies in the tested fluid. (For more on electrophoresis, see chapter 4.)
- *Radial Immunodiffusion.* Measures proteins in blood or urine. Serum or urine is placed on a special film, and the antibodies are allowed to diffuse, or float freely, until they bind with monoclonal antibodies (see below). Bound antibodies form characteristic patterns that can be detected.
- *Indirect immunofluorescence.* Most frequently employed to detect antibodies. Blood is placed on slides with antigens that bind with the antibody being tested. Bound antibodies are tagged with fluorescein (a light-sensitive substance), and the slide is exposed to special light. Antibodies present in the blood show up as tiny dots of fluorescent light. This test does not precisely measure antibodies; their amount can only be assessed approximately, depending on the strength of the light they produce.
- *Flow cytometry.* Measures the levels of different lymphocytes in the blood. An antibody known to bind with a particular type of lymphocyte is added to the blood sample, and the amount of binding is recorded.
- *Monoclonal antibodies.* Produced in a laboratory and designed to interact with a specific antigen. Often used as tags in ELISA tests, and may also be used in tests that detect infection.

inherited immunity problems, he or she will ask about other family members with autoimmune disease, allergy, or early cancer.

The physical exam may show a characteristic combination of symptoms that points to the proper diagnosis. For example, newborns with recurrent infections, tetany (muscle spasms and convulsions), peculiar facial features, and congenital heart disease may have an immunodeficiency disorder known as DiGeorge syndrome.

Your history and the doctor's observations may be supplemented by one or more of the following tests:

- *Complete blood count,* which measures the cells vital to immunity (see chapter 4).
- *ELISA,* which measures the levels of common antibodies (see chapter 14).

- *Complement assays*, which are used to detect complement deficiency.
- *Delayed-type hypersensitivity*, which tests cellular immunity (see chapter 14). If cellular immunity is found to be malfunctioning, a more specific test, such as lymphocyte typing, may be performed to determine the exact location of the malfunction.

SEDIMENTATION RATE

General information

Where It's Done	Who Does It	How Long It Takes	Discomfort/Pain
Doctor's office, hospital, or commercial laboratory.	Doctor, nurse, or lab technician.	5 minutes for drawing blood.	Minor discomfort associated with drawing blood.
Results Ready When	**Special Equipment**	**Risks/Complications**	**Average Cost**
2–3 hours or next day.	Supplies for drawing blood.	None.	$

Other names Sed rate or erythrocyte sedimentation rate (ESR).

Purpose To help detect autoimmune disorders, particularly vasculitis, but may also be used to detect any hidden infection or inflammation and a large number of other conditions.

How it works Various inflammatory conditions, including autoimmune conditions, increase the rate at which the red blood cells (erythrocytes) sink in a test tube and form a sediment.

Preparation None.

Test procedure The blood sample is drawn from a vein in your arm and sent to a laboratory for analysis.

After the test Follow procedure for drawing blood (see chapter 4).

Factors affecting results

- Age.
- Menstruation and pregnancy.
- Anemia.
- Kidney and thyroid disease and connective tissue disorders.
- Certain infections.

- Hormone disorders.
- Cancer.

Interpretation Although rates vary with measurement methods, in general normal sedimentation rates are considered to be up to 10 millimeters an hour in men and up to 20 an hour in women and the elderly.

Advantages There's no risk.

Disadvantages

- It detects infection or inflammation but not its cause.
- It cannot confirm a specific diagnosis.
- False-positive results may occur in healthy people.

The next step

- If rate is elevated and appropriate symptoms are present, the test confirms inflammation. If vasculitis is suspected, a skin or blood vessel biopsy may be done. In other generalized autoimmune conditions, the test confirms inflammation, and treatment may be initiated.
- If rate is normal, the test indicates an absence of general inflammation, and no further tests are necessary.

C-REACTIVE PROTEIN (CRP)

General information

Where It's Done	Who Does It	How Long It Takes	Discomfort/Pain
Doctor's office, hospital, or commercial laboratory.	Doctor, nurse, or lab technician.	Less than 5 minutes for drawing blood.	Minor discomfort associated with drawing blood.
Results Ready When	**Special Equipment**	**Risks/Complications**	**Average Cost**
1–3 days.	Supplies for drawing blood.	None.	$

Other names Acute phase reactant.

Purpose

- To check for severity of inflammatory disease and effectiveness of anti-inflammatory treatment.
- To help diagnose rheumatoid arthritis, which is characterized by high levels of CRP.
- Used for early detection of postoperative infection.

How it works Blood test detects blood levels of C-reactive protein, or CRP, which appears in the blood during inflammatory diseases.

Preparation None.

Test procedure Blood is drawn from a vein and analyzed for CRP. Several methods may be used for the analysis, including radioimmunoassay and agglutination.

After the test Follow procedure for drawing blood (see chapter 4).

Factors affecting results Pregnancy may increase CRP levels.

Interpretation CRP levels higher than 8 micrograms per milliliter may indicate presence of infection or inflammation.

Advantages

- There's no risk.
- It may be more sensitive than the sedimentation rate in detecting early- and late-stage infection.

Disadvantages

- It detects inflammation but not its cause (cannot be used to confirm a specific diagnosis).
- It's more complicated and expensive than sedimentation rate.

The next step

- If levels are elevated and arthritis is suspected, a rheumatoid factor test may be done. In other conditions, the test confirms the presence of systemic inflammation, and therapy may be started.
- If levels are normal, the test indicates lack of systemic inflammation, and no further tests are necessary.

AUTOANTIBODY TESTING

General information

Where It's Done	Who Does It	How Long It Takes	Discomfort/Pain
Doctor's office, hospital, or commercial laboratory.	Doctor, nurse, or lab technician.	Less than 5 minutes for drawing blood.	Minor discomfort associated with drawing blood.
Results Ready When	**Special Equipment**	**Risks/Complications**	**Average Cost**
1–7 days.	Supplies for drawing blood.	None.	$

Other names Antibody testing.

Purpose

- To help diagnose autoimmune disorders by detecting and measuring the levels of autoantibodies.
- To monitor the course of an autoimmune disorder.

How it works The presence of autoantibodies, detected by immunofluorescence or ELISA methods, means the body is making antibodies that are fighting its own tissue.

Preparation None.

Test procedure A sample of your blood is drawn and analyzed for the presence of particular antibodies.

After the test Follow procedure for drawing blood (see chapter 4).

Factors affecting results

- Drugs such as alphamethyldopa, chlorpromazine, diphenyl hydantoin, hydralazine, isoniazid, procainamide, and quinidine (even several months after they are stopped) may trigger production of antinuclear antibodies (ANAs) and produce false-positive results.
- Other drugs may lead to the production of other antibodies.
- ANAs may be found in the blood of healthy people aged 60 or older or occasionally in some younger people.

Interpretation This test may detect the following antibodies:

- *Antinuclear antibody (ANA),* which may be present in autoimmune disorders, particularly lupus, scleroderma, Sjögren's syndrome, polymyositis, and certain types of chronic active hepatitis.
- *Anti-DNA antibody,* which may be present in lupus but is usually not found in other autoimmune diseases. Levels generally decrease when treatment of lupus is successful.
- *Antiphospholipid antibody,* which may be found in lupus and certain other conditions. Associated with clots and miscarriages.
- *Anti–smooth muscle antibody,* which may be present in chronic active hepatitis. Testing helps distinguish between this type of hepatitis and other forms of liver disease.
- *Antimitochondrial antibody,* which is present in most cases of primary biliary cirrhosis and (rarely) with other types of chronic liver disease.
- *Rheumatoid factor,* which is often found in the blood and joint fluids of people with rheumatoid arthritis (see chapter 13).

Advantages There's no risk.

Disadvantages

- Presence of antibodies does not lead to a definitive diagnosis, while absence does not always rule out a disease.
- Levels of antibodies do not always correspond to severity of disease.
- Test sometimes produces false-positive and false-negative results.

The next step

- If antibodies are present along with appropriate symptoms, they are indicative of an autoimmune disorder, and treatment may be initiated.
- Absence of antibodies suggests a condition other than an autoimmune disorder; other tests may be ordered.

SCHIRMER'S TEST

General information

Where It's Done	Who Does It	How Long It Takes	Discomfort/Pain
Doctor's office, hospital, or commercial laboratory.	Doctor, nurse, lab technician, or optometrist.	10 minutes.	Minor discomfort associated with paper touching eye.
Results Ready When	**Special Equipment**	**Risks/Complications**	**Average Cost**
Immediately.	Filter paper; sometimes, anesthetic eyedrops.	None.	$

Other names Schirmer tearing test.

Purpose

- To measure amount of tears in people with suspected Sjögren's syndrome, an autoimmune disorder characterized by dry eyes and mouth.
- To evaluate the severity of dry-eye syndrome, which may be a side effect of medications or a result of allergies and other conditions.

How it works Tears are collected from the eye to see if a sufficient amount of moisture is being secreted.

Preparation

- Do not use eyedrops for 24 hours before the test.
- Do not wear contact lenses on the day of the test.

Test procedure

- A strip of filter paper is placed inside the lower eyelid and left for five minutes.
- Sometimes, a cotton swab may be inserted high into your nose to trigger a tear reflex.
- The test may be repeated after you are given anesthetic eyedrops.
- The paper is removed, and the amount of moisture absorbed is evaluated.

After the test

- You are free to return to normal activities.
- If anesthetic eyedrops were used, avoid rubbing your eyes for at least 30 minutes to prevent damage to the cornea, and do not reinsert your contact lenses for at least two hours.

Factors affecting results Use of anesthetic eyedrops, and wearing contact lenses.

Interpretation The moistened area on the filter paper is measured. A spot at least 8 millimeters (about ⅓ of an inch) in diameter is considered normal.

Advantages It's quick and simple.

Disadvantages

- It provides only a rough evaluation of tear secretion.
- It's unreliable in measuring moisture in moderately dry eyes.
- It measures the severity of eye dryness but does not establish its cause.

The next step

- If results are positive, a lip lower biopsy will be ordered.
- If results are negative, no further tests are necessary.

LOWER LIP BIOPSY

General Information

Where It's Done	Who Does It	How Long It Takes	Discomfort/Pain
Doctor's office or hospital.	Surgeon.	1 hour.	Soreness after anesthesia wears off.
Results Ready When	**Special Equipment**	**Risks/Complications**	**Average Cost**
7 days.	Surgical instruments and local anesthesia.	None.	$$$

Other names Minor or labial salivary gland biopsy.

Purpose To confirm the diagnosis of Sjögren's syndrome, an autoimmune disorder characterized by dry eyes and mouth.

How it works Salivary glands are removed and inspected for signs of Sjögren's syndrome or a tumor.

Preparation

- Do not take any aspirin or aspirin-containing drugs for about a week before the test.

- Avoid taking nonsteroidal anti-inflammatory drugs for at least two to three days before the biopsy.

Test procedure

- You sit in a dental chair, and local anesthesia is administered to your lower lip.
- The doctor cuts into the mucous lining of the inner part of your lip and removes at least five salivary glands.
- The glands are sent to a laboratory for analysis.

After the test

- It may be hard to eat or talk for two to three hours after the test until the anesthesia wears off.
- Do not eat solid foods for several hours after the test.
- The doctor may schedule a follow-up exam to check the incision.

Factors affecting results

Mouth sores and infections in lining of the mouth can produce false-positive results.

Interpretation

- If inflammatory cells in large clusters are found in the glands, you have Sjögren's syndrome.
- Abnormal cells in the biopsy sample may indicate a tumor.

Advantages

It's reliable in diagnosing Sjögren's syndrome.

Disadvantages

It's invasive.

The next step

- If results are positive, treatment for Sjögren's syndrome.
- If results are negative, another cause, such as medication, may be considered for dry eyes and mouth.

HLA TYPING

General information

Where It's Done	Who Does It	How Long It Takes	Discomfort/Pain
Doctor's office, hospital, or commercial laboratory.	Doctor, nurse, or lab technician.	5 minutes.	Minor discomfort associated with drawing blood.
Results Ready When	**Special Equipment**	**Risks/Complications**	**Average Cost**
7 days.	Needle, syringe, collecting tubes, and equipment for analyzing sample.	None.	$

Other names Human leukocyte antigens, organ donor or transplant tissue typing, lymphocyte cross match, and histocompatibility testing.

Purpose

- To identify surface groups of proteins known as human leukocyte antigens (HLAs), which are unique in each person.
- To match HLA types of organ donor and recipient, which lowers the risk of organ rejection.
- To help determine paternity, since HLA systems are inherited.
- To help diagnose ankylosing spondylitis and sacroiliitis, which are often associated with an HLA called HLA-B27.

How it works HLAs detectable in blood provide clues to immune conditions.

Preparation None.

Test procedure A blood sample is drawn and sent to a laboratory for analysis.

After the test Follow procedure for drawing blood (see chapter 4).

Factors affecting results None.

Interpretation

- If done for organ transplantation, HLA type will be compared to those of available organs.
- Blood may be analyzed for particular HLAs that indicate disease.
- To determine paternity, a child's HLA type is compared to that of a possible father.

Advantages

- There's no risk.
- It improves results of organ transplantation.

Disadvantages None.

The next step

- After a positive test, if done to confirm ankylosing spondylitis or sacroiliitis, X-rays of the spine or sacroiliac joints may be done and treatment begun.
- If done for donor matching, transplant can proceed if match is good.

COMPLEMENT ASSAY

General information

Where It's Done	Who Does It	How Long It Takes	Discomfort/Pain
Doctor's office, hospital, or commercial laboratory.	Doctor, nurse, or lab technician.	5 minutes.	Minor discomfort associated with drawing blood.
Results Ready When	**Special Equipment**	**Risks/Complications**	**Average Cost**
7 days.	Needle, syringe, collecting tubes, and equipment for analyzing sample.	None.	$$

Other names Total serum or hemolytic complement, CH_{50}, and complement components.

Purpose

- To detect immunodeficiency.
- To help diagnose certain autoimmune disorders.
- To predict flare-ups of disease in lupus patients or monitor the effectiveness of treatment for lupus.

How it works Abnormal levels of complements—the immune system's blood proteins—can signify disease.

Preparation None.

Test procedure A sample of your blood is drawn from a vein and analyzed in the laboratory for the amount of complement and its components.

After the test Follow procedure for drawing blood (see chapter 4).

Factors affecting results Genetic factors. You may inherit a particular set of complements.

Interpretation

- Normal levels of total complement amount to 40 to 100 hemolytic units (CH_{50} units).
- Above-normal complement levels may signal infection or inflammation.
- Below-normal complement components (called C_1, C_2, etc) may be associated with various disorders. For example, deficiency of C_3 leads to severe recurrent infections; deficiencies in C_1, C_2, and C_4 components are often found in rheumatic diseases, such as lupus or blood vessel inflammation.

- Drops in complement sometimes precede flare-ups of kidney inflammation in people with lupus.

Advantages There's no risk.

Disadvantages Although this test may show a normal level of complement components, it cannot detect whether or not they are functioning properly.

The next step

- If lupus is suspected, ANA testing may be ordered.
- If blood vessel inflammation is suspected, a biopsy may be done.

IMMUNE COMPLEX DETECTION

General information

Where It's Done	Who Does It	How Long It Takes	Discomfort/Pain
Doctor's office, hospital, or commercial laboratory.	Doctor, nurse, lab technician, or optometrist.	5 minutes.	Minor discomfort associated with drawing blood.
Results Ready When	**Special Equipment**	**Risks/Complications**	**Average Cost**
7 days.	Syringe, collecting tubes, and equipment for analyzing sample.	None	$$

Other names Immune complex assay, Raji cell assay, and circulating immune complexes.

Purpose To help diagnose and monitor disorders such as lupus, glomerulonephritis, and rheumatoid arthritis. Since immune complexes are common, however, their presence cannot always be linked to a particular disease.

How it works Blood or joint fluid is analyzed for the number and type of immune complexes present. These complex molecules, which are formed when an immune system protein binds with an antigen, can damage joints and tissues.

Preparation None.

Test procedure Blood or joint (synovial) fluid is drawn for analysis.

After the test Follow procedure for drawing blood (see chapter 4).

Factors affecting results Steroids and certain other anti-inflammatory medications.

Interpretation

- The presence of immune complexes, rarely seen in healthy blood and joint fluids, may indicate disorders in which they play a role.
- Fluctuating immune complex levels may correlate with a worsening or improvement of disease.

Advantages It's noninvasive.

Disadvantages

- It doesn't lead to a specific diagnosis.
- False-positive and false-negative results are common.

The next step This test is nonspecific. If results are positive, more definitive blood tests (eg, ANA or rheumatoid factor) or tissue biopsy need to be performed.

LYMPHOCYTE TYPING

General information

Where It's Done	Who Does It	How Long It Takes	Discomfort/Pain
Doctor's office or hospital.	Doctor, nurse, or lab technician.	5 minutes.	Minor, from drawing blood or taking tissue sample.

Results Ready When	Special Equipment	Risks/Complications	Average Cost
2 weeks.	Supplies for drawing blood and equipment for removing tissue sample and analyzing it.	None.	$$

Other names T and B lymphocyte subset assay or lymphocyte marker studies.

Purpose

- To detect immunodeficiency.
- To distinguish between inflammatory skin diseases and leukemias or lymphomas that cause rashes.
- To diagnose and distinguish between certain cancers, particularly leukemias and lymphomas.
- To diagnose skin allergies that may be due to abnormal activity of certain T cells.

How it works A blood or tissue sample is analyzed for its level of immune cells known as lymphocytes. The two principal types are T cells and B cells.

Preparation Do not eat or drink for several hours before the test.

Test procedure Blood is drawn or a tissue sample is taken and then analyzed for the presence of lymphocytes.

After the test Follow procedure for drawing blood (see chapter 4).

Factors affecting results

- Steroids and immunosuppressive therapy may significantly change amounts of various cells in blood and body tissues.
- The levels of lymphocytes vary daily.

Interpretation

- Immunodeficiency is associated with low levels or absence of T or B cells. For example, in congenital agammaglobulinemia, a genetic disease that affects only boys, no B cells are present. In HIV infection (see chapter 21), one type of T cell is decreased.
- An increase in T cells may signal leukemia or lymphoma.
- In a person with reddened skin, increased T cell levels may signal cutaneous T-cell lymphoma, a cancer that causes a skin rash, rather than an inflammatory skin condition.

Advantages It's noninvasive.

Disadvantages

- It's expensive.
- It detects an abnormality but not its cause.
- Results may be difficult to interpret and to correlate with symptoms.

The next step Additional tests are usually required and depend on the results. These may include HIV, bone marrow, or skin biopsy.

PHAGOCYTIC CELL ASSAY

General information

Where It's Done	Who Does It	How Long It Takes	Discomfort/Pain
Doctor's office, hospital, or commercial laboratory.	Doctor, nurse, or lab technician.	5 minutes.	Minor, associated with drawing blood.
Results Ready When	**Special Equipment**	**Risks/Complications**	**Average Cost**
7 days.	Syringe, collecting tubes, and equipment for analyzing sample.	None.	$$

Other names Phagocytic cell immunocompetence profile.

Purpose To evaluate the number and function of phagocytic cells. A deficiency may lead to recurrent bacterial infections, particularly staphylococcus.

How it works Phagocytic cells in the blood can be counted and compared to healthy levels.

Preparation None.

Test procedure Blood is drawn and analyzed for number of phagocytes as well as their ability to ingest bacteria.

After the test Follow procedure for drawing blood (see chapter 4).

Factors affecting results None.

Interpretation

- Results are correlated with symptoms and other blood tests. In the absence of other abnormalities, low level of phagocytic cells may help explain recurrent infections and other symptoms.
- Results showing impaired ability of phagocytes to ingest bacteria may explain immunodeficiency when level is normal.

Advantages There's no risk.

Disadvantages

- It's only available in a limited number of medical centers.
- Few laboratories have experience with this test because it is performed rarely.

The next step No specific follow-up. Treatment with prophylactic antibiotics may be appropriate.

Thomas P. Duffy, MD

16 The Blood and Lymphatic Systems

Tests Covered in This Chapter

The case of John G., a 33-year-old computer software consultant:

> *It was actually follow-up testing for lupus, a type of arthritis, that led to my being diagnosed with leukemia. I've had lupus for four years, and although the steroids I take have kept my symptoms under control, I have blood tests every three months to check my condition. When my doctor got the results from one of these tests, he immediately knew something was wrong: My red blood cells and platelets were abnormally low, and my level of white blood cells, unusually high—all indicators of leukemia.*
>
> *This really bowled me over. I'd experienced none of the fever, joint pain, or swelling of the lymph nodes, spleen, or liver that leukemia can bring on, although looking back, I realized that I had been feeling tired, which is another symptom. At the time, I attributed it to stress.*

The Tests Myelogenous leukemia results in an excessive accumulation of white blood cells in the peripheral blood and in the marrow, the spongy material in the bone cavities that manufactures blood cells. These white blood cells fail to mature, so they cannot adequately combat infection. Leukemia also affects the red blood cells and the platelets. John's first test was a complete blood count, in which the various types of cells in a blood sample are counted. He then had a bone marrow aspiration, in which a needle was used to withdraw a sample of bone marrow from his pelvic bone. Once leukemia was confirmed and its type established, John's doctors prepared for the possibility of a marrow transplant with a test to identify the proteins on the surface of John's cells. Called a human leukocyte antigen (HLA) test, it helps to match the HLA types of organ donor and recipient, which lowers the risk of organ rejection (see chapter 15).

The Outcome John was admitted to the hospital immediately and started on chemotherapy. His leukemia went into remission, but then he had a relapse that required another round of chemotherapy. The relapse convinced John to have a bone marrow transplant, which was successful in eliminating the leukemia.

INTRODUCTION

In the average adult, 10 pints of blood move constantly throughout the body's circulatory system, delivering oxygen and nutrients to 300 trillion cells. At the same time, the blood removes cellular waste products, helps to regulate body temperature, aids in healing wounds, and fights disease.

Blood is made up of different types of cells suspended in plasma, a watery, yellow-tinged fluid that carries the cells through the bloodstream and helps maintain the acid-base balance of the body. The majority of blood cells are erythrocytes, which get their red color from the pigment hemoglobin. Their main function is to carry oxygen from the lungs to the rest of the body. White blood cells (leukocytes) are larger but less numerous—there is only one for every 500 red blood cells. There are five specialized kinds of white blood cells, but all work to fight infection or promote healing. Platelets, the smallest components of blood, work together with blood vessel walls and coagulation factors in the plasma to control blood clotting.

The body's other circulatory system, the lymphatic system, is a complex network of ducts, organs, nodes, valves, and vessels that produces lymph (tissue fluid) and performs various filtering and transporting functions. Fats, proteins, and other substances reach the blood through the lymphatic system. The bone marrow—the soft, fatty, inner part of the bone—is considered part of the lymphatic system. It is here that the red blood cells and platelets, and most of the white blood cells, are produced. Thus, the lymphatic system plays a vital role in the body's defenses against cancer and infection.

DISORDERS OF THE BLOOD AND LYMPHATIC SYSTEMS

Disorders that affect the blood range from minor infections to serious malignancies. Early diagnosis and treatment can reverse many conditions and improve most others. The most common disorders are described below.

Red Blood Cell Disorders

Anemia, the most common red blood cell disorder, results from a deficit of red blood cells, which lowers the amount of hemoglobin, and thus oxygen, in the blood. Anemias range from those caused by vitamin or mineral deficiencies, which are easily treated, to incurable inherited disorders.

Erythrocytosis is characterized by an abnormal increase in red blood cells, which is the body's attempt to compensate for a decrease in oxygen in the arterial blood (hypoxemia). Cigarette smoking is a common cause. (For primary erythrocytosis, or polycythemia vera, see Component Proliferation [Myloproliferative] Disorders below.)

White Blood Cell Disorders

Leukopenia, an abnormal decrease in white blood cells, may be precipitated by factors such as overexposure to radiation or a reaction to a drug; while *granulocytopenia (neutropenia)* is an abnormal decrease in granulocytes, which may result from an infection (usually viral), nutritional deficiency, drugs, or other conditions.

Leukemoid reaction is an abnormal increase in white blood cells in response to an allergic condition, infection (such as tuberculosis), inflammatory disease, hemorrhage, or other physical trauma, while *leukocytosis* is an elevation in white blood cells, usually in response to infection.

Leukemia is a cancerous proliferation of white blood cells, which spreads through the body and interferes with its function. Although it is the leading cancer in young children, several types primarily affect adults. The most common leukemias, categorized by their course and the kind of white blood cells involved, are *acute lymphocytic, chronic myelocytic, acute myelocytic,* and *chronic lymphocytic.*

A benign condition sometimes mistaken for acute leukemia is *infectious mononucleosis,* an abnormal increase in the lymphocyte count, associated with the Epstein-Barr virus.

Lymphomas refer to tumors of the lymph tissues, which are usually cancerous. They include *Hodgkin's lymphoma,* which involves steadily enlarged lymph glands, and *non-Hodgkin's disease,* the general name for any other cancer of the lymph tissue.

Platelet Disorders

Thrombocytopenia is an abnormal reduction in the number of platelets, which is usually a result of an autoimmune response (see chapter 15), but may occur in response to a drug or viral infection. *Thrombocytosis* is an abnormal increase in platelets, usually as a result of excessive bleeding, hemolytic anemia, iron deficiency, spleen removal, or primary disease of the bone marrow.

Coagulation/Clotting Disorders

Hemophilia is the best known of these disorders. Most hemophilias, which are characterized by excessive and uncontrolled bleeding, are inherited and primarily affect males. In *acquired hemophilia,* the body develops an antibody against a normal clotting factor.

Disseminated intravascular coagulation occurs when the coagulation system overreacts to disease or injury, resulting first in excessive clotting, then in a decrease in coagulation factors. *Hypercoagulable state* is characterized by excessive clotting caused by a tumor or inherited disorder affecting coagulation factors.

Blood Protein Content Disorders

These conditions, called *dysproteinemias*, are characterized by excessive amounts of serum proteins, the products of lymphocytes or plasma cells in the blood. They include *Waldenstrom's,* a condition in which a proliferation of lymphocytes within the marrow secretes immunoglobulin molecules, and *multiple myeloma,* a bone marrow cancer in which plasma cells (antibody-producing cells) multiply rapidly, taking over the marrow, destroying the bone tissue, and frequently causing kidney failure.

Myeloproliferative Disorders

These conditions, characterized by an abnormal increase or proliferation of one or more blood or connective tissue components, often overlap so that a person experiences more than one disorder. They include *myelofibrosis (agnogenic myeloid metaplasia)*, a progressive condition in which the normal components of the bone marrow are replaced by fibrous tissue and the blood-forming (hematopoietic) tissue normally found there develops in other sites, and *polycythemia vera,* a disorder characterized by an abnormal proliferation of blood-forming tissue in the bone marrow resulting in an increased red blood cell mass. Chronic myelocytic leukemia (see white blood cell disorders, above) and primary thrombocytosis (see platelet disorders, above) also are classified as myeloproliferative disorders; some hematologists include acute leukemia in this category.

HOW YOUR DOCTOR DIAGNOSES DISORDERS OF THE BLOOD AND LYMPHATIC SYSTEMS

Although some diseases of the blood and lymphatic systems produce symptoms such as fatigue with anemia that may bring a patient to the doctor, most are uncovered by a standard blood test during a routine examination. Blood drawn from a vein in your arm (a procedure called a venipuncture) is sent to a laboratory for a complete blood count (CBC), where it is analyzed for factors such as the red blood cell count (RBC); white blood cell count (WBC); the hematocrit (HCT), which is the ratio of red blood cells to plasma; and the amount of hemoglobin (HGB) in the red blood cells. Women generally have fewer red blood cells than men and thus a lower hematocrit and hemoglobin level as well.

The first sign of a disease such as anemia is a drop in the red blood cell count, hematocrit, or hemoglobin. An increase in white blood cells often indicates that your body is fighting an infection. Your platelet count determines a problem in your clotting process. If there is any abnormality in complete blood count, your doctor may recommend additional tests (see table 16.1), usually done on the same blood sample. In many cases, however, your medical history, a review of your symptoms, and CBC results give all the information necessary to make a diagnosis and begin treatment.

Red Blood Cell Disorders

A physician examining a woman who has excessive menstrual bleeding and a low red blood cell count would suspect iron-deficiency anemia. A simple measurement of the iron level in her blood would confirm the diagnosis. Other types of anemia are differentiated with a variety of tests. For instance, the symptoms of pernicious anemia and folic acid deficiency anemia are similar but can be distinguished by checking the levels of B_{12} and folic acid in the blood.

An abnormal increase in the red blood cell count and hemoglobin concentration is called erythrocytosis. It may be due to a number of causes—including congenital heart disease, high altitude sickness, and some tumors, for instance—which must be considered in making a diagnosis.

White Blood Cell Disorders

White blood cell disorders must also be distinguished from each other. Infectious mononucleosis is sometimes confused with leukemia, but in acute leukemia, anemia and decreased platelets commonly accompany a high white blood cell count. A bone marrow aspiration may be done to diagnose leukemia or blood may be drawn to look for atypical lymphocytes, which characterize infectious mononucleosis.

Often the complete blood count gives an accurate picture that leads to a diagnosis. For example, leukemia and leukocytosis are both characterized by a high white blood cell count, but in leukemia there is also a simultaneous reduction in red blood cell and platelet counts in addition to the presence of immature leukemic cells.

A bone marrow aspiration may be performed if your physician suspects leukemia. In the case of acute leukemia, there may be an increased number of immature, abnormal white blood cells called blast cells. Tests for certain enzymes in the blood also help to differentiate between leukemias.

If you are experiencing recurrent, prolonged swelling of the lymph nodes in your neck, chest, and armpits—the first signs of Hodgkin's disease—and your blood tests pointed to that diagnosis, you might have to undergo a bone marrow and lymph node biopsy. Non-Hodgkin's lymphoma may have the same symptoms, and would require a biopsy for proper diagnosis.

TABLE 16.1 Tests Most Commonly Done on Blood Samples*

Test	Use
Activated partial thromboplastin time (APTT)	Measures the time it takes plasma to clot. Used to detect deficiencies in many clotting factors. Results will be abnormal in most hemophiliacs. The test is also used to monitor heparin therapy.
Antibody test	Identifies antibodies that, due to a malfunctioning immune system, attack cells of the patient's own body. Presence of these antibodies may indicate disorders such as collagen vascular disease (lupus, rheumatoid arthritis), thyroid disorders, and adrenal disorders.
Carboxyhemoglobin (carbon monoxide measurement)	Measures levels of carbon monoxide. A toxic level can be one cause of erythrocytosis. (This measurement is sometimes included in a blood gas test.)
Coagulation factors screening	Identifies congenital and acquired coagulation factor deficiencies. (Some factors may be increased in patients taking oral contraceptives.)
Coombs' test (antiglobulin test)	Detects immune antibodies that may cause anemia. (Drugs such as penicillin, cephalosporins, methyldopa, quinidine, and mefenamic acid may cause a positive result.)
Erythropoietin (EPO) measurement	Tests for some types of anemia and erythrocytosis. As the hematocrit (ratio of red blood cells to plasma) falls, EPO is released by the kidney to stimulate the marrow to produce more cells.
Ferritin level	Indicates iron stores in the body, used to diagnose iron deficiency anemia and iron overload states. High levels may also be associated with other types of anemia, inflammation, liver disease, leukemia, and lymphoma. Also used to monitor adequacy of iron replacement in iron-deficiency anemia and iron removal in hemochromatosis.
Fibrinogen test	Diagnoses blood disorders involving too much or too little fibrinogen, a key component in the clotting process.
Immunoelectrophoresis (IEP)	Diagnoses myeloma and serum protein disorders. Low levels of antibody proteins suggest immunodeficiency states, while elevated homogenous antibody protein suggests myeloma. About 3% of elderly people have elevated antibody protein levels that turn out to be benign.
Leukocyte alkaline phosphatase	Measures the degree of activity of this enzyme in white blood cells, which helps differentiate between chronic myelocytic leukemia (CML) and a leukemoid reaction. The latter is characterized by a marked elevation in the white blood cell count (usually as a result of infection, drugs, or tumors) that leads to confusion with leukemia.
Philadelphia chromosome screen	Helps diagnose chronic myelocytic leukemia by identifying this chromosome abnormality, which occurs in 90% of people with this disorder.
Prothrombin time (PT)	Measures the time it takes plasma to clot under selected conditions. Used to detect deficiencies in certain clotting factors produced by the liver. It monitors the effects of the anticoagulant drug coumarin. Results are frequently abnormal in patients with liver disease.
Reticulocyte count	Measures young or not quite mature red blood cells as an indication of production of red blood cells from the bone marrow. Evaluates ability of bone marrow to produce new red blood cells. Helps to distinguish between different types of anemia.
Serum viscosity	Measures the flow rate of plasma relative to water. An increased plasma viscosity is associated with macroglobulinemia and other blood protein content disorders (dysproteinemias).

*In addition to routine red blood, white blood, and platelet counts.

Platelet Disorders

A drop in platelet count may lead to black and blue spots (ecchymosis) or frecklelike tiny red spots (petchiae) on your skin. If these symptoms occur with a normal platelet count, your physician may recommend a bleeding time test.

Coagulation/Clotting Disorders

Coagulation factor deficiencies are detected by measuring their level in the blood. Disseminated intravascular coagulation (DIC) is characterized by a decreased level of coagulation factors and platelets, which have been consumed in the abnormal clotting process.

Blood Protein Content Disorders

A combination of anemia, susceptibility to infections, and bone pain or easily occurring fractures, especially of the vertebrae, might indicate further tests, such as immunoelectrophoresis, which identifies abnormal proteins produced by the malignant cells.

Myeloproliferative Disorders

Symptoms vary according to the specific type of disorder but may include weakness, visual disturbances, an enlarged spleen and perhaps enlarged liver, abnormal bleeding, headache, dizziness, and general malaise. Blood tests will show abnormal numbers of the affected blood cells; additional tests, such as chromosome studies and various other laboratory tests, are needed to identify the specific myeloproliferative disorder.

BONE MARROW ASPIRATION

General information

Where It's Done	Who Does It	How Long It Takes	Discomfort/Pain
In hospital as in- or out-patient procedure.	Hematologist or nurse-clinician.	About 30 minutes.	Discomfort at area of insertion.
Results Ready When	**Special Equipment**	**Risks/Complications**	**Average Cost**
1–2 days.	Large-bore aspiration needle.	Bleeding and discomfort at insertion site, and possible hematoma or infection.	$$

Other names Bone marrow sampling.

Purpose

- To determine cause of an abnormal result in a complete blood count or peripheral blood smear.
- To confirm diagnosis and evaluate severe unexplained anemia, leukemia, leukocytosis, multiple myeloma, leukopenia and/or thrombocytopenia, problems with the body's storage of iron, or an abnormality in production or maturation of blood elements.
- To obtain a sample for a culture to check for fungi, bacteria, or parasites, or for a chromosome analysis.
- To evaluate response to cancer therapy.

How it works A sample from the bone marrow (where blood cells are produced) is removed for laboratory analysis.

Preparation You are given a sedative if you choose.

Test procedure

- You receive a local anesthetic at the needle puncture site (in adults, the hip bone or the sternum; in children, a vertebra or long bone in the leg).
- The needle is rotated and forced through the outer cortex of the bone (see figure 16.1).

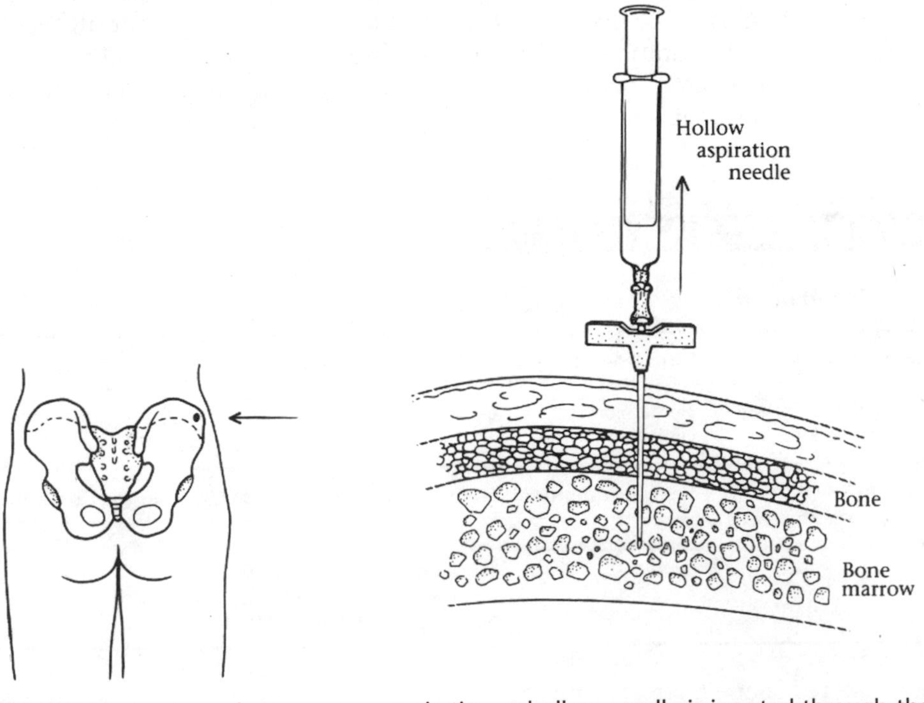

FIGURE 16.1 During a bone marrow aspiration, a hollow needle is inserted through the subcutaneous tissue and bone to withdraw a sample of marrow, the pulpy substance on the inside of the bone in which blood cells are manufactured.

- A syringe is attached, and about ½ teaspoon of bone marrow is extracted. Additional samples may be obtained for chromosomal analysis or cultures of the marrow.
- The marrow is checked immediately by a technologist to ensure that it is an adequate sample. If not, the needle is redirected slightly and another syringe is attached to obtain another sample.

After the test

- The needle is removed, direct pressure is applied to control bleeding at the needle site, and the area is covered with a dry, sterile dressing.
- Some pain or soreness will occur at the site, but you should be able to resume normal activities within a few hours.
- If possible, the site should be examined by a nurse or physician about 24 hours later.
- Because of the anesthesia used, you should arrange to be driven home after the test.
- If you notice any bleeding at home, lie on your back and apply pressure to the site with a rolled-up towel.
- Persistent bleeding, fever, or signs of infection such as redness or discharge are extremely rare, but should be reported to your doctor at once.

Factors affecting results

- Moving during the procedure.
- Radiation therapy at the insertion site.
- Severe coagulation or other clotting or bleeding disorders.

Interpretation

- The sample is examined microscopically and analyzed for iron stores, red blood cell and white blood cell production and maturation, and number of megakaryocytes (which produce platelets).
- If abnormalities (leukemia, lymphoma, etc) are detected, flow cytometry analysis is performed to identify abnormal cell populations and to classify the types of cells.
- Chromosomal analysis is performed in the genetics laboratory; this takes several days.
- Culture of the marrow, usually for tuberculosis, provides an additional means of detecting a hidden infection as the cause of an unexplained fever.

Advantages

- It's quick.
- There are relatively few complications.

Disadvantages

- It's an invasive procedure that can cause some discomfort.
- It yields only a small sample of marrow.

The next step

Once the cause of symptoms is identified, treatment can begin.

BONE MARROW BIOPSY

General information

Where It's Done	Who Does It	How Long It Takes	Discomfort/Pain
In hospital as in- or out-patient procedure.	Hematologist or nurse-clinician.	About 30 minutes.	Discomfort at area of insertion.

Results Ready When	Special Equipment	Risks/Complications	Average Cost
Within 3 days.	Large-bore bone marrow needle.	Bleeding and discomfort at insertion site, and possible hematoma or infection.	$$

Other names None.

Purpose

- To obtain a piece of bone containing intact marrow to study for abnormalities.
- To help diagnose erythrocytosis, thrombocythemia, and some kinds of anemia.
- To diagnose or determine the stage of tumors or lymphoma.
- To determine the underlying cause of an unexplained fever.
- To diagnose fibrosis of the marrow and myeloma when aspiration attempts have failed (called a "dry tap").

How it works Cellular relationships to other cells and the cellular makeup of the marrow can be determined under a microscope with a biopsy because the architecture of the sample is maintained (as opposed to an aspiration, in which the sample is smeared in its preparation).

Preparation You are given a sedative if you choose.

Test procedure

- You receive a local anesthetic at the needle puncture site (in adults, the hip bone; in children, a vertebra or long bone in the leg).
- A large-bore needle is forced through the outer cortex of the bone, about ¾ of an inch deep. The needle is rotated clockwise and counterclockwise, withdrawn slightly, reintroduced at a slightly different angle, and rotated again. This process continues until the core is sheared off.
- The needle is removed, again in a rotating motion, and wire is pushed through the tip of the needle to force the specimen onto sterile gauze. A slide is then made.
- Sometimes a biopsy is done immediately preceding or following an aspiration.

After the test

- Direct pressure is applied to control bleeding at the needle site, and the area is covered with a sterile dressing.
- Depending on the location of the biopsy, you may have to lie on your back for at least 30 minutes before getting dressed.
- Some pain or soreness will occur at the site, but you should be able to resume normal activities almost immediately.
- If possible, the site should be examined by a nurse or physician about 24 hours later.

Factors affecting results

- Obesity.
- Moving during the procedure.
- Radiation therapy at the insertion site.
- Severe coagulation or other clotting or bleeding disorders.

Interpretation The sample is analyzed under a microscope for the makeup of cells, the distribution and maturation of cell constituents, and the ratio of red to white blood cells. Arrested development of blood cell precursors or abnormal numbers of cells may indicate leukemia; while a markedly depleted marrow supply may indicate hypoplastic or aplastic anemia, which is incapable of producing sufficient blood cells.

Advantages

- It's quick.
- There are relatively few complications.

Disadvantages

- It's an invasive procedure that may cause pain.
- It's difficult to do in very obese people.
- It yields a small sample of marrow.

The next step Treatment for the problem identified by the biopsy can begin.

BLEEDING TIME TEST

General information

Where It's Done	Who Does It	How Long It Takes	Discomfort/Pain
Hospital room or outpatient clinic.	Medical technologist.	15–20 minutes.	Discomfort at incision or puncture site.
Results Ready When	**Special Equipment**	**Risks/Complications**	**Average Cost**
15 minutes to 2 hours.	Lancet, blood pressure cuff, and filter paper.	Possible formation of scar tissue.	$

Other names Duke, Ivy, Mielke, simplate, or template bleeding time tests.

Purpose To test for a bleeding problem.

How it works Surface bleeding is induced, and the time from initial blood flow until clotting is measured.

Preparation You must not take aspirin for ten days before the test.

Test procedure

- The test site is cleaned with alcohol.
- The earlobe or forearm is punctured or lanced. (If the forearm is used, a blood pressure cuff is placed above the elbow and slightly inflated.)
- A stopwatch is started, and the wound is blotted with filter paper every 30 seconds. When the blood flow stops, the stopwatch is stopped.

PATIENT TIP

About 20 different medications, including antihistamines and nonsteroidal anti-inflammatory drugs such as aspirin and ibuprofen, impair the platelets' ability to stick to wounds, and therefore produce a longer bleeding time. Ask your doctor for a list of these drugs, which should be discontinued one week before the test.

After the test The test sites are cleaned and bandaged. You return to normal activities.

Factors affecting results

- Anti-inflammatory drugs and antihistamines.
- Low platelet count.
- Skin problems.

Interpretation The normal bleeding time range is two to seven minutes (shorter in men than in women and shorter in people over 50). A longer time can indicate a disorder involving platelets or fibrinogen (a protein required for clot formation). Blood vessel diseases (scurvy) also produce an increased bleeding time.

DID YOU KNOW?

Bleeding time is shorter in men than in women by an average of about 30 seconds. This is probably because men have slightly more red blood cells than do women, and the higher the red cell count, the more efficient the platelets.

Advantages It's a quick procedure that provides immediate results.

Disadvantages

- It involves minor pain from puncture or incision.
- There is variation in test results because of an inability to strictly standardize the depth of the incision.

The next step

- If results are normal, no further testing is necessary.
- If results are abnormal and a clotting factor problem is suspected, coagulation tests (clotting factor assays) are done to confirm or rule out such disorders as Von Willebrand disease. If these assays are normal, platelet aggregation testing is recommended.
- If an abnormality in the blood vessel walls is suspected, a capillary fragility test is done.

Philip E. Shapiro, MD

17 The Skin

Tests Covered in This Chapter

The case of Justine B., 26, an accountant and bookkeeper:

I was watching a TV documentary that showed unusual moles as a risk factor for malignant melanoma. I thought, "That looks too familiar." I had spots on my body that resembled what they were showing. One dark, penny-sized mole on my groin especially concerned me, so I went to a dermatologist. I was really scared: An uncle of mine had melanoma on his forehead a few years before, and I knew that skin cancer can run in families.

The growth proved to be an atypical nevus, not a melanoma, but the dermatologist removed it and told me to come back in six months. Because the scare turned out not to be serious, I figured I was safe and didn't go back for a year. This time she discovered a suspicious spot in the middle of my torso. Although a definitive diagnosis can be made only by biopsying a sample of tissue, the dermatologist was so certain I had melanoma, she said, "I'm not taking any chances. This comes out right now." Before I had time to digest the news, the lesion was cut out and the wound stitched closed.

The Tests Justine's tissue sample was examined in the laboratory and proved to be malignant. Using a measurement known as Breslow's depth, it was measured to be 0.52 millimeters thick, indicating that it had burrowed through the epidermis and partway through the underlying dermis layer. To help determine if the cancer had spread to other parts of the body, a blood test and a chest X-ray were ordered. They were negative and no chemotherapy was necessary.

The Outcome A plastic surgeon reexcised Justine's skin around the biopsy site, a routine procedure used to ensure that all the malignant cells are removed. Justine now examines her skin regularly in front of a well-lighted full-length mirror. She has brought two more spots to the attention of her dermatologist. Both turned out to be early melanomas and were easily treated.

INTRODUCTION

Although most people don't think of the skin as an organ at all, it is in fact the largest organ in the body, and one of the most complex in the variety of roles it plays. It shields other organs from injuries, toxic substances, and infectious organisms, regulates body temperature, and transmits the sensations of heat and touch to the body. It also helps keep fluids inside the body, and plays a role in the immune system.

The skin consists of two major layers: a paper-thin outer layer known as the epidermis and a thicker inner layer called the dermis. The surface of the epidermis is made up of a horny layer of dead cells that are constantly sloughed off through wear and tear and replaced by new cells that move up from underneath. The dermis, which is primarily composed of collagen, water, and elastic tissue, harbors numerous living elements of the skin. In addition to blood vessels, lymph channels, nerve fibers, and muscle cells, one square inch of the dermis contains approximately 600 sebaceous glands, 1,000 sweat glands, and 400 hairs. Below the dermis, a layer of connective tissue and fat called the subcutis, or hypodermis, affects the body's contours, buffers it against blows, provides insulation against heat and cold, and stores fat for energy.

Although most of our skin appears hairless, it is actually covered by millions of hairs that grow everywhere except the palms, soles, nails, lips, tip of the penis, and nipples and areolae of the breasts. Each hair shaft is rooted below the surface of the skin in a sheath called a follicle. Baldness usually occurs when the follicle shrinks until it can produce only small, hardly visible hairs.

COMMON SKIN DISORDERS

Although skin problems are usually not life-threatening, their visibility can make even minor disturbances a source of concern. They can also reflect more generalized illness. Some of the major skin disorders are described below.

Basal and squamous cell skin cancers. The most common types of skin cancer are basal cell carcinoma and squamous cell carcinoma. Basal and squamous cell cancers appear mostly in lighter-skinned individuals over the age of 30, and their frequency increases with age. They occur principally on parts of the body that are regularly exposed to the sun—the face, neck, forearms, back of the hands, and upper trunk. Any skin lesion that is growing irregularly, changing shape or color, crusting, or bleeding frequently should be examined by a doctor. When detected early, these skin cancers have a high cure rate and are usually relatively easy to remove without disfiguring treatment.

Keratoses. These are growths that typically appear after age 30. Actinic keratoses are pink, tan, or brown, irregular, slightly raised, rough areas, usually found on the face, forearms, and back of the hands, that are caused by chronic exposure to the sun. A small percentage of them develop into squamous cell carcinomas. Seborrheic keratoses are most common on the trunk and are completely benign. They tend to be brown or tan, uniform, and raised above the skin surface, appearing as if they had been "stuck on."

Moles and melanomas. Moles are usually brown or black because they contain a large amount of the dark pigment melanin, produced by cells called melanocytes. The vast majority of moles are benign, but in rare cases they may turn malignant, producing a melanoma. Melanomas can also begin on their own without starting in a benign mole. Although melanomas are a less common type of skin cancer than a basal or squamous cell skin cancer, they are potentially more lethal. However, melanomas that are detected early are almost always curable. Any moles that look unusual because they are large, irregular, very dark, or growing rapidly should be examined by a physician (see the accompanying box).

Dermatitis. A variety of skin conditions marked by red and scaly or crusted skin are referred to as dermatitis and sometimes as eczema. These include atopic dermatitis, which tends to develop in front of the elbows and behind the knees, contact dermatitis, and seborrheic dermatitis, which is characterized by scaling of the skin around the nose, ears, eyebrows, and scalp. (For additional information on atopic dermatitis and contact dermatitis, see chapter 14.)

Psoriasis. Characterized by sharply demarcated areas of red and scaly skin, psoriasis affects more than 3 million Americans. Lesions typically appear on the scalp, elbows, knees, legs, and nails, but may affect other parts of the body.

Detecting Melanoma Early

Early detection is crucial for successfully treating malignant melanoma. The cure rate for this cancer is 100% when it is confined to the epidermis, but it declines as the melanoma grows deeper into the dermis. Most melanomas grow on clear skin, but up to one-third may develop from existing moles. Any changes in an existing mole should always be examined, and any new, unusual-looking brown spots should certainly be checked out.

Melanoma usually differs from benign growths in shape, borders, color, and size. Its distinguishing features are sometimes summed up as the ABCDs of melanoma:

A—asymmetry. While benign moles are often symmetrical, melanomas tend to be asymmetrical: if a line were drawn through the middle of the growth, its two halves would not be mirror images of one another.

B—borders. The borders of benign moles are usually smooth and even, while the edges of early melanomas are more likely to be uneven or notched.

C—color. The presence of different shades of brown or black (or even red, white, and dark blue) may be the first sign of malignant melanoma, while benign moles usually have a uniform color.

D—diameter. Melanomas tend to grow larger than 6 millimeters in diameter, about the size of a pencil eraser.

The risk of having malignant melanoma increases with age: it is very rare before puberty, but the risk rises steadily thereafter. Other risk factors include a family history of this cancer and the presence of numerous or large and irregular moles. Melanoma is more common in light-skinned, blue-eyed people who tend to burn rather than tan in the sun. The darker a person's skin, the lower the risk of melanoma, although even very dark-skinned individuals occasionally develop the cancer, especially on the palms, soles, and nails. Dark moles that are present from birth, especially large ones, also increase the risk of melanoma.

Infections and infestations. Viral infections can produce warts or small growths called molluscum contagiosum. Cold sores on the lips, caused by a herpesvirus, and shingles, caused by the same virus as chicken pox, are other examples of viral skin conditions. Bacterial infections of the skin include impetigo, which tends to affect children, and folliculitis, which starts in hair follicles. The skin may also be infected by fungi, as in athlete's foot and ringworm, and infested by lice, mites, and other parasites.

Hair and nail disorders. Hair shafts may become abnormal, and follicles may shrink or become deformed. Hair loss can be caused by illness, stress, pregnancy, drugs, and severe skin diseases that affect the scalp. Nail deformities may be caused by trauma, psoriasis, and fungal infections, among other things.

HOW YOUR DOCTOR DIAGNOSES A SKIN CONDITION

The doctor often starts with questions about your symptoms (see the accompanying box) and the history of the problem: When and where did your symptoms first appear? Is there anything that makes them better or worse? How long does each lesion last? Do you have any diseases or symptoms unrelated to the skin? Do you use any medications? Does your skin itch?

Because the signs of skin disorders are so readily apparent, however, the doctor may examine your skin first. Often a magnifying glass is the only equipment needed, and in the majority of cases, the physician can make a diagnosis and prescribe treatment simply by looking at the diseased skin.

Your doctor may examine the skin all over your body—the scalp, the trunk, and limbs down to the fingernails and toes. The distribution of the skin condition may be crucial to diagnosis, as some diseases have a predilection for certain areas. For example, psoriasis tends to affect the elbows, knees, and scalp, and the skin around the navel, lower spine, and genitals.

The number, shape, and arrangement of the abnormalities may help the doctor make the diagnosis. For example, blisters arranged in a line may be a sign of contact dermatitis caused when a substance such as poison ivy brushes along the skin in a linear fashion. Whereas in ringworm, the disease may be arranged in a circle.

The single most important test in the diagnosis of skin disorders is a biopsy, in which a piece of skin is removed for examination. This test may be done to diagnose skin diseases that involve inflammation

Signs and Symptoms of Skin Disorders

- Itching
- Erythema (reddening)
- Scaling
- Wheals (hives)
- Crusts
- Purple spots (purpura)
- Ulcers
- Blisters
- Skin thinning (atrophy)
- Skin hardening

Because the visible signs of skin abnormalities are so varied, numerous terms are used to describe them. For example, small flat areas of abnormal skin are called macules, while abnormal areas that are flat and large are referred to as patches. Small raised abnormalities are known as papules, while those that are raised and broad are called plaques. Large firm growths under the skin's surface are referred to as nodules, cysts are balls in the skin that are usually soft, and pustules are tiny bumps on the skin that are white because they contain large numbers of white blood cells called neutrophils.

and to determine if growths are benign or malignant. How soon a biopsy is performed depends on the urgency of establishing a diagnosis. If the disease is a growth, the biopsy is often done immediately. If the condition is due to inflammation rather than a growth (eg, contact dermatitis or psoriasis), the doctor may prescribe treatment and wait a month or two to see if the problem resolves. If it doesn't, a skin biopsy may be necessary (see below for the various types).

Another common test is the potassium hydroxide (KOH) examination, used to diagnose fungal infections. If an allergy is suspected as the cause of dermatitis, a patch test may be used to identify which substance or substances produce allergic reactions. A blood test may be ordered to diagnose an underlying disease, such as Lyme disease, syphilis, or systemic lupus erythematosus, that first manifests itself as a rash on the skin.

SKIN BIOPSY

General information

Where It's Done	Who Does It	How Long It Takes	Discomfort/Pain
Doctor's office or clinic.	Dermatologist, plastic surgeon, or other MD.	5–10 minutes; up to 60 minutes if complex.	Minor discomfort associated with injection of local anesthetic.
Results Ready When	**Special Equipment**	**Risks/Complications**	**Average Cost**
1–14 days, usually within 7.	Skin punch, scalpel, curette, scissors, sutures, and dressings.	Scarring, ranging from barely perceptible to obvious, depending on the type, size, and site of the biopsy; infection (rare); and underlying nerve damage if deep biopsy (very rare).	$$

Other names None.

Purpose Skin biopsy is a multipurpose test used to diagnose growths, such as skin cancers and keratoses, or inflammatory skin disorders, such as psoriasis, contact dermatitis, and insect bites. Biopsy can also be a treatment when it is used to remove warts, moles, skin cancers, or other growths.

How it works A small sample of cells is taken for examination under a microscope.

Preparation Usually none. For large biopsies, medications that can promote bleeding (such as aspirin and ibuprofen) should be stopped a few days beforehand.

Test procedure The skin is cleansed, and local anesthesia is usually administered. Depending on the type of disorder suspected, one of the following forms of skin biopsy is performed:

- *Punch biopsy*, illustrated in figure 17.1, is used to diagnose most inflammatory diseases and many tumors. It provides a tissue sample of cells from the full thickness of the skin. The sample is obtained with a punch, an instrument that resembles a small cookie cutter with a sharp circular edge that can be pushed through the skin. When the punch is removed, it yields a core of tissue that is cut from its base with scissors or a scalpel.
- *Shave biopsy*, illustrated in figure 17.2, is used to remove raised noncancerous growths, such as seborrheic keratoses, and for diagnosing abnormalities suspected of being nonmelanoma cancers. The technique involves shaving the skin with a scalpel or razor blade to remove the upper layer. It is not the preferred method if melanoma is strongly suspected because the tissue sample obtained may be inadequate for thorough examination.
- *Fusiform, or elliptical, biopsy*, illustrated in figure 17.3, removes unusual moles or growths suspected as cancerous. The sample it yields is larger than that provided by a punch biopsy. It can be excisional, meaning that the entire growth is removed, or incisional, meaning that a portion of the growth is removed.

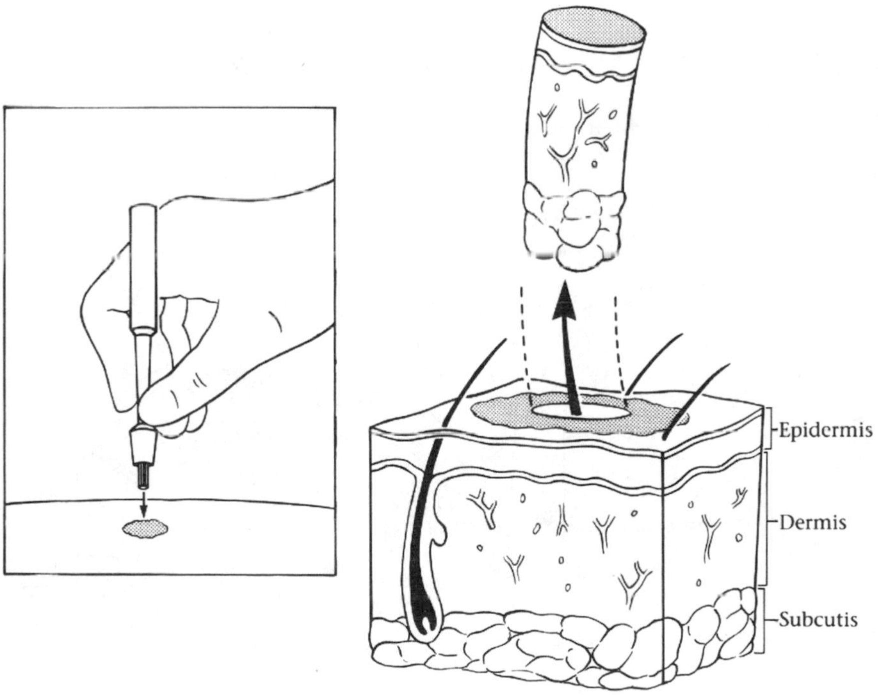

FIGURE 17.1 Punch Biopsy
A core of tissue is obtained by using a sharp, circular instrument.

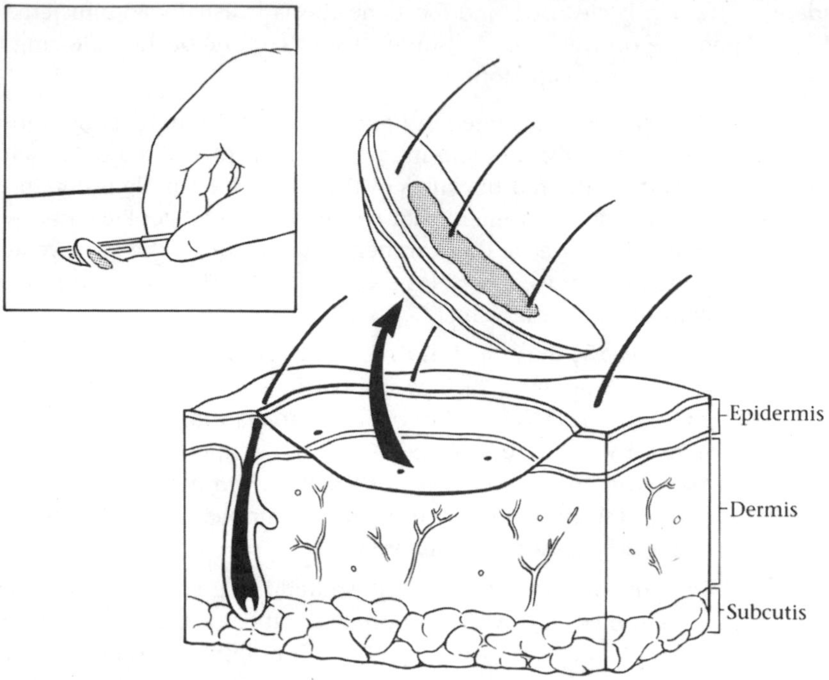

FIGURE 17.2 Shave Biopsy

A surgical knife is used to remove the upper layer of skin.

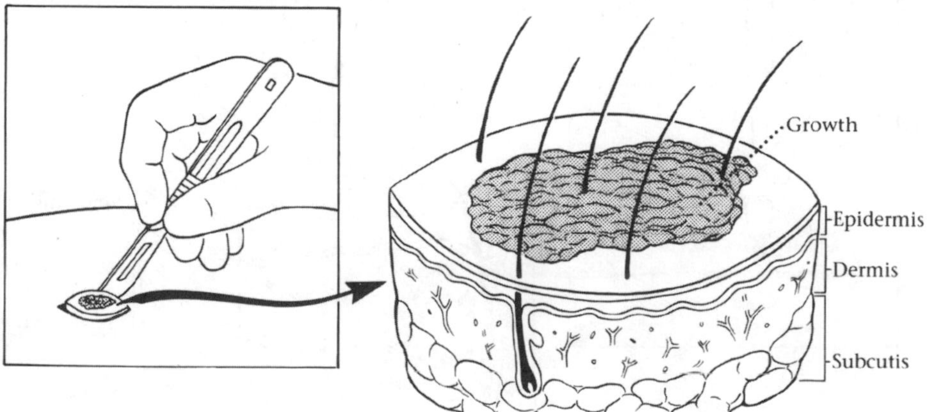

FIGURE 17.3 Fusiform Biopsy

A surgical knife is used to remove a tissue sample that is larger than can be collected with a punch instrument.

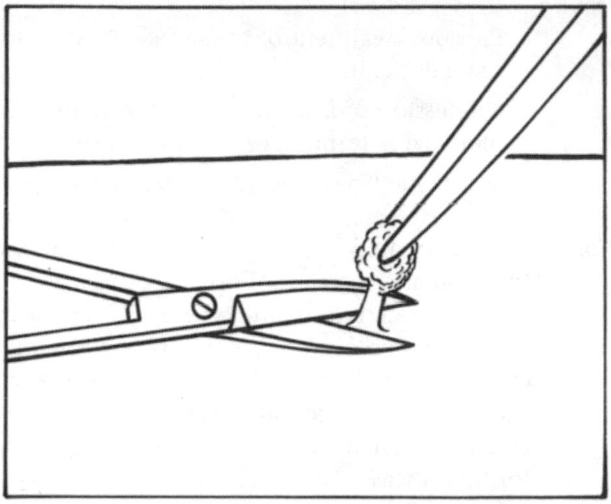

FIGURE 17.4 Scissors Biopsy

This procedure entails snipping off a growth that is attached to the skin with a stalk.

- *Scissors biopsy,* illustrated in figure 17.4, is used when a growth is attached to the skin by a short stalk. The growth is removed with a snip of the scissors.
- *Curette biopsy* involves scraping off a lesion with a curette, an instrument with an oval or round blade attached to a handle. This approach is less commonly used for diagnosis because it has a greater likelihood of producing an inadequate sample (ie, it breaks the specimen into pieces, sometimes precluding microscopic evaluation of structural features that are helpful in diagnosis). More often it is used to remove growths—such as warts or basal cell carcinomas—that have been biopsied and diagnosed by another means.

After the test

- If no stitches were used, as is the case with almost all shave, scissors, curette, and some punch biopsies, a dressing (and often an antibiotic ointment) will be placed over the biopsy site. You may be told to cleanse the site, reapply the ointment, and change the dressing once or several times a day until the area heals (usually in five to 28 days, depending on the size and location of the biopsy).
- If stitches were used, the dressing is usually left in place or periodically changed until the stitches are removed, five to 14 days later, depending on the size and location of the incision. You may be told to keep the area dry during that time and to report any bleeding, swelling, or unusual redness or pain. Also, your activity may be restricted (eg, no exercising or heavy lifting) for several weeks.

Factors affecting results

- Previous treatment of inflammatory skin diseases makes diagnosis more difficult.
- Submission of a small sample (for example, to minimize scarring) is more likely to produce an inconclusive result.
- Scar tissue from a previous biopsy makes diagnosis more difficult.

Interpretation The tissue sample is examined under a microscope to determine the type and arrangement of cells. If cancer is detected, microscopic examination can determine the type of malignant cells involved.

The presence of cells that play a role in inflammation, along with characteristic changes in the upper and lower levels of the skin, helps the doctor diagnose inflammatory disease. Depending on its stage, a disease may have a variety of appearances, only some of which are specific for that disease. Therefore, biopsy may be required at two or more stages to diagnose an inflammatory disorder.

Advantages

- It's highly informative.
- It sometimes provides both diagnosis and treatment.

Disadvantages

- It's invasive.
- It's expensive.
- Follow-up care of the biopsy site is often required.

The next step

- If the biopsy was for a growth and it was benign, usually no further therapy is necessary.
- If the biopsy yielded cancerous cells, treatment to completely remove the cells will be recommended (if not done with the first biopsy).
- If the biopsy was to diagnose an inflammatory condition, treatment can be initiated or altered based on the results. If the findings from a biopsy are inconclusive, another biopsy may be ordered.

KOH PREPARATION

General information

Where It's Done	Who Does It	How Long It Takes	Discomfort/Pain
Doctor's office or clinic.	Doctor.	About 1 minute.	Minor discomfort when sample is collected.
Results Ready When	**Special Equipment**	**Risks/Complications**	**Average Cost**
Usually within 10 minutes.	Scalpel or other instrument for scraping; sometimes, forceps or nail clippers.	None.	$

Other names Fungal scraping or potassium hydroxide examination.

Purpose To diagnose scaly or pustular conditions of the skin, hair, and nails suspected of being caused by fungi.

How it works Heat and potassium hydroxide (KOH) are used on a tissue sample to dissolve keratin (a hard protein substance) and keratinocytes, the keratin-making cells of the epidermis. This makes it possible to detect the microscopic presence of a fungus that would otherwise be obscured by these substances.

Preparation None.

Test procedure

- If the infection affects the scalp, the doctor plucks diseased or broken hairs. The scalp may also be scraped with a scalpel.
- In nail infections, the inner surface of the nail below the tip is scraped, or the part of the nail tip that appears abnormal is clipped off.
- In skin infections, the outer layer of the abnormal skin is scraped.

After the test You are free to resume normal activities.

Factors affecting results

- The sample may be too small or taken from an area where there is no fungus.
- Previous treatment with antifungal medications may produce false-negative results.

Interpretation If the abnormality is caused by a fungus, the infectious organism may be identified under the microscope. If no fungus can be seen, the test is considered negative. However, a single negative sample cannot rule out fungal infection because the organism may have been missed.

Advantages

- It's noninvasive.
- It provides results faster than skin fungus culture.

Disadvantages False-negative results are more common than with skin fungus culture and may occur in about one-quarter of cases.

The next step

- If the test is positive, appropriate antifungal medication can be prescribed. Sometimes a fungal culture is ordered to confirm the result or further classify the fungus.
- If the test is negative, a second sample may be taken or a fungal culture may be done.

SKIN FUNGUS CULTURE

General information

Where It's Done	Who Does It	How Long It Takes	Discomfort/Pain
Doctor's office or clinic.	Doctor.	About 1 minute.	Minimal discomfort when sample is collected.
Results Ready When	**Special Equipment**	**Risks/Complications**	**Average Cost**
5 days to 3 weeks.	Scalpel or other instrument for scraping; sometimes, forceps or nail clippers.	None.	$

Other names None.

Purpose To diagnose scaly or pustular conditions of the skin, hair loss, or nail disease suspected of being caused by fungi.

How it works Fungus sample is grown in a culture medium and then may be identified under a microscope.

Preparation None.

Test procedure Same as for KOH preparation.

After the test You are free to resume normal activities. The sample is sent to a commercial laboratory or cultured in a doctor's office.

Factors affecting results

- Previous treatment with antifungal medications may cause false-negative results.
- Some types of fungi found under the nails may not be the cause of the disease.

Interpretation If a fungus is present, it may be cultured and identified. The time required varies with the organism and may take up to a month. If no fungus appears by then, the test is considered negative. However, a single negative sample cannot rule out fungal infection because the organism may have been missed during the collection of the sample or may have failed to grow. False-negative results occur in about 10% of cases.

Advantages

- It's noninvasive.
- It's more reliable than a KOH.

Disadvantages

- Negative results do not completely rule out fungal infection.
- Results may take a long time.

The next step

- Once the fungus is identified, appropriate antifungal medication can be prescribed.
- If the test is negative but the problem persists, a second sample may be taken.

TZANCK SMEAR

General information

Where It's Done	Who Does It	How Long It Takes	Discomfort/Pain
Doctor's office or clinic.	Doctor.	1–2 minutes.	Minor discomfort when sample is collected.
When Results Ready	**Special Equipment**	**Risks/Complications**	**Average Cost**
10 minutes to 1 week, depending on where results analyzed.	Scalpel or other instrument for scraping.	None.	$

Other names Cytodiagnostic smear.

Purpose To diagnose infections caused by several types of herpesviruses, particularly shingles, chicken pox, and herpes simplex.

How it works The herpesvirus can cause certain skin cells to become abnormally large or develop other abnormalities. These cells, taken from a blister caused by the virus, can be seen under a microscope.

Preparation None.

Test procedure A blister that is typical of the infection is burst, and its bottom and top are scraped and smeared onto a microscope slide.

After the test You are free to resume normal activities. The slide is stained with dyes and examined under a microscope, either in the doctor's office or in a hospital or commercial laboratory.

Factors affecting results The stage of the blister. If the sample is taken when the blister is healing, the likelihood of detecting the virus decreases.

Interpretation Although the virus itself is not detected with this test, the presence of certain abnormally large cells can confirm the diagnosis. When results are negative, however, herpes cannot be ruled out.

Advantages Results are received faster than with the culture test.

Disadvantages False-negative results occur in about one-third of cases.

The next step The presence of certain cells definitively diagnoses herpes, which can then be treated. If the results are negative, a culture may be done, or the doctor may use that information to support a conclusion that a herpesvirus infection is not present.

ECTOPARASITIC DEMONSTRATION

General information

Where It's Done	Who Does It	How Long It Takes	Discomfort/Pain
Doctor's office or clinic.	Doctor.	1–2 minutes.	Minor discomfort or pain when skin is scraped.

When Results Ready	Special Equipment	Risks/Complications	Average Cost
Usually within 10 minutes.	Scalpel, immersion oil, and magnifying glass.	None.	$

Other names Arthropod identification.

Purpose To determine whether a skin abnormality marked by itching is caused by ectoparasites—parasites that live on the surface of the skin (in contrast to endoparasites, which live inside the body). These include mites and ticks. Most commonly used to diagnose scabies, which is caused by a mite.

How it works Examination of the parasite under a microscope allows identification and diagnosis.

Preparation None.

Test procedure The procedure used for collecting a specimen depends on the suspected cause of the problem.

- For scabies, a condition in which mites burrow into the skin and cause intense itching, the doctor will scrape out one of your sores with a scalpel. Prior to scraping, a drop of immersion oil is placed on the sore or the scalpel, which helps the mite stick to the scalpel blade.

- A magnifying glass and forceps will be used to locate and pick up lice, which may infest the head (head lice), pubic area (crab lice), or other parts of the body (body lice). Lice eggs may be picked up by plucking or cutting the hairs to which they are attached.
- Chiggers (harvest mites, red bugs) attach themselves to humans around the ankles, legs, and waist, where they cause itching and swelling. The doctor may first examine the skin to identify a lesion that contains a chigger, then collect it by scraping the affected area with a scalpel.

After the test You are free to resume normal activities.

Factors affecting results The test may be performed on a sore that contains no parasites. In scabies, only a small percentage of the bumps contain mites.

Interpretation Ectoparasites are identified on the basis of their size and shape.

Advantages It provides a definitive diagnosis when a parasite is found.

Disadvantages Failure to find a parasite may not rule out parasitic infestation.

The next step

- If a parasite is found and identified, treatment can begin.
- If no parasite is found, but scabies is still suspected, a trial treatment may be prescribed anyhow.

MICROSCOPIC HAIR SHAFT EVALUATION

General information

Where It's Done	Who Does It	How Long It Takes	Discomfort/Pain
Doctor's office or clinic.	Doctor.	2–5 minutes.	Minor discomfort if hair is plucked.
Results Ready When	**Special Equipment**	**Risks/Complications**	**Average Cost**
About 10 minutes in doctor's office; up to 7 days if hair is sent to laboratory.	Scissors.	None.	$

Other names Hair examination.

Purpose

- To evaluate the structure of hair in people with excessive hair loss or hair that has abnormal texture or fails to grow beyond a certain length.
- To help determine whether such problems are genetic or the result of trauma (such as excessive hair care practices or compulsive twisting of the hair).

How it works The hairs are examined under a microscope for certain distorted shapes or alterations of their bases that can identify several causes of abnormal hair growth.

Preparation None.

Test procedure The doctor cuts approximately 25 hairs as close to the scalp as possible from a representative area. If hair roots are to be examined, the hairs may be pulled or plucked. Alternatively, you may be asked to collect some hairs that have fallen out and bring them to the doctor's office.

After the test You are free to resume normal activities.

Factors affecting results None.

Interpretation Various abnormalities may be detected by examining the appearance of the hair roots, shafts, and ends or by calculating the proportion of hairs in a growing phase to those in a resting phase.

Advantages It's simple and noninvasive.

Disadvantages None.

The next step

- If an abnormality is found, it can help the doctor identify the cause of the abnormal hair growth or loss.
- In some such circumstances, a treatment can be recommended. If no abnormality is found, the test can help exclude from consideration some causes of hair loss or abnormal growth.

PATCH TEST (AND PHOTOPATCH VARIATION)

General information

Where It's Done	Who Does It	How Long It Takes	Discomfort/Pain
Doctor's office or clinic.	Doctor or nurse.	Less than 30 minutes to apply patches.	Occasional itching.

Results Ready When	Special Equipment	Risks/Complications	Average Cost
3–4 days.	Aluminum cups or paper disks, tape, and allergen extracts.	Occasional mild irritation at test site. Uncommonly, dermatitis may worsen temporarily, or the entire back may become red (known as "angry back").	$$

Other names Contact dermatitis skin test or epicutaneous patch test (also see chapter 14).

Purpose To identify the substance causing allergic contact dermatitis (eg, nickel in jewelry, preservatives in cosmetics, or rubber).

How it works The skin is exposed to various allergens (substances that cause an allergic reaction in susceptible people) to determine what produces the contact dermatitis.

Preparation You will be asked not to apply steroid cream or ointment to the area of skin that will be used for the test. Whenever possible, you should bring suspected allergens, such as cosmetics or items of clothing, to the doctor's office.

Test procedure

- Small amounts of suspected allergens are placed on cups or disks and taped to your back.
- The site of each patch (usually about 24) is marked on the skin with a pen for later identification.
- The patches remain in place for about 48 hours, during which time they must remain dry (you must therefore avoid strenuous exercise to prevent heavy sweating).
- If any of the patches causes severe itching or pain, remove it and inform your doctor immediately.

Variations If you are suspected of having a photocontact allergy—contact dermatitis that develops under the joint influence of contact with an allergen and exposure to ultraviolet light—a photopatch test may be conducted. In this test, two patches are used for each allergen and held in place with opaque material. After 24 to 48 hours, the patches are removed, and one of the test sites from each pair is uncovered and exposed to an ultraviolet lamp while the other remains protected from light. If you have photoallergic contact dermatitis, a reaction will subsequently develop at the site that was exposed to the ultraviolet light but not at the corresponding protected site.

After the test

- You remove the patches approximately 48 hours after they were placed. You can shower or take a bath but you should avoid rubbing the test sites.
- The doctor or nurse examines the test sites 24 hours later.
- Alternatively, the patches are removed in the doctor's office after 48 hours, and you are examined then and in another one to five days.
- Some test sites may remain somewhat dark for several weeks but will fade eventually. If they itch, a steroid ointment or cream may be prescribed.

Factors affecting results

- Use of excessively high or low concentrations of allergen extracts, or impurities in the extracts.
- Placing patches on inflamed skin or after cleaning the skin with an irritating substance.
- Examining the patch sites too early or too late.
- Failing to seal the patches tightly.
- Taking steroids in high doses or using a steroid ointment over the tested area.
- The absence of real-life conditions, such as sweating and friction.
- The development of "angry back," in which hypersensitivity of the skin can cause excess reactivity at patch sites where there is not a true allergic reaction, can make interpretation of results impossible.

Interpretation

The presence of redness, swelling, blisters, or other skin abnormalities at a test site indicates that you may be allergic to the tested substance.

Advantages

- It's an objective test for determining the cause of allergic contact dermatitis.
- It's generally safe.

Disadvantages

- Skin irritation can be confused with an allergic reaction.
- Bathing is prohibited for two days.

The next step

- A positive test for an allergen can identify the cause of contact dermatitis, and the offending substance can then be avoided.
- A negative test does not exclude the diagnosis of allergic contact dermatitis, but it suggests that the dermatitis is not being caused by one of the substances that was tested. Also, some positive tests may occur to substances other than those causing the current symptoms.

DARK-FIELD EXAMINATION

General information

Where It's Done	Who Does It	How Long It Takes	Discomfort/Pain
Doctor's office (rarely) or health department clinic.	Doctor.	Less than 5 minutes.	Minimal discomfort associated with scratching.

Results Ready When	Special Equipment	Risks/Complications	Average Cost
15 minutes.	Special microscope; glass slide and coverslip.	Negligible.	$

Other names Dark-field microscopy.

Purpose To diagnose syphilis. Used mostly to diagnose its early stage, when a single ulcerous sore first appears.

How it works Syphilis bacteria cannot be seen well with an ordinary microscope but can be detected with a special dark-field microscope in which light rays do not shine directly through the slide. A sample of fluid from the syphilis sore is smeared on a slide. The way the light passes through the slide causes the spirochetes (*Treponema pallidum*, the spiral-shaped bacterium that causes the disease) to appear as bright spiral objects against a black background. The test provides a quick way of distinguishing syphilis from other disorders but is rarely used these days because the special microscope equipment is not available in most doctor's offices and because currently available blood tests offer a reliable, more efficient alternative.

Preparation Usually the decision to perform the test is made during an office visit and there is no advance preparation. If you have advance notice, on the day before the test, remove with soap and water any ointments you have used on the affected area. Do not wash the affected skin on the day of the test.

Test procedure First, the infected area may be cleansed with a saline solution. The doctor obtains serous fluid from the ulcerous sore by pressing a microscope slide against the affected skin.

After the test You are free to resume normal activities.

Factors affecting results

- Oral antibiotics or an antibiotic ointment used before the test may kill the spirochetes.

- Nonsyphilitic bacteria that cause no disease can also be found, and these may be difficult to distinguish from the syphilis spirochetes, especially in samples taken from the mouth.
- Ointments used on the skin interfere with the examination.
- Healing syphilis sores may contain no spirochetes.

Interpretation The presence of characteristic spirochetes suggests that the skin abnormality is due to syphilis, which is caused by these organisms. The bacteria are identified by their corkscrew shape and characteristic bending movements.

Advantages Positive results help make a quick diagnosis.

Disadvantages

- Negative results do not rule out syphilis.
- The test does not work well on dry sores.

The next step

- If the results are positive, a blood test may be ordered to confirm it or to establish a baseline result to monitor treatment, and antibiotic therapy will be started.
- If the test is negative, a blood test may be ordered or treatment initiated anyway, depending on the doctor's degree of suspicion that the sore is caused by syphilis.

Craig Friedman, MD ■ Kathleen M. Stoessel, MD

18 The Sensory Organs

Tests Covered in This Chapter

The case of Sophia M., a 30-year-old mother of an 8-year-old daughter:

You wouldn't think that a 3-year-old could break your nose, but my daughter did just that. She was bouncing on the couch when she fell backward. Her head struck my nose and broke it in three places.

I had surgery by a specialist whom I liked and trusted; he was also a friend of the family. When the bandages came off, I looked in a mirror and I was sick. I hated the way my nose looked, and I couldn't breathe. He reassured me that the swelling would go down and the nostrils would even up. But they didn't, even though he tried three times over the next two years to fix the problem under local anesthesia.

My whole life changed. I went into a depression. I quit my job and slept most of the day. I became sick all the time. I developed chronic bronchitis. I coughed constantly, had a low-grade fever, and was extremely weak and lethargic, and my chest always hurt. Then finally I found another doctor I could trust.

The Tests Sophia's new doctor examined her nasal passages for obstructions by feeling her nose and peering inside with a nasal telescope (a lighted magnifying instrument that allowed him to see deep into the nose). The exam revealed that the cartilage that forms the structure of the nose had healed poorly, blocking more than half of Sophia's nasal passageway. What's more, cartilage had been removed in the nasal valve area, resulting in a lack of support. Each time she took a breath, the skin would collapse and obstruct the valve.

The Outcome Because the damage was so extensive, reconstructive surgery was the only option. During an operation lasting almost six hours, Sophia's surgeon took cartilage from deep inside her ear and used it to rebuild the inner structure of her nose, which was not only damaged but covered with scar tissue.

The surgery was a success—physiologically, aesthetically, and emotionally. Sophia no longer has any problem breathing. All her physical symptoms have disappeared, and so has her depression. She is happy with her nose and feels that she has been given her life back.

THE EYE

Vision is a special sense, and one of the body's most complex systems. The eye is the organ of vision and, like a camera, it adjusts to changes in lighting, distance, and head position to focus the images that we look at for good vision. Each eye sits in a bony socket and is connected to the brain by an optic nerve, which extends from the back of the eye. Each eye has six specialized muscles attached to its wall that allow proper alignment and eye movement with varying head positions. The eyes are protected by eyelids, behind which are tear glands that make a tear film to lubricate the front of the eye. A continuation of the tissue on the inside of the eyelid covers the white of the eye; this tissue is the conjunctiva, the cellophane-like tissue that contains blood vessels and can become pink or red when irritated (ie, "pink eye").

The eye is a sphere, or "ball" that has a specialized anterior (front) and posterior (back) segment. The sclera is the white fibrous coat of the posterior eye that gives its shape, and has its own inner wall circulation called the uvea. The anterior extension of the uvea forms a ring of tissue around the pupil, called the iris, which gives the eye its color. Just behind the iris is a specialized muscle to change the pupil diameter, and ligaments to hold a crystalline lens in place behind the pupil. Changes in the pupil size and in the shape of the lens occur in response to differences in lighting and image distance and give different focusing powers for vision. For example, reading vision requires more focusing power of the lens than distance vision.

Also behind the iris are ciliary processes containing cells that make "aqueous fluid," a clear liquid that fills the anterior chamber, the space between the iris and the clear anterior coat of the eye, the cornea. The intraocular pressure is maintained in a normal range by aqueous movement out of the eye through the trabecular meshwork, or eye filter, at the outer edge of the iris.

Behind the iris and lens, the posterior segment of the eye is filled with a clear vitreous gel that attaches to the lining of the retina. The retina is a specialized tissue that covers the entire back wall of the eye and is often compared to the "film" of a camera. The retina contains blood vessels and is made of tissue similar to the brain. In fact, the innermost layer of the retina contains cells that make up the fibers of the optic nerve, which extend into the brain.

The images that we "see" are transmitted through the clear front of the eye and focused on the retina. These visual images set off photochemical impulses deep in the retinal photoreceptors (rods and cones) that travel through the optic nerves to visual pathways in the brain and are interpreted by the brain as "vision." The visual system has a major influence on the development of the brain, and its function is more intricate and precise than the most advanced computer.

HOW YOUR DOCTOR DIAGNOSES EYE DISORDERS

There is often confusion about the differences among eye care professionals—ophthalmologists, optometrists, and opticians. An ophthalmologist is a medical doctor (MD) who has graduated from medical school and has completed a residency in the specialty of ophthalmology. Ophthalmologists are trained to diagnose and treat diseases of the eye, which often are manifestations of a more general systemic disease such as diabetes, hypertension, stroke, inflammation, or cancer. The ophthalmologist may prescribe corrective lenses, medications (ocular, oral, or intravenous), laser procedures, or surgery.

An optometrist is a doctor of optometry (OD) who has graduated from a school of optometry. Optometrists are primarily trained to diagnose refractive disorders (near-sightedness, for example) and prescribe corrective lenses. The optometrist is also trained to detect signs of other eye disorders although these may require the attention of an ophthalmologist for treatment. Finally, an optician does not examine the eyes but is trained to fill prescriptions for corrective lenses.

Most children have their first formal vision test by a pediatrician at about the age of three, when children can respond to simple questions and describe what they see. However, premature babies and full-term babies with any developmental or medical problems have initial eye examinations within the first few weeks of life. Any children with a turned or wandering eye (strabismus), nystagmus, or asymmetry of eye size, color, etc, should have early eye exams to determine if ocular disease or amblyopia is present so that early treatment can be recommended.

Adults should have a complete eye examination every two years. If there is a family history of ocular diseases such as glaucoma or macular degeneration, or any retinal degeneration, or if there is a chronic medical condition that can affect your eyes such as diabetes, at least annual exams are recommended, and sometimes eye exams every few months are needed.

Regular visits are important not only because vision can sometimes change gradually over time so that it may go unnoticed but also because some serious eye diseases do not show symptoms until they are far advanced. Permanent vision loss may result if timely treatment does not occur. For example, glaucoma, a disease in which the eye pressure is too high, is a leading cause of blindness. It is also one of the most easily diagnosed and treated diseases, yet only about half of the people who have it are aware of it until very late when vision is already compromised. Another example is age-related macular degeneration, an aging disorder of the central retina, which does not usually cause blindness but can cause blurred central vision. Some types of macular degeneration can be helped by laser treatment.

THE EYE EXAM

Although the eye examination may vary from doctor to doctor, it should begin with a complete history. Some eye disorders are hereditary, so it would help the doctor to know about any problems that run in your family. Furthermore, some eye disorders may develop slowly so that it is important to tell the doctor about any symptoms or changes in vision, even if they seem insignificant to you. Sometimes symptoms may occur abruptly, such as the appearance of floaters or flashes of light, or a shade coming across the peripheral vision, or even a change in the central vision. These symptoms should always be reported to the eye doctor immediately. Usually, the doctor will ask that you come into the office promptly for a thorough eye examination.

During the eye examination, the doctor will conduct a number of tests designed to assess the ability of your eyes to move independently, focus at near and far, adjust for a moving object, and adjust to different light conditions. Your peripheral vision and your ability to see and distinguish between different colors may also be tested.

Usually, a test called the Snellen visual acuity chart is used to measure your vision. Letters, numbers, or symbols are arranged from the largest at the top to the smallest at the bottom. You are asked to stand or sit 20 feet from the chart or screen and identify the figures line by line from top to bottom until you can no longer recognize them. The doctor will check each eye alone while covering the alternate eye and usually both eyes together are also tested. Your vision is described with a fraction, such as 20/40.

With the preliminary data of your visual acuity, the ophthalmologist or optometrist will continue to diagnose potential refractive problems by providing corrective lenses. You are asked to look through a series of corrective lenses, identifying the ones that help you see the vision chart better. Using a trial frame, the doctor can change lenses for each eye until the proper combination is found. You should not worry about giving a "wrong" answer, since the doctor is trained to distinguish subtle differences in how you are able to see with the various lenses.

A slit lamp microscope is used to shine light into your eyes to examine the lids and anterior eye surface, and some of the inner eye structures at high magnification. This may entail putting a contact lens containing mirrors on the eye to evaluate the eye filter and the posterior eye structures. Eye drops are sometimes used to temporarily anesthetize the front of the eye, and often eye drops are used to dilate the pupils for the complete retinal evaluation. An ophthalmoscope is used to evaluate the vitreous and retina. The indirect ophthalmoscope is a hat with a light and mirror attachment, worn by the eye doctor, who can focus the light with a special lens through the pupil of the eye, to evaluate the entire retina including the extreme peripheral retina where holes or other lesions are sometimes found. The direct ophthalmoscope is a smaller handheld light that the doctor may use to look at the central retina only.

Using a device called a tonometer, the doctor measures the pressure inside of the eyes. Tonometry is a quick and painless test that can diagnose potentially serious conditions such as glaucoma.

Finally, in addition to the details about the eyes and the best corrected vision, the doctor examines for any underlying health condition that may show itself in the eye. For example, diabetes is a condition that can cause changes in the retinal blood vessels, called diabetic retinopathy. Sometimes diabetic retinopathy can include swelling in the central retina, or abnormal blood vessel growth with bleeding in the eye: in both cases laser treatment can be helpful in preserving vision.

Some other tests that the eye doctor may recommend are listed in table 18.1. These tests can be helpful in diagnosing specific eye disorders.

THE HEAD AND NECK

The ears, nose, mouth, and throat control our ability to hear, smell, breathe, speak, taste, swallow, and keep our balance. Whenever one part of the system has problems, it can upset the entire complex, leading to a loss of several sensory experiences.

The Ear

The ear, the primary organ of hearing, is made of three parts—outer, middle, and inner. The outer ear, called the auricle or pinna, is the part that protrudes from the head. Cartilage gives it shape and support. The outer ear canal is the first part to receive sound, and it focuses sound waves on the eardrum, or tympanic membrane. This thin

TABLE 18.1 Function Tests

Test	Description
Eyes	
Amsler-grid test	Measures your central vision using a checkerboard grid with a dark spot in the middle. The grid is shown to you as you alternately cover your right or left eye. If the grid appears distorted, there may be a problem with central vision for that eye. The test is commonly used to detect subtle central vision changes in patients with macular degeneration.
Color-vision tests	Tests your color vision using panels with primary-colored patterns juxtaposed against a multicolored background. Other more detailed color-vision tests require you to match color saturations.
Electro-oculogram (EOG)	Measures a constantly present resting potential between the cornea (positive) and the retinal pigment epithelium (negative) on the back wall of the eye. This test is helpful in evaluating some of the hereditary retinal disorders.
Electroretinogram (ERG)	The full-field, light-evoked ERG records a diffuse electrical response from different cells within the retina to a light stimulus. The ERG response of the retina can vary with many situations, including your refractive error, pupil size, age, dark adaptation, etc. This test is used often to help diagnose retinal dystrophies, such as retinitis pigmentosa.
Exophthalmometry	A device called an exophthalmometer measures how much one eye may protrude out of its socket compared to the other eye, and compared to the rim of the orbit. Prominent eyes may sometimes indicate a thyroid disorder, inflammation, or tumor.
Gonioscopy	Direct or indirect examination of the "filter" or chamber of the eye, using special contact lenses to diagnose types of diabetes.
Lancaster red–green test	This test is used to accurately measure and map out eye muscle deviations (strabismus). This test can be helpful in documenting the muscle deviations prior to any surgical correction and also post-surgery to show the improvement. During this test you are asked to wear glasses consisting of red color over one eye and green color over the other eye, depending on which eye is the fixing eye. With the help of the doctor any muscle deviations can be mapped out either on a computerized test, or on a large screen in front of you.
Ophthalmoscopy	*Direct*: Handheld light allows the doctor to examine only the center retina. *Indirect*: Dilating eye drops are first used to dilate the pupils. The doctor wears a headlight instrument and focuses light with a magnifying lens, through the dilated pupil to examine the central and peripheral retina and vitreous.
Refraction test	Detects focusing disorders of the eye. Dilating eye drops are sometimes used for this test, and if so, you may have trouble focusing close vision for two to four hours after the test. The eye care specialist may use a retinoscope to measure reflexes in the back of the eyes, as well as using a standard visual acuity (Snellen) chart and sample lenses to determine the amount of any needed correction. These tests determine your eyeglass or contact lens prescription.
Schirmer tearing test	Measures your eyes' tearing ability using a strip of filter tape placed between the lower eyelid and the eye for about five minutes. This test is used to detect dry eye syndrome.
Slit-lamp examination	An eye doctor examines the lids and front surface of the eyes as well as some of the inner eye structures. You sit with your head in a brace, chin in a chin rest, and forehead leaning against a padded bar. A narrow beam of light is focused on your eye while the doctor looks into the area through the special microscope. This test is used to evaluate the eyelids, cornea, conjunctiva, anterior chamber and angle, iris, lens or cataracts, vitreous, and retina.

TABLE 18.1 (continued)

Test	Description
Eyes (continued)	
Visual-acuity tests	Tests to assess near and distant vision using the standard visual-acuity charts.
Visual-evoked potential (VEP)	A gross electrical signal is generated in the visual cortex portion of the brain in response to visual stimulation with either a flash of light or a pattern. This test is used to evaluate the central visual field, and the time taken for an impulse from the retina to travel through the optic nerves and visual pathways to the visual cortex in the brain.
Visual-field tests	These tests measure peripheral and paracentral vision by tangent screen, Goldmann perimetry, or automated (computerized) perimetry such as the octopus perimetry. You are given the proper eyeglasses to use and each eye is tested separately. Each eye focuses on a special spot or light, while test objects or lights come in from the side. You are asked to press a handheld button whenever you see an object coming in from your side vision. This test is used for diagnosis and monitoring of glaucoma, pituitary tumors, and retinal degenerations, etc.
Head and Neck	
Auditory brain stem response (ABR)	This test is used to track nerve signals from the inner ear as they travel through the auditory nerve to the brain region responsible for hearing, and to determine where along the path the hearing loss has occurred. A small speaker, which produces clicking sounds, is placed near the ear. Special electrodes automatically record the nerve signal. The test may be used in young children because it does not require direct participation.
Dynamic platform posturography (DPP)	DPP is a computerized test system used to evaluate all aspects of balance function. You stand on a platform that measures body sway and the forces you exert to remain stable. It also provokes balance reactions by changing its grade or angle. A computer isolates each of your sensory inputs and identifies where a balance problem exists.
Electronystagmometry (ENG)	This is a special test of the balance mechanism of the inner ear. It helps diagnose some types of hearing loss and determine reasons for dizziness, "ringing in the ears,," or vertigo. The test involves running a cool liquid and then a warm liquid through a small tube through the ear canal. The temperature change stimulates the inner ear, which in turn causes rapid reflex movements of the eyes, which are observed to evaluate the balance mechanism.
Pure-tone audiometry	See full description below.
Tympanometry	The tympanogram measures vibrations of the eardrum. The middle ear is normally filled with air at a pressure equal to the surrounding atmosphere. If it is filled with fluid, the eardrum will not vibrate, and the tympanogram will be flat. If it is filled with air at a different pressure than that of the atmosphere, the tympanogram will be shifted in position. The tympanogram is a quick and easy test: A special probe is placed up against the ear canal, like an earplug, and in 15 seconds a printout of a graph is obtained.
Video stroboscopy	Stroboscopic exam allows careful video evaluation of the function of the vocal tract and cords with a telescope or fiber-optic laryngoscope. Useful for identifying the reasons for hoarseness or voice dysfunction.

membrane between the outer and middle ear conducts sound vibrations through the three connected bones of the middle ear: the hammer (malleus), the anvil (incus), and the stirrup (stapes); these bones then conduct sound to the inner ear.

The eustachian tube, lined with mucous membranes, connects the middle ear to the back of the nose (nasopharynx) and serves to equalize the air pressure in the inner ear with that of the outside air.

The inner ear consists of the cochlea, a snail-shaped bony hearing organ that carries signals to the acoustic nerve, and the labyrinth, a fluid-filled canal that helps you maintain your balance.

The Nose and Sinuses

The nose—the primary organ of smell—is also one of the organs of taste. The internal part of the nose lies just above the roof of the mouth. The external part is divided into two chambers by the septum, each chamber developing into a nostril. The septum is made up primarily of cartilage and bone covered by mucous membranes. Cartilage also gives shape and support to the outer part of the nose.

The nasal passages are lined with mucous membranes and tiny hairs (cilia) that help filter the air. These open into four pairs of air-filled cavities called sinuses, which are also lined with mucous membranes.

The Mouth and Salivary Glands

Besides the teeth, gums, and tongue, the mouth contains three pairs of salivary glands that help digestion by secreting saliva, which helps break up food and keeps the mouth wet.

The Throat

The throat (pharynx) is a ringlike muscular tube that acts as the passageway for both air and food or liquid and helps in forming speech. It contains the openings of the eustachian tubes, the nasal passages, the larynx (voice box), the esophagus (which connects the mouth to the stomach), and the tonsils.

The larynx is crucial to speech and breathing. It houses the vocal cords and is the gateway to both the trachea (windpipe), which leads to the lungs, and the esophagus, which leads to the stomach. Above the larynx is the epiglottis, which works with the larynx and vocal cords during swallowing to push food into the esophagus and keep it from entering the windpipe. When food goes "down the wrong pipe," the extremely sensitive larynx produces a violent cough that is designed to clear the pathway so that air can reach the lungs.

Tonsils and adenoids are lumps of lymph tissue at the back and sides of the mouth. They are designed to protect against infection but have little purpose beyond childhood. Tonsils start out rather large but eventually shrink to almond size. Adenoids shrink so much that they are almost nonexistent in adulthood.

HOW YOUR DOCTOR DIAGNOSES HEAD AND NECK DISORDERS

The area of medicine devoted to diagnosing and treating disorders of the ear, nose, throat, and nearby parts of the head and neck is otolaryngology (and sometimes head and neck surgery). The doctor trained in this specialty is called an otolaryngologist, ENT (ear, nose, and throat) specialist, or head and neck specialist.

Whether you are examined by your family doctor or an ENT specialist, the exam is likely to begin with a complete history of your symptoms and then the familiar "Open your mouth and say, 'Ahhhh.'" This simple maneuver gives your doctor a good view of the structures in the back of the mouth, the throat, the tonsils, and any unusual nasal discharge. The doctor may also use a device called a speculum to look into your ears and nostrils. Other special instruments, used to examine the larynx, include the nasopharyngoscope, a flexible fiber-optic tube that can be passed through the nostrils and through the pharynx, allowing a good view of the vocal cords. Another tool otolaryngologists use is the 90-degree telescope, a scope that is angled so that it can be inserted into the mouth and used to look down the throat, projecting images to the eyepiece.

In addition to observing the easily visible structures, your doctor will also palpate (feel) parts of the head and neck to assess the health of internal organs. These techniques are often all that is necessary for an initial diagnosis.

Additional tests may help confirm the diagnosis, but your doctor may opt for treatment before the results are available. The doctor may also postpone any further tests to see if an easy treatment solves the problem. For example, if you have signs of a sinus infection, the doctor may start an antibiotic without doing a culture of the sinus fluid (see chapter 22). On the other hand, if your doctor suspects that your nasal passages are blocked and cannot see them adequately during a physical exam, he or she will probably order a nasal endoscopy to find out the cause, especially if you are having trouble breathing.

A second component of a head and neck exam is a hearing test. Usually the easiest and most comprehensive way to assess hearing is with pure-tone audiometry, in which tones of differing magnitude and frequency are played for you to identify. The test is usually performed by an audiologist, who is specially trained to give and score the hearing test. The test is so widespread that it is often performed outside a doctor's office, at schools and at some job sites.

Many people go to an otolaryngologist when they experience reductions in taste and smell. These closely related senses can be evaluated using booklets that have "scratch-and-sniff" labels. Problems identified by this test may be related to malfunction of the taste and smell receptors that are part of the oral-nasal system, or may have roots in the structures in the brain that interpret sensory information.

Major eye disorders, along with their symptoms and diagnostic tests are summarized in table 18.2; table 18.3 provides similar information on ear, nose, and throat disorders. An overview of imaging studies for the eyes, head, and neck can be found in table 18.4.

TABLE 18.2 The Eye: Major Disorders, Symptoms, and Diagnostic Tests

Disorder	Description	Symptoms	Tests
Amblyopia ("lazy eye")	Blurred vision in one or both eyes due to an uncorrected visual problem early in life.	Trouble focusing, turned eyes (strabismus), tilting head to try to focus. (A full-term infant should be able to focus by 3 months.)	Eye examination to observe how eyes move and focus as they follow an object, visual acuity test, tests for depth perception, and ophthalmoscopy.
Cataracts	Clouding of the lens loses its transparency, becoming visibly opaque.	Gray-white film behind pupil; blurred or reduced vision.	Eye exam including tests for visual acuity, side (peripheral) vision, sensitivity to glare, and eye movement; ophthalmoscopy; slit-lamp examination; and tonometry.
Color blindness	Inability to perceive one or more colors, especially reds and greens.	Seeing grays and browns when looking at reds and greens.	Color-blindness tests to determine color saturation and color discrimination.
Conjunctivitis ("pink eye")	Irritation of the eyelid lining caused by infection or allergy.	Red, irritated, burning eyes; sometimes a mucus discharge.	Eye exam and culture for severe cases.
Corneal injury or infection	Damaged cornea due to excessive exposure to ultraviolet light, improper use of contact lenses, a blow to the eye, or infection.	Red, painful, swollen eyes; bacterial infection may cause pus.	Eye exam and culture for severe infectious cases.
Diabetic retinopathy	Retinal damage caused by diabetic changes in small blood vessels.	Blurred vision from retinal swelling, more severe vision loss from bleeding in the retina, vitreous gel, or retinal detachment.	Visual acuity test, tonometry, slit-lamp biomicroscopy, indirect ophthalmoscopy, fundus photography, fluorescein angiogram.
Glaucoma	Damage to the optic nerve and visual field caused by increased pressure of the fluid in the eyes.	Vary according to type of glaucoma; may include decreased peripheral vision progressing to tunnel vision, pain, redness, and blurred vision.	Eye exam including visual acuity and refraction, pupil exam, ophthalmoscopy, slit-lamp examination, tonometry, gonioscopy, and optic nerve head photography.

Macular degeneration	Pigment abnormalities caused by aging that may be dry (atrophic) or wet (exudative). Wet degeneration develops from abnormal blood vessels in the back wall of the eye that may bleed or leak fluid.	Blurred central vision that may range from mild distortion to more severe loss of central vision.	Amsler-grid test, visual acuity tests, refraction, fluorescein angiography, fundus photography, and sometimes indocyanine green angiography.
Refractive errors	Images coming through the eye do not focus properly on the retina.	Inability to focus clearly on distant objects (myopia, or nearsightedness) or near objects (presbyopia, or farsightedness) or vision (astigmatism).	Visual acuity tests, refraction test for proper eyeglasses or contact lenses.
Retinal detachment	Fluid accumulates under the retina, separating it from the back of the eyeball. Most often caused by a tear or hole in the peripheral retina.	Seeing flashes or floaters; shadow over the visual field; blurred vision.	Visual acuity, tonometry, indirect ophthalmoscopy, ultrasound.
Retinal hemorrhage	Blood from a broken retinal blood vessel seeps into the retinal tissue.	May cause a dark spot in the central vision if the hemorrhage happens in the macula. A peripheral hemorrhage may cause a dark spot in the side vision.	Indirect ophthalmoscopy, fundus photography.
Scleritis	Inflammation of the sclera, the outer white coat of the eye.	Redness and swelling of the white portion of the eye; pain; blurred vision; sometimes associated with inflammation in the body.	Visual acuity, tonometry, slit-lamp biomicroscopy; ophthalmoscopy.
Uveitis	Inflammation of the inner anterior part of the eye, including the iris and ciliary body. Inflammatory cells can be seen in the anterior chamber and often the vitreous.	Painful, red, light-sensitive eyes; blurred vision.	Visual acuity, tonometry, slit-lamp biomicroscopy; ophthalmoscopy.
Vitreous hemorrhage	Bleeding from the retinal or choroidal vessels into the vitreous chamber.	Sudden vision loss, and "floaters" in visual field; cloudy vision.	Visual acuity tests, indirect ophthalmoscopy, and ultrasound.

TABLE 18.3 Ear, Nose, and Throat: Major Disorders, Symptoms, and Diagnostic Tests

Disorder	Description	Symptoms	Tests
Ear			
External otitis	Ear infection called "swimmer's ear" because it often occurs after swimming in bacteria-filled water.	Inflammation of ear canal, itching, pain, pus discharge, and poor hearing in the affected ear.	Physical exam, and culture in severe cases.
Otitis media	Infection of the middle ear.	Inability to "pop" the ear, fluid in the ear, poor hearing, fever, and pain.	Physical exam, and culture in severe cases.
Meniere's disease	Disease of the inner ear.	Period of dizziness (vertigo), ringing in the ears (tinnitus), nausea, and sensitivity to sound.	Physical exam and history, pure-tone audiometry, electronystagmometry, dynamic platform posturography, and auditory brain stem response.
Hearing loss	May be due to interference or to changes in the inner ear, nerve, or brain.	In cases of interference, such as earwax buildup, sounds are muffled. If loss is due to degeneration of inner ear, sounds may be heard but are hard to precisely identify; hearing sounds of higher frequencies becomes limited with age.	Pure-tone audiometry.
Nose			
Deviated septum	The septum or center section of the nose moves to one side.	May cause infection, repeated cases of sinusitis, breathing problems, increased nosebleeds, and differences in cosmetic appearance.	Physical exam and nasal endoscopy.
Epitaxis (nosebleeds)	Can be caused by minor irritation or a long list of underlying complaints.	Bleeding from nose, dizziness, and breathing problems.	Physical exam and history; which tests used depend on possible underlying causes.

Rhinitis	Inflammation of the mucous membranes of the nose.	May be caused by a sinus infection or allergic reaction and, thus, display symptoms of those problems; in all cases, nasal discharge.	Physical exam; possibly allergy tests, culture, and nasal endoscopy (may be called rhinoscopy).
Sinuses			
Sinusitis	Inflammation of nasal sinuses from numerous causes.	Breathing problems from blocked sinuses, pain, headache, and fever.	Physical exam and history; possibly culture, nasal endoscopy, and CT scan.
Nasal polyps	Benign protruding swellings of tissue lining the sinuses.	Breathing problems from blocked nasal cavities.	Physical exam, nasal endoscopy, and CT scan.
Throat and Neck			
Pharyngitis	Inflammation or infection of the throat; may be strep throat.	Sore throat, difficulty swallowing, pain, and possibly fever.	Physical exam and culture; possibly nasal endoscopy (may be called rhinopharyngoscopy).
Tonsillitis/adenoiditis	Inflammation or infection of the tonsils or adenoids.	Sore throat, difficulty swallowing, and possibly fever	Physical exam, and culture in severe cases.
Laryngitis	Inflammation of the mucous membranes of the larynx; may be a symptom of a more serious problem such as vocal cord cancer.	Sore or hoarse throat, cough, loss of voice, and breathing problems.	Physical exam and history; possibly fiber-optic laryngoscopy.
Neck mass	Swelling in the neck; may be caused by a tumor of lymph nodes, parotid gland, or thyroid gland.	Sore throat, hoarseness, and coughing up blood.	Fiber-optic laryngoscopy and fine-needle aspiration.

TABLE 18.4 Imaging Tests*

Test	Description
Eye	
Fluorescein angiogram	A diagnostic tool to study the retinal and choroidal circulation, and the retinal pigment epithelium of the eye as well as any diseases affecting them. Prior to this test, your doctor would discuss your medical history, medications, and the test procedure. The doctor would question you about any allergies. After your visual acuity is obtained and your pupils are dilated, photographs are taken of the back of the eye, and special camera filters are used to take photographs of the retina as a small amount of sterile fluorescein dye is injected into the vein of the arm or hand. This dye allows the camera to capture on special film the timing of blood flow coming into the eye, as well as any alterations in the retinal blood vessels, the choroidal vessels in the wall of the eye, and any alterations in retinal pigment.
Indocyanine green digital videoangiography	Similar to the fluorescein angiogram test but uses a different "indocyanine green" dye that will give a better picture of the choroidal circulation in the wall of the eye. This test is sometimes helpful in diagnosing macular degeneration.
Keratoscope	A handheld instrument the doctor uses to measure the corneal astigmatism after cataract or corneal surgery.
Orbital computed tomography (CT)	A noninvasive imaging procedure often used to localize intraocular foreign bodies, and evaluate eye muscles and certain intraocular or orbital inflammations or tumors.
Magnetic resonance imaging (MRI)	Often used to differentiate intraocular and/or orbital inflammation and infection from certain tumors. Helpful in evaluating the orbit and sinuses, and helpful in diagnosing choroidal malignant melanomas in the eye.
Ocular ultrasonography	A small transducer is placed on your closed eyelids as ultrasound waves are sent out and reflected back from within the eye to create an image of your eye structures. This can help in the diagnosis of several internal eye disorders.
Pachymetry	Measurement of the corneal thickness done by the doctor as you sit at the slit-lamp microscope.
Scanning laser ophthalmoscope	A noninvasive test that can quantitatively measure the topography of the retina and optic nerve.
Head and Neck	
Computed tomography of pharynx and temporal bone	See above. Allows images of bone and soft tissues. Very good for sinus evaluation.
Magnetic resonance imaging (MRI)	See above. Good for seeing the brain and soft tissues of the head and neck.
Modified barium (cookie) swallow	See full description below.

*See also chapter 3.

ELECTRO-OCULOGRAPHY (EOG)

General information

Where It's Done	Who Does It	How Long It Takes	Discomfort/Pain
Ophthalmologist's office.	Ophthalmologist or ophthalmic technician.	45 minutes.	None.
Results Ready When	**Special Equipment**	**Risks/Complications**	**Average Cost**
Immediately.	Electrodes and electrophysiology machine to measure impulses.	Patients with narrow-angle glaucoma may have an increase in eye pressure from pupil dilation.	$$

Other names Electro-oculogram.

Purpose

- To evaluate the function of the retinal pigment epithelium (RPE), the layer of cells between the retina and eye wall.
- To help diagnose certain retinal discorders that cause blurred vision.

How it works Measures electrical impulses generated by the RPE in both light and darkness as the eyes move from side to side.

Preparation Your pupils may be dilated prior to the test.

Test procedure

- Electrodes are placed at the junctions where your upper and lower eyelids meet (called the canthi) and on your forehead.
- When your eyes have adapted to normal conditions, the doctor gives you two objects to focus on, thereby moving your eyes horizontally back and forth. The electrical impulses generated by your eyes are measured.
- Then your eyes are allowed to adapt to the dark for about 20 minutes, and the test is repeated.
- Your eyes are again exposed to light for another ten minutes, and the test is performed a final time.

After the test

- Because your pupils may still be dilated, for three to four hours, you should arrange for a ride home from the doctor's office.
- Wearing dark glasses may make your eyes more comfortable.

Factors affecting results Pupil size, refraction, age, certain medications, and proper dark or light adaptation.

Interpretation The ratio of peak voltages generated in the light compared to the minimum voltages generated in the dark (called the Arden ratio) is about 2:1

in people with normal function. If you have a reduced ratio, you may have a disorder affecting the retinal pigment epithelium (RPE), or there may be a more generalized disorder of the retina or choroid such as retinitis pigmentosis or choroideremia.

Advantages It is noninvasive.

Disadvantages It may not give an expert diagnosis.

The next step Test results need to be correlated with a clinical examination, and with other eye tests, such as fluorescein angiogram and visual field.

ELECTRORETINOGRAPHY (ERG)

General information

Where It's Done	Who Does It	How Long It Takes	Discomfort/Pain
Ophthalmologist's office.	Ophthalmologist or ophthalmic technician.	30–45 minutes.	None.

Results Ready When	Special Equipment	Risks/Complications	Average Cost
Immediately.	Electrodes and machine that measures impulses.	None. However, caution is advised for patients with narrow-angle glaucoma.	$$

Other names Electroretinogram.

Purpose

- To measure the electrical response of the entire retina to light.
- To diagnose disorders of the photoreceptors, such as retinitis pigmentosa.

How it works A flash of light induces responses from the photoreceptors and from the retina under both light- and dark-adapted tests. These responses are measured against a standard for the time it takes the response to occur.

Preparation Eye drops are used to dilate your pupils, along with administration of a topical anesthetic.

Test procedure

- Electrodes in the form of a contact lens are applied directly to your eyes. Other electrodes are applied to your forehead and earlobe.
- After your eyes have become adapted to dark (after about 10 to 20 minutes), you look at a flashing light. The contact lens measures the

response. The test may also be performed when your eyes are adapted to light conditions.

After the test

- Your pupils may be dilated for three to four hours; you should arrange for someone to drive you home.
- Wearing dark glasses may provide some comfort until your eyes return to normal.
- You should refrain from rubbing your eyes for at least 30 minutes after the test because of the anesthetic.

Factors affecting results Refractive error, pupil size, age, certain medications, amount of dark or light adaptation, comfort with contact lens electrode, among others.

Interpretation The levels of response are supernormal, normal, subnormal, and nonrecordable. The response consists of two components—one from the photoreceptors and another from cells in the inner retina. Because of this separation of responses, ERG testing is sometimes helpful in distinguishing retinal disorders, such as retinitis pigmentosis from abnormal retinal blood vessels. However, the overall ERG is a mass response of the entire retina.

Advantages

- It's noninvasive.
- The test allows separate evaluation of the different layers of the retina.

Disadvantages It provides good information only when large areas of the retina are affected and thus is not useful in diagnosing conditions that affect only discrete areas of the retina such as the macula.

The next step Correlation is needed with a clinical exam and other diagnostic tests, such as visual field and fluorescan angiogram.

FLUORESCEIN ANGIOGRAPHY

General information

Where It's Done	Who Does It	How Long It Takes	Discomfort/Pain
Ophthalmologist's office or hospital.	Ophthalmologist, nurse, and ophthalmic photographer.	30 minutes.	There may be mild discomfort when the fluorescein dye is injected.
Results Ready When	**Special Equipment**	**Risks/Complications**	**Average Cost**
Immediately (or when film is developed).	A fundus camera and optical filters.	Though rare, an allergic reaction to the contrast dye is possible.	$$

Other names None.

Purpose To evaluate the retinal blood vessels, circulation in the choroid, and the retinal pigment epithelium (RPE).

How it works As the fluorescein dye is injected into an arm vein, photographs are taken of the back of the eye with special camera filters that show the blood flow coming into the eye, and any alterations in retinal vessels, choroid, or retinal pigment epithelium.

Preparation Prior to the test, the doctor will obtain a full medical history including use of medications and any allergies. After the doctor does a visual acuity test, the pupils are dilated with eye drops.

Test procedure

- You place your head in a brace that holds your chin in a chin rest and your forehead against a padded bar.
- The sterile fluorescein dye is then injected into a blood vessel in your arm.
- Over the next 30 to 60 seconds, pictures are taken using a special camera that shows the progress of the dye as it goes through your retinal and choroidal vessels in the back of your eye. Sometimes, late photographs are taken after five or ten minutes.

After the test

- The pupils will be dilated for three to four hours; you should have someone drive you home.
- The dye may cause some temporary and harmless discoloration of your skin and urine for about 24 hours.

Factors affecting results Ability to keep eyes steady for the camera; pupil dilation.

Interpretation The photographs are observed for any dye leakage or staining that might indicate an abnormal choroidal vessel, or disease of the retinal pigment epithelium.

Advantages Areas of retinal disease, such as diabetic retinopathy, are detected, even when they may not be seen during a doctor's examination. Allows precise evaluation of retinal capillaries and pigment layer.

Disadvantages Need for intravenous dye injection.

The next step Observation or laser treatment, depending on the findings.

TONOMETRY

General information

Where It's Done	Who Does It	How Long It Takes	Discomfort/Pain
Doctor's office, optometrist's office, or hospital.	Ophthalmologist or optometrist or ophthalmic nurse or technician.	1–2 minutes.	None.

Results Ready When	Special Equipment	Risks/Complications	Average Cost
Immediately.	One of three kinds of tonometers: indentation, applanation, and noncontact or air puff.	The indentation or applanation (contact) tonometers can cause corneal abrasions.	$

Other names None.

Purpose

- To help diagnose glaucoma or high eye pressure.
- The test is often part of a routine eye exam.

How it works The pressure of the aqueous fluid inside the eyes is measured.

Preparation A topical anesthetic is applied to the eyes.

Test procedure

- The tonometer in the form of a contact lens is applied directly to your eye's surface.
- During indentation tonometry, you lie on a table while the tonometer is placed on your eye, and a pressure reading is taken.
- During applanation tonometry, you sit with your head in a brace that has a chin rest and a padded bar for your forehead. The tonometer is then placed against your anesthetized cornea.
- In noncontact tonometry, the tonometer does not touch your eye. Instead, it blows a puff of pressurized air into your eye and records the amount of pressure.

After the test

- You are free to leave and resume normal activities.
- You should avoid rubbing your eyes for at least 30 minutes after the test.

Factors affecting results An irregularly shaped cornea requires a special tonometer.

Interpretation Pressure readings are in millimeters (mm) of mercury (Hg). A normal reading is about 20 mm Hg or lower. Higher readings may indicate either glaucoma or ocular hypertension.

Advantages

- It's a quick, easy test for glaucoma.
- It's noninvasive.

Disadvantages Other tests may be necessary to diagnose glaucoma; these include visual field tests and ophathalmoscopy to evaluate the optic nerve.

The next step Repeat tonometry or other tests may be necessary to distinguish between glaucoma and ocular hypertension or to assess borderline cases.

VISUAL-FIELD TEST (PERIMETRY)

General information

Where It's Done	Who Does It	How Long It Takes	Discomfort/Pain
Ophthalmologist's office.	Ophthalmologist or ophthalmic technician.	30 minutes.	None.

Results Ready When	Special Equipment	Risks/Complications	Average Cost
Immediately.	Perimeter (manual or automated).	None.	$

Other name Tangent screen perimetry, Goldmann perimetry, octopus computerized perimetry, Humphrey perimetry.

Purpose To check for problems in the paracentral vision and side vision. This test evaluates the visual field for blurred or missing spots due to glaucoma, and to monitor these spots for stability or progression over time. It may also be used to detect visual field loss from brain tumors or strokes, from various retinal or optic nerve diseases, and sometimes to check the eyelid for orbital disorders.

How it works When the eye looks at an object either in central or side vision, the object's image is focused on a spot on the retina, and is sent through the optic nerve into the visual pathways of the brain, eventually to the "visual cortex" at the back of the brain. If there are abnormalities anywhere along this visual pathway, a trouble spot may show up in your visual field with careful testing, even if you do not notice a problem.

Preparation Both eyes are refracted to the best corrected vision. Pupils are not usually dilated.

Test procedure

- You sit at a table and place your head in a chin rest, so that your head is comfortable and steady.
- Each eye is tested separately, and the eye not being tested is covered with a patch.
- The proper focusing lens (eyeglass) for your eye is placed in front of your eye for the best vision, but you do not need to wear your own glasses.
- Your eye looks straight ahead into a large bowl that has a fixed spot in the center (usually yellow or green light) on which you focus.
- The perimetrist (person doing the test) may move objects or lights of different size and brightness from the side in toward a spot where you "see" the object in your side vision. As soon as you "see" the object, you press a button to record your visual field. The same test may also be done using stationary objects of light that "blink" on and off in various parts of the visual field.
- The same test is repeated for the other eye.

After the test Resume normal activity.

Factors affecting results Your level of vision and attentiveness; background lighting; experience of the perimetrist; your level of vision.

Interpretation An ophthalmologist can immediately assess the results.

Advantages It is noninvasive, and the results are immediate.

Disadvantages It may be difficult to concentrate during the test.

The next step

- Depending on results, further followups, evaluation, or treatment may be recommended.
- For glaucoma testing, special photography of the optic nerve can be done using a scanning laser ophthalmoscope to measure the nerve tissue and check for problems from eye pressure.

MODIFIED BARIUM SWALLOW

General information

Where It's Done	Who Does It	How Long It Takes	Discomfort/Pain
Radiology clinic or hospital.	Otolaryngologist/ radiologist and speech therapist together.	About 30 minutes to 1 hour depending on findings.	Swallowing the barium is not pleasant.
Results Ready When	**Special Equipment**	**Risks/Complications**	**Average Cost**
Immediately.	Fluoroscopy tube and video screen.	None.	$

Other names Cookie swallow or videofluoroscopy. (Also see chapters 3 and 8.)

Purpose To evaluate the swallowing process for people who are having problems speaking or swallowing food without aspirating it into the windpipe (a variation of the upper gastrointestinal series).

How it works By using a swallowed contrast material which can be seen using X-rays, the physician is able to see all structures involved in swallowing (from the oral cavity to the esophagus) on a video screen while the test is taking place.

Preparation

- You will be asked to refrain from eating or drinking for several hours before the test.
- You undress and don a hospital gown.
- The radiologist or technician will strap you to a table that tilts vertically.
- The fluoroscopic tube, attached to a video monitor, will then be placed to give the examiners the desired view.

Test procedure

- You will be given small amounts of a barium preparation of varying consistencies from thin liquids to paste to a piece of coated cookie.
- Varying the amounts and consistency of the contrast material allows your doctor to determine which types of food are difficult for you to swallow and to locate the structure responsible for the trouble. The fluoroscopic screen allows the physician to view the results as the test takes place.
- The test is usually performed with a speech pathologist present who can assess your swallowing ability and devise a strategy to correct the problem. You may be asked to change your head position, breathing pattern, chewing habits, or the consistency of your food.

After the test You are free to leave and resume normal activities.

Factors affecting results Inability to remain still while the test is performed.

Interpretation The otolaryngologist/radiologist and speech pathologist look directly at a video monitor to see a magnified view of swallowing structures. If possible, they will continue the test with modifications until the abnormality is detected and resolved.

Advantages

- It allows both diagnosis and treatment in some cases.
- It provides a direct view of structures.
- It's relatively painless.
- It's inexpensive.

Disadvantages

- It provides a low level of detail for examining structural damage.
- You must swallow the contrast material, which some people are unable to tolerate.
- You must remain very still during the test.
- The stage of swallowing involving the esophagus is not adequately studied using this method.

The next step

- If the speech pathologist is able to recommend strategies during the test to resolve the problem, no further testing or treatment is needed.
- If test results are not definitive, endoscopy may be recommended.

NASAL ENDOSCOPY

General Information

Where It's Done	Who Does It	How Long It Takes	Discomfort/Pain
Doctor's office or hospital.	Otolaryngologist or allergist.	10–15 minutes.	Possible gag reflex, but this can be alleviated with anesthetic spray.
Results Ready When	**Special Equipment**	**Risks/Complications**	**Average Cost**
Immediately.	Fiber-optic nasal endoscope.	Nosebleed, nasal discomfort, spasms, and cough.	$$

Other names Rhinoscopy, rhinolaryngoscopy, and rhinopharyngoscopy. (Also see chapters 7 and 8.)

Purpose

- To provide direct observation of the nasal passages, larynx, pharynx, and other surrounding structures.
- To help diagnose or delineate problems such as nasal polyps, nasal blockage, recurrent sinusitis, or laryngeal trauma.

How it works

- A flexible fiber-optic tube called an endoscope or a metal telescope is threaded through the nasal passages.

Preparation

- You sit in a comfortable chair with a head support while an anesthetic spray or liquid is applied to your throat area.

Test procedure

- After the area is numb, your doctor threads the endoscope into a nostril and through the nasal passages as far as the vocal cords in the throat.
- The doctor observes internal structures as the endoscope is introduced and withdrawn.

After the test

- Once the endoscope is removed, you may return to most normal activities immediately.
- You should refrain from eating or drinking until your gag reflex returns.

Factors affecting results People with a tendency for nosebleeds may not be able to undergo this test.

Interpretation Direct observation allows immediate assessment of the problem.

Advantages

- It's quick.
- It's safe.
- It's an easy way to view the nasal passages, throat, and vocal cords.

Disadvantages Endoscopy does not provide treatment, only diagnosis.

The next step

- Depending on the findings, surgery or other treatment can usually be recommended.
- A CT scan or MRI may be recommended.

PURE-TONE AUDIOMETRY

General information

Where It's Done	Who Does It	How Long It Takes	Discomfort/Pain
Doctor's office or hospital audiology department.	Audiologist.	30–45 minutes.	None.
Results Ready When	**Special Equipment**	**Risks/Complications**	**Average Cost**
Immediately.	Soundproof testing room, headphones, special headband, and audiometry equipment.	None.	$$

Other names None.

Purpose To diagnose hearing problems that result from such conditions as acoustic trauma, sudden hearing loss, or rock-and-roll deafness.

How it works Your ability to hear tones at different volumes and pitches is measured when the sound is transmitted through bone and through air. A comparison between these two types of conduction can help determine which part of the hearing mechanism is responsible for the loss.

Preparation Your ears are checked to be sure wax is not blocking the ear canal. If so, you will be sent to a doctor for removal of the wax.

Test procedure

- If the test is being performed in a hospital audiometry department, you enter a special soundproof metal room.
- You don headphones and are instructed to raise your hand when you hear a tone.
- Tones (steady or beeping) are played at six different pitches, representing the range of human hearing.
- Each time you raise your hand, the volume is dropped 10 decibels (dB) until you can no longer hear it. The test is repeated in the other ear.
- You remove the headphones and put on a headband with a small plastic rectangle that fits behind your ear and conducts sound to your bone. The tones are repeated.
- If either ear tests poorly with earphones but normally with the bone conduction piece, crossover (the good ear "helping out" the poor ear) is suspected. The good ear will then be covered with a headphone, background masking noise played, and the test resumed.
- To test your ability to discern speech, you will put on the earphones again and listen to and repeat 25 common words.

After the test You are free to leave and resume normal activities.

Factors affecting results Ambient sound when the test is not performed in a soundproof room, as is common in screening tests.

Interpretation The results of audiograms are most often displayed in grid form, showing the amount of hearing loss expressed in decibels at different sound frequencies (also called hertz or Hz). High frequencies correspond to high tones, and low frequencies to low tones. Most audiograms range from around 250 to 4,000 Hz, and normal hearing is considered 0 dB to 20 dB. The failure to pick out any tone of 20 dB or louder indicates a degree of hearing loss. On the speech test, a score of 85% or better is deemed normal.

Advantages It's quick, painless, and accurate.

Disadvantages None.

The next step

- If responses are normal, no additional testing or treatment is needed.
- If the bone test indicates a conductive hearing loss, a tympanogram (see table 18.1) may be recommended.
- An unexplained difference between the two ears in the tone test or the speech segment may warrant a test, called an auditory brain stem response (ABR) or a brain stem evoked response (see chapter 23), to look for an acoustic tumor.

FIBER-OPTIC LARYNGOSCOPY

General information

Where It's Done	Who Does It	How Long It Takes	Discomfort/Pain
Hospital or outpatient surgery clinic.	Surgeon.	About 45 minutes (but you may spend the entire day and possibly the night).	Your throat will be anesthetized, so you should feel no discomfort.

Results Ready When	Special Equipment	Risks/Complications	Average Cost
Immediately unless a lab report is needed. In that case, 3–5 days.	Fiber-optic laryngoscope, X-ray equipment, and video monitor.	There is risk of injury to the mouth and throat structures, but this is relatively rare.	$$$

Other names None.

Purpose

- To locate a mass, such as a polyp or tumor.
- To obtain a tissue sample for laboratory analysis.
- To determine the severity of an already diagnosed malignancy.

How it works A flexible fiber-optic tube is used to directly assess the structures of the oral cavity and throat, and a rigid tube may then be used to obtain the tissue sample. (Also see chapters 7 and 8.)

Preparation

- Several days before the test, you may have a routine chest X-ray, a barium swallow, and a CT scan.
- Avoid taking aspirin and acetaminophen at least two weeks prior to the scheduled procedure. If you are taking a blood-thinning drug such as Coumadin, you may also need to discontinue it.
- You will be asked to refrain from eating or drinking for several hours before the test.

- On the day of the test, you undress and don a hospital gown.
- You may be given general anesthesia, or a topical anesthetic may be sprayed into your throat to numb it and limit the gag reflex.

Test procedure

- The surgeon will use a laryngoscope to examine your mouth and throat.
- A dye called toluidine blue, which stains abnormal cells, may be applied to indicate areas for biopsy.
- If a biopsy is warranted, a rigid scope may be used to help remove the tissue sample.
- Photographs of any suspicious areas may also be taken.

Variation

Panendoscopy encompasses the use of direct laryngoscopy, bronchoscopy, and esophagoscopy in the evaluation of the head and neck–cancer patient.

After the test

- You may be kept for 24-hour observation after a laryngoscopy.
- You should be able to return to normal activities within a few days, although you may have a lingering sore throat and you may cough up blood.
- If you notice an excessive amount of blood or if you develop a high fever or any other signs of infection, call your doctor immediately.

Factors affecting results

Inadequate sample.

Interpretation

The surgeon is able to see the structures directly. Tissue samples are examined by a pathologist.

Advantages

- It allows for direct examination and biopsy in the same procedure.
- It provides quick results.

Disadvantages

- It's invasive.
- It's expensive.

The next step

- The test is considered definitive, and surgery may be recommended.
- If the mass is cancerous, radiation or surgery may be recommended.

FINE-NEEDLE ASPIRATION OF A NECK MASS

General information

Where It's Done	Who Does It	How Long It Takes	Discomfort/Pain
Outpatient surgery clinic or hospital.	Surgeon.	About 1 hour.	Just a needle stick when anesthetic is administered.

Results Ready When	Special Equipment	Risks/Complications	Average Cost
In about 3–5 days.	Large-core needle and imaging equipment.	There is some risk of puncturing other structures in the neck, but this is rare.	$$$

Other names None.

Purpose To test whether a neck mass is malignant or benign.

How it works A sample of the tissue from a neck mass is withdrawn and analyzed in a laboratory.

Preparation

- Before the day of the test, you will have routine preoperative tests as well as imaging tests to determine the exact location of the mass.
- You undress and don a hospital gown.
- You will usually receive a local anesthetic. Since it is important that you remain still during the procedure, you may receive a sedative or general anesthesia if any problems are anticipated.

Test procedure With computed tomography or ultrasound as a guide to find the neck mass, the surgeon uses a large-core needle to withdraw a sample from the mass.

After the test

- The sample is sent to a laboratory for analysis.
- As soon as the anesthesia has worn off and you are able to walk around, you may dress and leave.
- You should arrange to have someone take you home.
- If you experience any excessive pain or bleeding at the site of the biopsy, or a high fever, which could indicate infection, call your physician immediately.

Factors affecting results

- Inadequate sample.
- Moving during the test.

Interpretation The doctor will receive a report from a pathologist indicating whether or not the cells from the sample are cancerous.

Advantages

- It avoids a surgical biopsy.
- It's quick.
- It's relatively inexpensive.

Disadvantages

- It's invasive.
- It may not provide an adequately sized sample.

The next step

- If biopsy sample is not adequate, surgical biopsy may be required.
- If biopsy is sufficient and cells are cancerous, surgery will be recommended.
- If cells are not cancerous, the recommendation of surgery will depend on the size of the mass.

Robert S. Sherwin, MD

19 Diabetes

Tests Covered in This Chapter

The case of Evelyn S., a 31-year-old oncology nurse:

> *Being a nurse, I was aware of the symptoms of diabetes, and I suddenly seemed to have all the classic ones: extreme thirst, increased urination, fatigue, and weight loss. In a short period of time, I dropped about 10 pounds—and not intentionally!*
>
> *Because an uncle of mine had diabetes, we kept a blood glucose meter around the house. I tested my blood and saw that my blood sugar level was over 300 milligrams per deciliter of blood, which is roughly three times the normal level.*
>
> *When I told my doctor this, she had me go to the emergency room immediately. They gave me fluids, did a blood test to confirm that my blood sugar, or glucose, level was indeed elevated, and kept me overnight. The next day I looked better, and my blood sugar had improved, so I went home and saw my regular doctor. In addition to a physical, she performed additional tests.*

The Tests Patients who are as ill as Evelyn routinely have their blood analyzed not only for glucose but also for levels of electrolytes, essential minerals that help maintain the body's balance of fluids. When blood glucose reaches 300 mg/dL, patients frequently lose electrolytes in their urine. This may cause weakness or possibly an irregular heartbeat or other disturbances in the body. Her blood was also tested for fat by-products called ketones. Since insulin greatly suppresses ketone production, a high ketone level often signals a lack of insulin. Because she was severely dehydrated, her kidneys were assessed for damage with blood and urine tests to monitor blood urea nitrogen (BUN) and creatinine.

The Outcome Evelyn's symptoms were so evident, and her blood sugar so high, that the diagnosis was made without any additional tests. She has Type I diabetes, which is typically controlled with insulin. She had always been healthy, so the concept of daily insulin injections came as a shock at first, but she soon adjusted. With nutritional counseling, she has modified her diet and is doing well.

INTRODUCTION

Diabetes mellitus is a disorder in which the body's metabolism of carbohydrates, as well as proteins and fats, is abnormal. It tends to run in families and is caused by a relative or total lack of insulin, a hormone formed in the beta cells of the pancreas. Insulin regulates glucose, the simplest form of sugar and the body's fuel. Depending on the type of diabetes, either the pancreas is unable to release enough insulin into the body or the body stops responding to the insulin appropriately and the pancreas cannot compensate for this resistance.

Without insulin, the body is forced to burn its own fat and muscle for energy, often with devastating consequences. Untreated diabetes can, over many years, damage the blood vessels and nerves and bring about serious complications such as kidney disease, blindness, and heart disease. Diabetes causes 40,000 deaths annually in the United States, the majority of them from heart attack.

TYPES OF DIABETES

Type I Diabetes

Also called insulin-dependent diabetes mellitus and, formerly, juvenile diabetes, Type I diabetes makes up about 5% to 10% of all known cases in the United States. It is the most serious form of diabetes and usually comes on abruptly, set off by an autoimmune attack that ultimately destroys the pancreas's beta cells and results in total insulin deficiency.

Type I diabetes typically develops in childhood or at puberty. It can occur later, but the vast majority of cases are diagnosed before age 30, making Evelyn's case unusual. People with this type of diabetes must have injections of insulin to live. The injections prevent an excessive buildup of glucose (or sugar) and ketones, substances that are generated by the liver from amino acids and fats and released into the bloodstream. Insulin deficiency in its most extreme form leads to a condition known as ketoacidosis or diabetic coma.

Type II Diabetes

Also called non-insulin-dependent diabetes mellitus, Type II diabetes makes up about 90% to 95% of all known cases in the United States. It typically develops after age 40, and although people who have it are often obese, they may have few symptoms or none at all. These people often produce adequate insulin, but they are unable to utilize it. Exercise and diet usually can control Type II diabetes, although some people may need oral antidiabetes drugs or even insulin to correct excess sugar in the blood (hyperglycemia) if diet and exercise are not adequate. Type II diabetes is diagnosed in 6 to 7 million people in the United States—about 2.5% to 3% of the population. Experts estimate that, due to its virtual lack of symptoms, an equal number of cases go undiagnosed.

Sometimes Type II diabetes is a secondary event resulting from another condition, such as a disease of the pancreas or a disorder of the endocrine system. Certain drugs and other chemical agents may also unmask diabetic tendencies. These include some antihypertensive medications, thiazide diuretics, hormones that interfere with carbohydrate processing while relieving inflammation (glucocorticoids), some birth control pills, some drugs used to treat epilepsy (dilantin), certain decongestants, and drugs used to treat low blood pressure (sympathomimetics). In addition, Type II diabetes has been associated with disorders characterized by defective binding of insulin to the tissues upon which it acts, genetic syndromes such as muscular dystrophies or Huntington's chorea, and other miscellaneous conditions such as malnutrition.

Gestational Diabetes

Some women who are not known diabetics develop gestational diabetes mellitus, a form of glucose intolerance or diabetes that occurs during pregnancy. After delivery, the impairment of glucose metabolism usually disappears, but in some cases, it does not. Gestational diabetes most commonly resembles a mild form of Type II diabetes and may require only diet modification. More severe forms may occur, however, and in rare cases, pregnancy may precipitate Type I diabetes.

Even if diabetes disappears after giving birth, if you have diabetes during pregnancy, you are more likely to be prone to it later in life. Gestational diabetes affects about 2% of all pregnant women, usually during the second or third trimester. Within five to ten years, about 30% to 40% of these women develop non-pregnancy-related diabetes mellitus, usually the Type II variety.

Impaired Glucose Tolerance

Impaired glucose tolerance refers to a disorder in which there is a high glucose level in the blood after meals but not enough to be considered diabetes mellitus. About 25% of the people with impaired glucose tolerance eventually develop full-blown Type II diabetes.

Signs and Symptoms of Diabetes Mellitus

The major sign of diabetes mellitus is a high level of sugar in the blood and urine. Classic symptoms include the following:

- Frequent need to urinate.
- Increased thirst.
- Weight loss.
- Increased appetite.
- Impairment of the eyes, kidneys, and nervous system.
- Being prone to infections.
- Accelerated hardening of the arteries that direct blood to the heart, brain, and lower limbs.

Although people with Type II diabetes have less overt symptoms or none at all, they are at risk for chronic complications of diabetes such as atherosclerosis and eye, kidney, and nervous system impairment.

Type II diabetes and impaired glucose tolerance are commonly associated with hypertension, high triglyceride and low HDL ("good") cholesterol levels, and accelerated atherosclerosis. This association is known as syndrome X, Reaven's syndrome, or insulin resistance syndrome. It has been suggested that the common link between these associated disorders is resistance of the body to the action of insulin. Researchers are trying to determine why insulin resistance develops, whether the syndrome can be treated, and whether atherosclerosis can be attenuated by strategies that improve the body's response to insulin.

HOW YOUR DOCTOR DIAGNOSES DIABETES

If you experience any of classic symptoms of diabetes mellitus (see the accompanying box), or if a routine urinalysis or blood test shows excessive sugar in your urine or blood, your doctor will want to test you further for diabetes. For nonpregnant adults, the most accurate diagnostic tool is a simple blood test to determine the level of glucose in your blood when you fast overnight. You can be considered a diabetic *only* if you have a random (nonfasting) plasma glucose level of 200 milligrams per deciliter (mg/dL) of blood or above in addition to symptoms; if you have a fasting plasma glucose level of 140 mg/dL or above on at least two occasions; or if you have a normal fasting glu-

DID YOU KNOW?

When the blood sugar level approaches 200 mg/dL, the kidneys can no longer reabsorb the sugar, which spills into the urine. Sugar is an osmotic agent, meaning it pulls water along with it as it passes out of the body. This is what causes the incessant urination, dehydration, thirst, and weight loss characteristic of diabetes.

cose level but sustained elevated plasma glucose levels (that is, over 200 mg/dL) during an oral glucose tolerance test (see below). Because of the possibility of false-positive test results, a single glucose tolerance test may not always be sufficient to establish a diagnosis.

Your diagnosis may be impaired glucose tolerance if you have normal results (below 140 mg/dL) on a fasting plasma glucose test, but have readings that rise to 200 mg/dL or above then level off to between 140 and 200 mg/dL within two hours during oral glucose tolerance testing. This classification means that your doctor is likely to monitor you because you have a higher than normal risk of developing diabetes and atherosclerotic heart disease in the future.

If you have a history of pregnancy that resulted in stillbirth or in babies that weighed more than 9 pounds at birth, or if you had impaired glucose tolerance in a prior pregnancy, you should be tested for diabetes mellitus, especially if you are planning another pregnancy. If you are already pregnant and a blood glucose test used to screen for gestational diabetes has shown an elevated result, your physician will order an oral glucose tolerance test, taking into consideration that fasting plasma glucose levels tend to fall and post-glucose-load levels tend to rise during a normal pregnancy.

For children, the most appropriate test for diabetes is the fasting glucose level, which, like the adult test, must exceed 140 mg/d L on at least two occasions to confirm a diabetes diagnosis.

Some factors that may adversely affect tests for diabetes mellitus are certain drugs, significant restriction of carbohydrate intake, low potassium levels, stress, and prolonged inactivity. Your doctor will give you a list of drugs that should be discontinued for a few days before testing.

EVALUATION BEFORE THERAPY

Once a diagnosis of diabetes mellitus has been established on the basis of plasma glucose tests, your doctor will want to evaluate you more thoroughly before beginning treatment. In addition to undergoing a routine history and physical examination, including weight and blood pressure measurements, you will be examined and tested for such complications as visual impairment, leg or foot ulcers, skin problems, nerve damage, and vascular disorders. The doctor may order a fasting plasma glucose (if you haven't had one already), a baseline glycosylated hemoglobin, and various tests to check for kidney disease,

TABLE 19.1 Lab Tests to Diagnose and Monitor Diabetes

Test	Description	What Measurement Means	Additional Information
Plasma glucose (sugar) level	A blood test that measures the body's ability to dispose of excess glucose.	Normal range for fasting test is 70–115 mg/dL (increases slightly over age 50). Between 115 and 140 mg/dL indicates impaired glucose tolerance. A measurement of 140 or above on two occasions confirms diagnosis of diabetes. Normal range for 2-hour postmeal test is less than 140 mg/dL. Between 140 and 200 mg/dL indicates impaired glucose tolerance. A measurement of 200 or above on two occasions confirms diagnosis of diabetes.	Fasting test requires at least an 8-hour fast before blood is drawn. Two-hour postmeal (postprandial) test requires that you ingest your usual meal or a physician-prescribed glucose load 2 hours before the test.
Creatinine clearance (24-hour urine collection and single simultaneous blood sample)	Creatinine is a chemical normally found in the blood and excreted in the urine. The filtration function of the kidneys can be assessed by comparing the amount of creatinine in the blood with the amount excreted by the kidneys over 24 hours.	Normal range: child—70–140 mg/dL; adult male—85–125 mg/dL; adult female—75–115 mg/dL. May be increased in the early stages of diabetes, especially in young people. Some people with long-term diabetes may have decreased levels.	Drink water before and throughout the testing time. See chapter 12 for a full description of the 24-hour urine collection procedure.
Glycosylated hemoglobin (also called glycated hemoglobin)	A blood test that reflects the success of glucose control in the diabetic patient over the past 100–120 days. Not normally used for diagnosis.	No good standardization procedures exist, so the normal range varies with the laboratory, but it is usually 4%–8% of total hemoglobin.	Type I diabetic patients are tested about every 3 months; Type II diabetics, every 3–6 months.
Lipid profile	Levels in blood of various lipids (fats)—total cholesterol, high-density lipoprotein cholesterol, low-density lipoprotein cholesterol, and triglycerides—are an indicator of coronary heart disease risk.	Normal values vary according to age and gender (see chapter 4). Higher-than-normal levels of triglyceride and lower-than-normal levels of HDL cholesterol are associated with diabetes mellitus.	Eat a stable diet (not extremely high or low in fat) for 2–3 weeks before test; fast for at least 12 hours before blood is drawn.
Urinary albumin excretion (microalbumin-urea test)	Albumin is one of the proteins that are normally found in blood and play a role in maintaining blood volume. This test is designed to detect subtle changes in the handling of albumin by the kidney, the earliest sign of diabetic kidney disease. Results may be altered by exercise, high blood pressure, or high glucose levels in the absence of kidney disease; thus interpretation may be clouded by other variables.	Normal values are up to 40 mg excreted in 24 hours.	Best done as an overnight collection or as a timed urine collection while activity is minimal.

TABLE 19.2 Selected Tests and Procedures to Evaluate Complications of Diabetes

Test	Use
Autonomic function tests	Examine variations in heart rate with deep breathing or when holding one's breath. Tested with special equipment that analyzes electrocardiogram (see below).
Blood urea nitrogen (BUN)	Evaluates kidney function (see chapters 4 and 12).
Electrocardiography (ECG)	Evaluates heart function, which may be associated with diabetes (see chapter 5).
Fluorescein angiography	Evaluates eye disease associated with diabetes (see chapters 3 and 18).
Nerve conduction tests	Evaluates nerve damage associated with diabetes; also called electromyography (see chapter 23).
Potassium	Evaluates kidney function or hormone balance (see chapters 4 and 12).
Retinal photography	Evaluates eye disease associated with diabetes (see chapter 18).
Thyroxine and TSH measurements	Evaluate other endocrine disorders (see chapter 9).

accelerated heart disease, and other endocrine disorders or potassium deficiency (see tables 19.1 and 19.2 for further descriptions of these tests).

Even if you do not have symptoms, your doctor may recommend a screening test for diabetes mellitus if you have a family history of the disease; are markedly obese; have a history of recurrent skin, genital, or urinary tract infections; or have evidence of premature hardening of the arteries, such as angina, heart attack, stroke, or poor circulation in the legs. The recommended screening test for nonpregnant adults and children is a fasting plasma glucose level. This is a simple blood test following an eight-hour fast (see table 19.1). Use of oral glucose tolerance testing is discouraged for routine screening. During a glucose tolerance test, you drink a glucose solution, and your body's ability to process the sugar is monitored through blood testing (see below for a full description).

If you test positive on a screening test or if you go to your doctor with obvious signs and symptoms of diabetes mellitus—excessive thirst, excessive urination, hunger, and weight loss—he or she will probably schedule you for further diagnostic testing. Also, if a routine urinalysis shows excessive sugar or your blood glucose level is high but not high enough to conclusively diagnose diabetes mellitus, you will undergo diagnostic testing.

Gestational Diabetes Screening

Many doctors recommend that all pregnant women have a blood glucose tolerance test between the 24th and 28th weeks of pregnancy (see chapter 25).

ORAL GLUCOSE TOLERANCE TEST (OGTT)

General information

Where It's Done	Who Does It	How Long It Takes	Discomfort/Pain
Laboratory or doctor's office.	Lab technician or nurse.	2–3 hours; up to 6 hours in rare cases.	Mild discomfort at needle insertion. Glucose solution can be unpalatably sweet.

Results Ready When	Special Equipment	Risks/Complications	Average Cost
Within 1 day.	Needle, blood collecting tubes, and sometimes a vena-access portal.	Bruising from needle sticks, and hypoglycemia (low blood sugar) after test is completed.	$$

Other names Glucose tolerance test.

Purpose

- To detect problems in the body's metabolism of glucose (sugar).
- Most commonly used to diagnose gestational diabetes.
- Also used to diagnose diabetes in people who exhibit symptoms but have high-normal results on blood glucose test.

How it works The pancreas releases insulin into the bloodstream to regulate the body's processing of glucose. By measuring the amount of glucose in the blood after a concentrated amount of glucose is ingested, it is possible to assess how well insulin is functioning.

Preparation

- Eat and exercise normally for three days prior to the test. Be sure to consume sufficient carbohydrates.
- Discontinue medication three days before testing when possible (ask your doctor for a list of drugs to avoid).
- Take nothing but water for ten hours before the test. Avoid smoking before the test.
- Bring reading material or something else to keep you occupied between blood drawings.
- Alert your family and/or employer that the test may last for up to six hours.

Test procedure

- An initial fasting blood sample is drawn from a vein in your arm. Sometimes a vena-access portal is inserted into the vein to provide access without repeated stickings.
- You drink several ounces of glucose solution.
- Blood will be drawn every hour for the duration of the test until your blood glucose level returns to normal. This is usually two hours for

nonpregnant adults and three hours for pregnant women (beginning when you drink the solution), but may in special cases be as long as five or six hours. Sometimes blood is drawn after the first 30 minutes or every 30 minutes.

- You must remain quiet in the testing area for the duration of the test.
- You may drink water but must refrain from eating, drinking coffee, or smoking during the test.
- You may be offered juice or a small snack to break your fast once the test is completed.

After the test

- You may return to normal activities and resume medications immediately.
- If you have discomfort from the needle sticks, you may apply warm compresses to the affected area.
- Although it is rare, some people develop a low blood sugar level about three to five hours after having ingested a large glucose load, so it is advisable to have a small meal immediately after the test.

Factors affecting results

- Failure to maintain normal exercise and dietary habits for three days before the test, especially restricting your carbohydrate intake to less than 150 grams per day.
- Illness.
- Anxiety about needle sticks.
- Smoking or consuming caffeine before or during the test.

Interpretation

- A sustained elevated plasma glucose level (above 200 mg/dL), if you have had a normal fasting glucose level, usually indicates diabetes.
- Results that rise to 200 mg/dL or above after you ingest the glucose, then drop to between 140 and 200 mg/dL after two hours, may indicate impaired glucose tolerance when you have had normal results (below 140 mg/dL) on a fasting glucose test.

Advantages

- It can detect very subtle disturbances in carbohydrate metabolism that are not apparent from a measurement of fasting glucose.
- It's valuable in pregnancy to protect the health and safety of the fetus.

Disadvantages

It may lead to an erroneous diagnosis, especially if the physician fails to take into consideration the many factors that can adversely affect test results.

The next step

- If the test indicates diabetes, treatment can begin.
- If the test has been used to screen, a fasting glucose test should be done or the glucose tolerance test may need to be repeated before diabetes is diagnosed.

- If the diagnosis is gestational diabetes, the condition may be controlled with increased exercise and diet modifications, but insulin treatment may be necessary.
- If the diagnosis is impaired glucose tolerance, your doctor will monitor you for the later development of diabetes by watching for symptoms and scheduling periodic fasting glucose tests. Also, you may be advised to modify your diet or increase physical activity to decrease your risk of developing diabetes or heart disease.

20

John F. Setaro, MD

Hypertension

Tests Covered in This Chapter

The case of Jo-Ann F., 39, a respiratory therapist:

> *I was diagnosed with hypertension a few years ago. I had been getting headaches at work, and I was also retaining fluid—almost overnight I gained 5 pounds, and my fingers got puffy. But it wasn't until I had a sudden nosebleed that I asked one of the physicians I work for to take my blood pressure. It was 200/120. (Normal for an adult is 120/80 millimeters of mercury, or mm Hg.)*
>
> *I'd already had angioplasty twice for clogged coronary arteries. I was afraid that my arteries were obstructed again, but when I went to my cardiologist, he determined that they were clear.*
>
> *Next I saw an endocrinologist, who, after ordering a 24-hour urine study and a thyroid function test, attributed my high blood pressure to stress. Finally, I saw a hypertension specialist, who felt that my history of artery disease warranted a test of my renal arteries for signs of blockage.*

The Tests Jo-Ann had a nuclear medicine scan called a captopril study. The test revealed a near-total blockage in her left renal artery. To confirm the diagnosis, she was given an arteriogram, in which a contrast medium is injected into the renal arteries, which can then be observed on an X-ray screen.

The Outcome Jo-Ann underwent renal angioplasty, in which a tiny balloon inside a catheter is inserted into an artery and inflated to increase the size of the arterial opening. Her blood pressure immediately dropped from 200/120 mm Hg to 120/80 mm Hg.

Unfortunately, her arteries soon reoccluded. Six months later, she underwent a renal artery bypass, in which a little-used vein was taken from near her ankle and surgically attached to the kidney, beyond the blockage—in effect constructing a new left renal artery.

Since her surgery, Jo-Ann's kidneys function normally, and her blood pressure has remained normal without any medication, although she does take a drug to help lower her cholesterol to prevent further artery blockages.

INTRODUCTION

High blood pressure, also referred to as hypertension, affects approximately 50 million Americans, putting them at increased risk of such serious disorders as coronary heart disease, congestive heart failure, stroke, and kidney disease. Most people who suffer from high blood pressure experience no symptoms at all, at least not until their problem is well advanced and has begun to damage their organs. This is what makes hypertension so insidious and gives it the nickname "the silent killer."

High blood pressure is usually discovered during a simple test using an inflatable cuff wrapped around the upper arm and a sphygmomanometer, a gauge that measures pressure. The average blood pressure measurement for a healthy adult is about 120/80 mm Hg (millimeters of mercury, corresponding to the height arterial blood would spurt if it weighed as much as mercury). The first number represents systolic pressure, the amount of pressure in your arteries when blood is pumped into them with each heartbeat. The second number is a measurement of diastolic pressure, the amount of pressure in your arteries between heartbeats, when the heart is at rest. Consistent high blood pressure readings—persistently greater than 140/90 mm Hg or, for people over 60, 160/90 mm Hg—define hypertension.

SIGNS AND SYMPTOMS OF HYPERTENSION

When high blood pressure does produce symptoms, they tend to be related to the organs or organ systems affected by the increased pressure. The most common one is early-morning headaches, usually in the back of the head. Other neurological symptoms may include weakness, vision loss, stroke, or "ministroke" (medically, a transient ischemic attack, or TIA). If the coronary arteries are affected, you may experience chest pain (angina) or difficulty breathing.

Your physician may notice other signs of hypertension-related damage: heart failure, hardening of the peripheral arteries, subtle damage to the blood vessels in the backs of the eyes, kidney failure, fluid buildup (edema) in the lungs, or a bruit (French for "noise"), which is a rushing sound heard in a kidney or other artery, indicating a possible blockage.

TYPES OF HYPERTENSION

Hypertension can be divided into two basic categories. Primary, or essential, hypertension is the diagnosis when the specific cause is currently unknown. The great majority of cases, approximately 90% to 95%, fit into this category. Experts believe that heredity plays a part in this type of high blood pressure. A high-sodium diet, obesity, and constant stress may also contribute to its development. Whatever the cause, there is no known cure. But fortunately, most cases can be kept in control with lifestyle modifications and, if necessary, medication.

Secondary hypertension is defined as high blood pressure caused by another health problem, a diagnosis that accounts for the remaining 5% to 10% of cases. Most secondary hypertension results from disease in the kidneys or the arteries that lead to them. Rarely, it is caused by tumors or other abnormalities of the adrenal glands, which control the balance of water and sodium in the body, or by a hormone imbalance or blood vessel abnormality.

HOW YOUR DOCTOR DIAGNOSES HYPERTENSION

Most cases of hypertension are diagnosed on the basis of medical history, a complete physical exam, a simple blood pressure test, and several basic laboratory tests.

History

The doctor will want to know if anyone in your family has had high blood pressure, premature coronary heart disease, stroke or cerebral hemorrhage, heart failure, kidney disease, diabetes, adrenal gland tumors, or blood lipid (cholesterol) disorders. You will be asked about your own history and symptoms: if you have any indicators of cardiovascular disease such as chest pain, disorders of the blood vessels that supply the brain (cerebrovascular disease), kidney disease, diabetes, elevated cholesterol, and gout; whether you have ever been treated for hypertension; and the details of your therapy. Your doctor will discuss any risk factors such as excess weight, tobacco use, alcohol consumption, sedentary lifestyle, and psychosocial or environmental influences on blood pressure control, such as a stressful workplace or home life. If your symptoms suggest secondary hypertension, those potential causes will be investigated.

The doctor will also ask you about any other medicines you are taking, because some may increase blood pressure or interfere with the effectiveness of medicine used to treat high blood pressure. These medications include female hormone replacements containing both estrogen and progestins, oral contraceptives, adrenal steroids, nonsteroidal anti-inflammatory drugs such as ibuprofen, some nasal decongestants and other cold remedies, appetite suppressants, cyclosporine, and certain drugs used to treat depression and anxiety.

Blood Pressure Measurement

The first step in diagnosis is a simple blood pressure test. For an accurate measurement, you should avoid consuming caffeine and tobacco for at least 30 minutes before the test. After you rest for at least three to five minutes, your doctor or other health care professional will check your blood pressure using a mercury sphygmomanometer with a cuff. The clinician will record both your systolic and diastolic pressure, using a stethoscope to listen for your pulse as the cuff is inflated and then slowly deflated.

The pressure should be checked in both arms. It may also be measured while you stand or lie down. If the first reading is high, the test should be repeated in a few minutes. If the second reading is also high, you will be scheduled for at least two more measurements over the following few weeks. Only if these readings are also high will you be treated for high blood pressure. Even if they are not, your doctor may still want to monitor you over the coming months, keeping in mind the potential for hypertension.

In some cases, the initial blood pressure reading is so high (above 150–160/105–110 mm Hg) that therapy is begun immediately. If the blood pressure measurement is markedly different from arm to arm, your physician may suspect a narrowing in the artery leading to the arm with the lower pressure.

Sometimes blood pressure readings taken in a doctor's office, clinic, or other medical setting are not representative of your normal

Home Blood Pressure Measurement

Taking your blood pressure at home is relatively easy. The blood pressure measuring device is called a sphygmomanometer. Any accurate device must have a cuff with an inflatable bladder that encircles at least two-thirds of your upper arm. The following procedure is for a nonautomatic sphygmomanometer and a stethoscope. With an automatic device, the blood pressure measurement will appear on a digital readout. You can measure your blood pressure alone, but you may find it useful to have assistance at first. Avoid consuming caffeine or tobacco for at least 30 minutes beforehand. Then do the following:

- Sit down with your arm supported, and place the cuff so that its lower edge is 1 inch above the inner crease of your elbow.
- Place the diaphragm of the stethoscope over the brachial artery (found in the crease area).
- Inflate the cuff until the sounds of your pulse disappear.
- Deflate the cuff slowly. The level at which sounds are first heard is the systolic blood pressure. The level at which all sounds, including soft muffled sounds, disappear is the diastolic blood pressure. You should note the time of day of the reading.

It may be useful to bring your home device to your doctor's office to compare blood pressure values, thereby checking the accuracy of the instrument as well as your skill in taking your own blood pressure.

blood pressure. If just being in this environment creates anxiety and stress, you may suffer from so-called white-coat hypertension. If your physician suspects this, you may be asked to monitor your blood pressure at home or work (see the accompanying box). Alternatively, your physician may request a continuous blood pressure recording over 24 hours (ambulatory blood pressure monitoring).

The Physical Exam

After measuring your height and weight, your doctor will examine your eyes with a light (called a funduscopic exam) to check for any hypertension-related damage to the tiny blood vessels in the retina. This is the only way of looking directly at your small blood vessels. The doctor will examine your neck, checking the thyroid gland for enlargement, measuring the pressure in the jugular vein to assess possible heart failure, and listening for bruits that may emanate from partially obstructed carotid arteries leading to the brain.

The doctor will also evaluate your heart for increased rate or size, abnormal rhythms, or unusual sounds. He or she will check your abdomen for bruits; enlarged liver, spleen, or kidneys; other kidney disorders; abnormal masses; or aortic pulsations. Your legs and arms may be examined for weak or absent pulses, bruits, or fluid buildup (edema). A reduction in leg pulse may indicate a narrowing of the aorta (coarctation) in the young, or disease of the outlying blood vessels (peripheral vascular disease) in older people. And finally, you may have a neurologic assessment for evidence of a stroke or nerve damage, especially if you have a history of diabetes or alcoholism.

Additional Testing

Before initiating therapy, your physician will probably recommend some routine tests, including urinalysis, a complete blood count, a fasting blood glucose, and an automated blood chemistry (see table 20.1). An electrocardiogram (ECG) and other tests may be used to help determine the severity of any risk factors for cardiovascular disease and any organ damage that is a result of hypertension. This not only helps define the nature of your treatment and its urgency, but also helps assess risk factors that can be modified to reduce your risk of coronary heart disease. Finally, these studies provide baseline information against which your doctor can judge the effects of treatment.

Some tests that were once a standard part of a hypertension evaluation are no longer recommended as routine, but in rare circumstances may still be necessary. These include chest X-rays (see chapter 7), intravenous pyelography (see chapter 12), and plasma renin activity studies (see below). An ambulatory measurement of blood pressure may be helpful in some cases—providing information about your blood pressure during daily activities—but is often unnecessary and may not be as useful because most of what is known about hypertension is based on office readings.

TABLE 20.1 Blood Tests: Markers for Hypertension

As part of a routine physical, your physician will likely take a sample of your blood for a complete blood count, measuring hemoglobin and hematocrit (see chapter 4 for more information). This information may be useful in diagnosing hypertension and determining secondary causes. In addition, the doctor may order an automated blood chemistry analysis to check the components listed below.

Blood Component	Meaning of Abnormal Value or Result
Calcium	An excess of calcium in the blood can result from a parathyroid gland disorder, which can cause hypertension.
Cholesterol (total)	May indicate increased general cardiovascular risk.
Creatinine	Can be a signal of kidney failure, which can cause hypertension.
Glucose (fasting)	May indicate that hypertension is caused by diabetes, a tumor of the adrenal gland, or overactive thyroid or adrenal glands. Abnormal results can also indicate a treatment-related alteration.
Phosphates	Closely linked with abnormal calcium level.
Potassium	May indicate a treatment-related alteration, or an excess of aldosterone.
Sodium	May indicate a treatment-related alteration.
Urea nitrogen	Can be a signal that hypertension is caused by kidney failure.
Uric acid	May indicate a treatment-related alteration that could aggravate a condition such as gout.

TESTS TO DETERMINE THE CAUSES OF HYPERTENSION

For many people, especially those in the most common age group for hypertension, the tests discussed above will be sufficient to diagnose and treat high blood pressure. This condition is uncommon in those under 15 and not likely to develop for the first time in those over 60. People with hypertension who fall into these groups and those who have symptoms characteristic of other diseases may be advised to undergo more sophisticated tests. Even though secondary hypertension is unusual, your health care team may investigate this possibility further in hopes of finding a reversible cause. Additional tests might also be advised when treatment does not control hypertension or when previously well-controlled hypertension becomes suddenly resistant to treatment.

If kidney disease is suspected, your doctor may order plasma renin activity (PRA) tests and/or a captopril renal scan (see below). If these tests prove inconclusive or suggest the possibility of a kidney disorder, arteriography would be the next step (see chapter 4). In the case of potential thyroid gland disorders, your physician would order thyroid function tests, while the overproduction of the adrenal gland's glucocorticoid hormone would be investigated via a plasma cortisol and dexamethasone suppression test (see chapter 9).

In some cases, the adrenal gland or other glandular tissue causes hypertension by producing too much of the hormone adrenalin (epinephrine). A 24-hour urine study (see chapter 12) may be ordered to

TABLE 20.2 Urine Tests and Hypertension

Urine Component	Meaning of Abnormal Value or Result
Certain adrenal gland horomones that can raise blood pressure (catecholamines)	Increased level could cause your doctor to suspect an adrenal gland tumor.
Protein	Presence of protein in the urine suggests some types of kidney disease as causes of hypertension.
Red blood cells and white blood cells	Can indicate infections or inflammatory diseases of the kidney that could be responsible for kidney failure or hypertension.

determine if levels are elevated, and if so, a CT scan or MRI scan may be recommended to find the source of the hormone. The problem with these scans is that they sometimes identify innocent masses, so your doctor may prefer a more specific test called an MIBG (meta-iodo-benzyl-guanidine) radioisotope scan (see chapter 4 for more information).

Your physician may also order additional blood and urine studies to see if your body is producing the adrenal gland's stress hormone, aldosterone, in excess (see chapter 4 and table 20.2). Too much aldosterone can cause the body to retain sodium and water, which can cause hypertension.

PLASMA RENIN ACTIVITY (PRA) TESTS

General information

Where It's Done	Who Does It	How Long It Takes	Discomfort/Pain
Hospital, doctor's office, or hospital surgical unit.	Lab technician, nurse, or doctor.	45 minutes for catheter test; 5–10 minutes for blood test.	Mild discomfort from needle insertion.
Results Ready When	**Special Equipment**	**Risks/Complications**	**Average Cost**
Within a few days.	For blood test: needle, syringe, and collecting tubes. For catheter test: needle, catheter, and fluoroscope.	For blood test: none. For catheter test: there is some risk of leakage from the vein in the leg.	$ (for blood test) $$$ (for catheter test)

Other names Renal vein renins.

Purpose To help determine the cause of hypertension in cases where signs of kidney disease are present.

How it works The test determines whether the kidneys are producing too much renin, an enzyme that can raise blood pressure. It may be a simple blood test or a catheterization procedure.

Preparation

- Do not eat licorice or salt your food for two days before the test.
- Your doctor will inform you of any medications that you must discontinue before the test. These may include diuretics, antihypertensives, vasodilators, and oral contraceptives, and you may have to stop taking them for as much as a month prior to testing.
- For the blood test, you will only have to roll up your sleeve.
- For the catheter test, you will disrobe and don a surgical gown. You may have to stand, sit, or lie down for as long as two hours before the test.

Test procedure

- For the blood test, a tourniquet or blood pressure cuff is wrapped around your upper arm, the vein is punctured, and blood is drawn and sent to a laboratory for analysis.
- For the catheter test, a local anesthetic may be applied to the groin area. A catheter is then passed into the femoral vein and threaded toward the kidneys under X-ray or fluoroscopic guidance.
- Blood samples are collected from the kidney vessels and the vena cava, the catheter is removed, and the samples are sent to a laboratory for analysis.

After the test

- After either procedure, pressure will be applied to the puncture site until the bleeding has stopped. This may last for ten to 20 minutes after the catheter procedure.
- If there is any discomfort, you can apply moist, warm compresses to the puncture site every two to four hours. You can return to normal activities and resume taking medications immediately.
- If you see blood in your urine or experience back pain, call your physician immediately.

Factors affecting results

- Not following dietary restrictions before the test.
- Taking medication that interferes with the test.

Interpretation

Test results are determined by radioimmunoassay. If the values are higher than normal, your hypertension may be caused by a disorder of the kidneys. If test results show lower-than-normal values, your hypertension may be primary and have no specific cause, or it may stem from overproduction of the hormone aldosterone. If you are being treated with sodium-retaining drugs, this might also cause the lower values.

Advantages

- The blood test is easy and relatively noninvasive.
- The catheter test gives specific information about the kidneys.

Disadvantages

The catheter test is an invasive, somewhat uncomfortable procedure and may be associated with slight bleeding complications.

The next step

- If the results are high, your doctor may recommend an imaging test, such as a captopril renal scan or arteriography.
- If the results are low and other test results normal, no further testing is necessary and treatment may begin or be continued.

RENAL SCAN

General information

Where It's Done	Who Does It	How Long It Takes	Discomfort/Pain
Hospital radiology suite or office of radiologist.	Radiology technician and physician.	About 4–5 hours.	Minor discomfort of injection and line insertion. Lying still for substantial period may cause numbness. Possible flush, burning sensation, or slight nausea during isotope injection
Results Ready When	**Special Equipment**	**Risks/Complications**	**Average Cost**
A few minutes to a few days.	An IV set, the radioisotope, a gamma scintillation camera, and an oscilloscope.	In rare cases, there may be renal system impairment and decreased urine output, but these are usually reversible.	$$$

Other names Renal scintigram or captopril renal scan.

Purpose To evaluate blood flow to the kidneys to help detect any narrowing or blockage of the renal artery.

How it works When blood flow to the kidneys is reduced, the kidneys attempt to improve their blood supply by producing angiotensin, which raises blood pressure and helps maintain their filtration function. In this test, an initial scan is followed by administration of the drug captopril, which suppresses angiotensin production. If a second scan shows a decrease in kidney function, it suggests that angiotensin had been at work as a result of a blockage. No change in function after administering captopril suggests that the renal arteries are not constricted and therefore that the kidneys are not dependent on angiotensin.

Preparation

- Your doctor may have you discontinue certain medications in the captopril family for several days prior to the test to improve the accuracy of the test.
- You disrobe and don a hospital gown.

Test procedure

- You will receive an injection of a very small quantity of a short-acting radioactive compound (less than the amount of radiation in two chest X-rays) into a vein, usually in your arm.
- You will lie still while a gamma scintillation camera or scanner detects the rays emitted by the radioactive dye. These rays are converted into a video image, and photographs or videotape of that image are taken over about a 20-minute period.
- Three hours later, you will be given a captopril tablet. After another hour, the process will be repeated, providing the same images as before to show any differences caused by the captopril.

After the test

- You will return immediately to normal activities.
- The radioisotope is excreted within about 24 hours. During that time, you should flush the toilet immediately after you urinate to limit your exposure.

Factors affecting results

If you move during the scan, the images may be inaccurate.

Interpretation

If there is a decrease in kidney filtration (as measured by changes in dye uptake by the kidney) on the scan after the captopril is given compared to the initial scan, there may be a renal artery blockage. If no decrease is present after the captopril is given, filtration is not under the influence of angiotensin, and it is likely that no renal artery blockage exists.

Advantages

This is a relatively noninvasive way of screening for renal artery blockage.

Disadvantages

- It's simply a screening procedure.
- It does not provide a specific image of the blood vessel.
- Any captopril family drug must be discontinued several days before the test.

The next step

- A positive test indicates a 90% chance that you have a blockage. Your physician will probably recommend renal arteriography (see chapter 3) for an actual view of the blockage.
- A negative test indicates a 90% chance that a renal artery blockage is *not* the cause of hypertension. In this case, you would be treated for primary hypertension with appropropriate drug therapy.

Michael O. Rigsby, MD ■ *Gerald Friedland, MD*

21 Human Immunodeficiency Virus (HIV) and Acquired Immunodeficiency Syndrome (AIDS)

Tests Covered in This Chapter

The case of Michelle W., 33, a single mother of a 6-year-old daughter:

Although I had no symptoms of the HIV virus, had never used intravenous drugs or had a blood transfusion, all the news about AIDS convinced me that no one was completely safe. Three years earlier, I had ended a difficult, five-year relationship. I was monogamous, but I never really knew what my partner was doing. If I were HIV positive—which I seriously doubted—I didn't want to give the virus unknowingly to someone else. So during my annual checkup, I asked my internist for an HIV test. My biggest worry was about my daughter. If I were HIV positive, would she have it too? How would I take care of both of us?

The Tests After Michelle received counseling, her blood was tested for antibodies against the human immunodeficiency virus (HIV), the virus responsible for AIDS. When the first ELISA test was positive, it was repeated and followed by a Western blot test in order to confirm that the results were accurate. Once Michelle was diagnosed, she underwent other tests to gauge the extent of the disease: X-rays of her lungs, a skin test for tuberculosis, and blood tests to detect signs of syphilis, viral hepatitis, and toxoplasmosis, a parasitic infection that causes abscesses of the brain. These diseases are called opportunistic infections—illnesses that occur most commonly in people with decreased immunity and the inability to fight infections.

The Outcome Although Michelle was HIV positive, she was healthy and her tests did not indicate any opportunistic infections. Based on the stage of her infection, Michelle's doctor prescribed didanosine (ddI) and zidovudine (AZT) to reduce the amount of virus in the body and delay the development of full-blown AIDS. She received counseling on ways to minimize the effects of the virus through diet, rest, exercise, and stress reduction, and she has joined a support group for HIV-positive women. She returns periodically for a physical exam to check for symptoms of infection, and blood tests to monitor the effects of the medication. Much to Michelle's relief, her daughter has tested negative.

INTRODUCTION

The human immunodeficiency virus, or HIV, is an infectious organism that invades cells of the immune system. People may live for many years after being infected with HIV, but the virus gradually destroys crucial elements of their immunity. The last and most devastating stage of HIV infection is the disease known as acquired immunodeficiency syndrome, or AIDS. People with AIDS eventually die of infections or other ailments because their failing immune system cannot mount a resistance against disease. At present, there is no cure for AIDS, but drugs are available that greatly reduce the amount of virus in the body and delay the progression of infection. Many of the infections and other diseases that result from HIV infection can also be treated effectively.

Transmission

HIV can be transmitted when an infected person has sex (especially vaginal or anal intercourse) or shares a hypodermic needle to inject drugs. An infected woman can pass the virus to her baby during pregnancy or breast-feeding. HIV infection can also result from the transfusion of blood contaminated with the virus, although now all blood donors are tested, and blood from infected donors is disposed of or used for laboratory research only.

Infection requires fairly large amounts of the virus and direct exchange of body fluids. People who have their blood or other fluids drawn for medical purposes using disposable needles are at no risk of infection. Nor is there a risk of contracting HIV by donating blood; through household contacts, including sharing dishes or towels; or via mosquito bites.

After entering the body, HIV inserts its genes into the genetic material of cells and uses the cell's machinery to make new copies of the virus. HIV may live in the body for many years without causing obvious damage, but gradually it destroys the infected cells. Its primary targets are immune cells known as helper T cells, or CD4 cells, which are an important part of the body's immune system.

Definition of AIDS

As the number of CD4 cells in the blood drops, the immune system deteriorates. Since the decline is gradual, the point at which a person is considered to have AIDS can be defined in different ways. The term "HIV-positive" refers to anyone who is infected with the virus. However, "AIDS" refers only to the clinical condition that is the most advanced stage of HIV infection. According to the latest definition from the Centers for Disease Control and Prevention (CDC), a person infected with HIV is considered to have AIDS when he or she develops one of the 26 opportunistic infections or conditions that characterize the syndrome, or has a CD4 concentration below 200 cells per microliter of blood, even in the absence of any of these infections.

The Course of HIV Infection

HIV infection typically has the following four stages (see also table 21.1):

1. *Initial infection.* Possible flulike illness (fever, joint and muscle aches, and sometimes a skin rash or hives) within two to six weeks of infection. In rare cases, infections that usually affect patients with impaired immunity may develop, last up to two weeks, and disappear. CD4 count may drop temporarily, then return to normal.
2. *Symptom-free stage.* The infected person is symptom-free for anywhere from two to ten years or even longer. (Some people have swollen lymph nodes in the neck and armpits.) However, the CD4 count is slowly falling, from the normal level of about 1,000 cells in a microliter of blood to about 500.
3. *Early symptoms.* Most people first experience symptoms (fatigue, weight loss, fever, night sweats, and unexplained diarrhea) when the CD4 count falls below 500. They may have various infections, including vaginitis, bacterial pneumonia, shingles, and oral thrush (a fungal infection), as well as seborrheic dermatitis, characterized by oily, scaly skin, or a blood disease called immune thrombocytopenic purpura (ITP).
4. *Full-blown AIDS.* Within ten years, about half of infected people develop full-blown AIDS. They usually have CD4 cell counts of less than 200, and their symptoms become more severe. One common sign is wasting, characterized by weakness and severe weight loss, sometimes accompanied by persistent diarrhea. Opportunistic infections, such as *Pneumocystis carinii* pneumonia, begin to occur. Women with AIDS are also prone to cervical cancer,

TABLE 21.1 The Course of HIV Infection in Adults

Average Time in Relation to Infection or Diagnosis	Symptoms and Characteristic Disorders	CD4 Cell Count (average number of cells in a microliter of blood)
When infection occurs	None.	Normal (approximately 1,000).
2–4 weeks after infection	Minor flulike illness: fever, joint and muscle aches, abdominal cramps and diarrhea; sometimes, skin rash or hives.	Temporary drop.
6–12 weeks after infection	None (antibodies to the virus appear in blood).	Normal.
0–10 years after infection	None (some people may have swollen lymph nodes).	Gradual decline, 50–80 a year on average.
4–10 years after infection	Early symptoms, formerly referred to as AIDS-related complex, or ARC: fatigue, weight loss, fever, night sweats, unexplained diarrhea, skin problems, blood diseases, and various infections, including oral thrush, vaginitis, bacterial pneumonia, and shingles.	50–300.
6–10 years after infection	AIDS: *Pneumocystis carinii* pneumonia, wasting, Kaposi's sarcoma, AIDS-related dementia, lymphoma, cryptococcal meningitis, CMV, TB, etc.	Less than 200.
6–24 months after diagnosis of AIDS	Death.	Less than 50.

Adapted from John G. Bartlett, MD, *1992–1993 Recommendations for the Medical Care of Persons with HIV Infection, A Guide to HIV Care from the AIDS Care Program of The Johns Hopkins Medical Institutions.* Published by Critical Care America.

while both sexes are prone to cancers of the lymphatic system, particularly non-Hodgkin's lymphoma, and to Kaposi's sarcoma.

HOW YOUR DOCTOR DIAGNOSES HIV

HIV testing is meant only for people at risk of having the infection. To help determine if you should be tested, your doctor or a counselor will likely ask about any behavior that may have put you at risk.

- Have you ever engaged in unprotected intercourse with a partner whose HIV status is unknown to you or who is in a risk group for HIV—for instance, gay or bisexual men and intravenous drug users?
- Have you injected drugs and shared a needle with other people?
- Did you receive a blood transfusion before March 1985, when the blood supply began being tested for HIV? (See the accompanying box.)

If you have even the slightest possibility of infection, you should find out your HIV status to make sure that you are not spreading the

Screening the Blood Supply

Since March 1985, all the blood used for transfusions in the United States has been screened for HIV. People at a high risk of being infected with the virus are discouraged from donating blood, and every unit of blood that is donated is tested for HIV-1 (the strain of the AIDS virus prevalent in the U.S.) and HIV-2 (the strain prevalent in parts of Africa). The two ELISA tests detect virtually all infected units of blood. However, in an extremely small number of cases, screening tests may produce false-negative results. This is believed to occur in less than one in every 500,000 units of blood tested. Sometimes the false-negative result occurs because the donor was infected so recently that antibodies had not yet developed. For this reason, a second type of test, which detects the virus itself rather than antibodies to the virus, has been recently added to the screening process. Although this is expected to reduce the risk even further, you can avoid even the remotest risk by arranging to donate your own blood in advance if you expect to undergo surgery in which you may need a blood transfusion (this is called an autologous blood transfusion).

virus, and because early detection grants a chance for a better and longer life through the use of drugs that fight opportunistic infections.

The common commercial tests for HIV detect the presence of antibodies against the virus in the blood. These antibodies are proteins produced by the body's immune system in response to the HIV invader. Although the majority of people infected will develop antibodies within five months, a test performed too soon after infection may fail to detect antibodies.

PATIENT TIP

Sometimes tests for HIV infections give ambiguous or "indeterminate" results. One of the causes may be a recent vaccination for influenza or tetanus. If you have an indeterminate result, wait two or three months to have the test repeated.

The test most commonly used to screen people for HIV infection is the ELISA (enzyme-linked immunosorbent assay). This test is very effective in detecting antibodies, but it can produce false-positive results—that is, it may sound a false alarm when no infection is present. Therefore, whenever the initial test is positive, it is usually repeated and then a more accurate (but more expensive and time-consuming) test, called Western blot, is also performed.

In the rare cases when the diagnosis remains uncertain, the Western blot is repeated, or your doctor may order a test known as polymerase chain reaction (also called PCR), which detects the virus itself. Testing may be repeated in three to six months.

Confidentiality

The highest level of confidentiality is available at anonymous testing sites (ATSs), where blood samples are labeled by codes. If the test is conducted at a hospital or in another setting that precludes anonymity, the law usually prohibits disclosure of results to anyone but the individual being tested. Most states have confidentiality laws to this

DID YOU KNOW?

In other parts of the world, the pattern of HIV transmission differs from that in the United States. In Africa, where the largest number of AIDS cases is believed to have occurred, most people become infected through heterosexual intercourse. This may be due to the prevalence of other sexually transmitted diseases that produce open sores on the genitals that make it easier for the virus to enter the body. HIV infection in Africa is as common in women as in men, whereas in the United States, men infected with HIV have outnumbered women, but this is changing with the rise in infection among intravenous drug users.

effect, as well as an informed-consent law, which makes it illegal to test a blood sample for HIV infection without consent. (See the accompanying box on where to get tested for HIV.) If the patient has health insurance, the test is recorded only as blood work, and the results are not reported.

Because of the grim prognosis of AIDS, as well as the stigma and potential discrimination that a positive diagnosis may carry, many people experience profound anxiety before the test and while awaiting results. People who test positive for the virus often experience depression or a feeling akin to mourning. For this reason, many states require that people who want to be tested see a counselor before the test and when the results are given, even if they are negative.

If your HIV infection is confirmed, your doctor may order other tests, depending on your symptoms (if any) to monitor your immune status and diagnose cancers and opportunistic infections. These may include X rays, sputum cultures, blood tests for syphilis and hepatitis, and skin tests.

Where to Get Tested for HIV

If you decide to have an HIV test, consider the date of your last potential exposure. If it was within three months, the infection may be missed. If you have had a single potential exposure, it would probably be best to wait two to three months before being tested. You can be very sure that a negative test six months or more after your last potential exposure means that you are not infected with HIV.

For completely anonymous testing, look for an anonymous testing site, or ATS; these are available in most states and provide free or low-cost testing. For locations, call the nearest AIDS support group, your local health department, or the hot-line run by the Centers for Disease Control and Prevention, (800) 342-AIDS.

You can also be tested for HIV at a doctor's office, hospital, or commercial laboratory, in which case you will have to rely on the test site to abide by the rules of confidentiality.

If you may have been exposed to HIV in Africa, you should also be tested for HIV-2, the strain of the virus that is prevalent there. To locate a site that performs this test, call the CDC hot-line mentioned above or have your doctor call the CDC laboratory research branch at (404) 639–3174.

Before going in for testing, ask whether the facility provides counseling or a referral to counseling. Most centers check all positive results twice, with a repeat ELISA followed by a Western blot, but it is wise to confirm this.

ENZYME-LINKED IMMUNOSORBENT ASSAY (ELISA) FOR HIV

General information

Where It's Done	Who Does It	How Long It Takes	Discomfort/Pain
Doctor's office, hospital, laboratory, or anonymous testing site (ATS).	Doctor, nurse, or lab technician.	Less than 5 minutes for drawing blood.	Minor discomfort associated with drawing blood.
Results Ready When	**Special Equipment**	**Risks/Complications**	**Average Cost**
2–14 days.	Supplies for drawing blood.	Negligible.	$

Other names Blood test for AIDS, AIDS screening, HIV antibody test, AIDS or HIV serology, and serologic testing for AIDS. (Also see chapter 14.)

Purpose To detect the presence of HIV infection and to screen blood for use in transfusion.

How it works When the body is infected with a virus, the immune system responds by producing antibodies—proteins that circulate in the blood and attempt to destroy the virus. If antibodies against HIV are present in a blood sample, they will stick to a plate coated with fragments of the virus. The ELISA reagent will detect the presence of the bound antibodies and will change color, denoting a positive result.

Preparation You will receive counseling about the test and possible results.

Test procedure A sample of blood is drawn from a vein in your arm. In the lab, ELISA technology (see chapter 4) is used to analyze for HIV antibodies in the blood serum.

After the test You will follow venous blood-drawing procedures (see chapter 4).

Factors affecting results A test performed too soon after exposure may fail to detect the infection because antibodies have not yet developed.

Interpretation A color change on the ELISA plate indicates the presence of HIV antibodies, and thus the presence of HIV infection.

Advantages

- It's faster, less expensive, and easier to perform than other blood tests for HIV infection, which makes it suitable for screening.
- It detects more than 99% of HIV infections.

Disadvantages

- It produces false-positive results in two out of 1,000 cases.

- It cannot detect HIV infection until antibodies develop, which may take six to 24 weeks from exposure.

The next step

- If results are negative, repeat test at three and six months if potential exposure was recent; otherwise, repeat only if you suspect subsequent exposure.
- If results are positive, confirm by repeat ELISA test, followed by Western blot.

WESTERN BLOT FOR AIDS

General information

Where It's Done	Who Does It	How Long It Takes	Discomfort/Pain
Doctor's office, hospital, laboratory, or anonymous testing site (ATS).	Doctor, nurse, or lab technician.	Less than 5 minutes for drawing blood.	Minor discomfort associated with drawing blood.
Results Ready When	**Special Equipment**	**Risks/Complications**	**Average Cost**
2–14 days.	Supplies for drawing blood.	Negligible.	$$

Other names Blood test for AIDS, HIV antibody test, AIDS or HIV serology, serologic testing for AIDS.

Purpose To confirm an HIV infection previously detected by ELISA.

How it works When the body is infected with a virus, the immune system responds by producing antibodies—proteins that circulate in the blood and attempt to destroy the virus. Exposing a blood sample to a special paper impregnated with selected virus fragments will cause any antibodies present to bind to the virus and produce a characteristic pattern.

Preparation You will receive counseling about the test and possible results.

Test procedure A sample of blood is drawn from a vein in your arm. In the lab, Western blot technology is used to analyze for HIV antibodies in the blood serum.

After the test You will follow venous blood-drawing procedures (see chapter 4).

Factors affecting results A test performed too soon after exposure may fail to detect the infection because antibodies have not yet developed.

Interpretation

- The appearance of the characteristic pattern, or blot, confirms the presence of the HIV virus.
- In rare cases, results are ambiguous: antibodies are bound to some fragments of the virus but not others. The test will then be repeated, but in people at low risk, it will usually be negative.

Advantages

- It definitively confirms or rules out HIV infection.
- It detects at least 96% of HIV infections.
- It produces very few false-positive results.

Disadvantages

- It's more expensive, complex, and time-consuming than ELISA, making it inappropriate for screening.
- It cannot detect HIV infection until antibodies develop, which may take six to 24 weeks after exposure.
- In rare cases, it may produce ambiguous results.

The next step

- If results are negative, repeat ELISA test at three and six months if potential exposure was recent; otherwise, repeat only if you suspect subsequent exposure.
- If results are positive, your doctor will recommend additional tests and possibly drug therapy.

CD4 COUNT

General information

Where It's Done	Who Does It	How Long It Takes	Discomfort/Pain
Doctor's office, hospital, commercial laboratory, or clinic.	Doctor, nurse, or lab technician.	Less than 5 minutes for drawing blood.	Minor discomfort associated with drawing blood.
Results Ready When	**Special Equipment**	**Risks/Complications**	**Average Cost**
7–14 days.	Supplies for drawing blood.	Negligible.	$$

Other names T-cell assay, studies, or analysis.

Purpose

- To establish the stage of HIV infection.
- To make treatment decisions and monitor the effects of treatment.

How it works

- CD4 cells are part of the body's defense against infection. Their numbers decline throughout the course of HIV infection, as the immune system becomes overwhelmed.

- Counting the CD4 cells in a blood sample by using monoclonal antibody technology and flow cytometry (see chapter 4) indicates the stage of infection.

Preparation None.

Test procedure

- Blood is drawn from a vein in your arm, and the concentration of CD4 cells in the sample is measured.
- Levels of other types of immune cells and the total number of lymphocytes may also be measured.

After the test You will follow venous blood-drawing procedures (see chapter 4).

Factors affecting results

- Illnesses.
- Antiviral, steroid, immunosuppressive, or other drugs.
- The type of cell-counting method used by the lab.

Interpretation A normal CD4 level is about 1,000 cells in a microliter of blood, or more than 20% of total lymphocytes. Some labs also report the ratio of CD4 to CD8 cells. A normal ratio is greater than 1—in other words, more CD4 than CD8 cells.

Advantages It reflects the disease process better than any other current laboratory measurement.

Disadvantages

- CD4 counts vary from hour to hour and must be evaluated in the context of symptoms. Even if they are higher than 200, the presence of symptoms indicates immunosuppression.
- There is no perfect correlation between CD4 cell count and the stage of HIV infection.

The next step Test will be repeated every four to six months to track the infection and predict its course (see table 21.1 above).

VIRAL LOAD TEST

General information

Where It's Done	Who Does It	How Long It Takes	Discomfort/Pain
Doctor's office, hospital, or laboratory.	Doctor, nurse, or lab technician.	Less than 5 minutes for drawing blood.	Minor discomfort associated with drawing blood.

Results Ready When	Special Equipment	Risks/Complications	Average Cost
7–14 days.	Supplies for drawing blood.	Negligible.	$$

Other names HIV-RNA PCR, HIV bDNA assay, viral burden.

Purpose To measure the amount of HIV in the blood stream, which helps to:

- Establish the stage of HIV infection.
- Determine when to begin anti-HIV medications.
- Monitor the effect of therapy.

How it works Throughout the course of HIV infection, the virus is present in the blood. The amount of virus in the blood is an important indicator of how fast a person is likely to develop complications from infection. The genetic material of the virus (RNA) can be measured using PCR or a technology known as branched-DNA (bDNA) assay. The two methods produce similar results.

Preparation You will receive counseling about the test and possible results.

Test procedure A sample of blood is drawn from a vein in your arm. In the lab, PCR or bDNA technology is used to measure the number of viral particles per milliliter (mL) of blood plasma.

After the test You will follow the venous blood drawing procedures (see chapter 4).

Factors affecting results The viral load is relatively stable over time but will fall rapidly after the patient starts taking effective medications. Other illnesses and some vaccinations will temporarily increase the viral load.

Interpretation The results are expressed as copies (of viral RNA) per mL of plasma. The higher the number, the greater the risk of disease progression, so the test can be used to identify patients most likely to benefit from treatment against HIV. Once treatment is started, the viral load test can be used to monitor how effective the treatment is. The lower the viral load, the better. Results range from "undetectable" (usually a few hundred copies per mL) to over a million copies per mL.

Advantages

- It's a very important and accurate test for predicting the risk of disease progression.
- It's the best test for predicting the efficacy of a particular treatment regimen in an individual patient.

Disadvantages It does not reflect the extent of existing damage to the immune system, so it must be used in conjunction with the CD4 cell count.

The next step The test may be repeated approximately every six months to monitor the course of the disease or the therapy.

22

Vincent Quagliarello, MD

Infectious Diseases

Tests Covered in This Chapter

The case of Jack T., 52, owner of a food-brokerage company:

> *Almost 20 years ago I broke my ankle during a softball game. The fracture was so severe, I had to have a stainless-steel plate implanted in the ankle. Through the years, arthritis set in, and the joint degenerated. I began having inflammation and pain, and in attempt to avoid surgery to fuse the ankle, I started having cortisone shots. The first two shots gave me months of being pain-free. Then my ankle really started hurting again, and it got so bad that I couldn't walk.*
>
> *The third shot was no help. My ankle swelled to five times its normal size, and the pain was intolerable. I went to see the doctor right away. One look and he said, "I hope this isn't an infection."*

The Tests Jack's doctor immediately ordered a blood culture and aspirated fluid from the ankle joint. Initially, the blood culture showed that the infection had not yet traveled into the bloodstream. Next, a bone scan was done to see if the infection had migrated from the joint space into the bone itself. For the bone scan, a radioisotope was injected into a vein, and X-rays of the leg and ankle were obtained (see chapters 3 and 13).

The Outcome The laboratory analysis of the fluid revealed an infection caused by *Staphylococcus aureus*, a normally harmless bacterium found on the skin that can enter your body through a cut or scratch. In most instances, your body's immune system clears up the infection, but if you have a steel plate such as Jack had, an artificial heart valve, or another foreign body, the infection can become serious.

By the time the bacterium was identified, the infection had entered the bloodstream and was raging throughout Jack's body, necessitating emergency treatment. The plate in his ankle had to be surgically removed. He was put on an intravenous antibiotic and remained hospitalized for eight days, during which time he ran a high fever. He continued on the IV at home, then switched to oral penicillin derivative (oxacilin) for several months before the infection was finally was cleared up completely.

INTRODUCTION

Infectious diseases are the world's leading cause of death. In the United States, where they have been on the wane since early in this century, they are on the rise again. A recent study from the Centers for Disease Control and Prevention shows an almost 40% increase in deaths from infectious diseases between 1980 and 1992. Although AIDS accounts for the majority of these deaths, fatal respiratory tract infections and septicemia (blood poisoning) have shown significant increases. Nevertheless, the vast majority of infections encountered in this country are relatively innocuous and either resolve on their own or are easily treated.

Respiratory tract infections are by far the most common infectious diseases—virtually all of us have suffered the common cold. But infections invade every organ system in the body, including the joints (Lyme disease), the heart (infective endocarditis), the nervous system (meningitis), and the skin (athlete's foot).

Infections occur when tiny, living entities, called microorganisms, attack a vulnerable host, such as a human being. These foreign invaders produce varying levels of infection based on their ability to upset the body's natural balance. Often our bodies are able to heal on their own. Symptoms such as fever, pus, and inflammation indicate the body's attempts to overpower the infection. But sometimes doctors need to find out what is causing the infection in order to offer appropriate treatment and limit our exposure to the offending organism in the future.

There are thousands of infectious agents—bacteria, viruses, fungi, and others—in our environment. It is nearly impossible to avoid them and still live an active, productive life. In fact, some of the bacteria and fungi that cause infections, as well as many that do not, are already present in the body and normally play a beneficial role in its healthy equilibrium.

TYPES OF INFECTIOUS AGENTS

Bacteria are one-celled organisms that are grouped according to shape: Cocci are round, bacilli are rod-shaped, and spirochetes look like spirals or corkscrews. Bacteria may also be classified according to whether they require oxygen to stay alive (aerobic) or can live and grow without it (anaerobic). Yet another way of identifying bacteria involves their reaction to a test called a Gram stain. Microorganisms that turn violet color are termed gram-positive bacteria; those that turn pink are called gram-negative bacteria.

Disease-causing, or virulent, bacteria have a difficult task: They must somehow enter the body and then fight with normal bacteria for control of healthy cells. They also must survive attacks from the body's other defenses. When enough cells are "taken over" by virulent bacteria, an infection is present and may cause illness.

Viruses also cause infection. They cannot live on their own, but instead can only grow in the cells of other living things. A virus enters a cell, takes it over, kills it, and moves on to the next cell. This continuous destruction explains why some viruses cause so much damage. There are a wide variety of viruses—more than 200 that are known to cause disease. They include those that are self-limiting and will eventually die off with no treatment—common cold viruses, for example—and those that cause serious, chronic diseases, such as human immunodeficiency virus (HIV), the virus that leads to AIDS (see chapter 21).

Two types of infectious agents—rickettsia and chlamydia organisms—resemble bacteria and viruses but differ enough to be classified separately. Rickettsia live within hosts such as ticks, which pass the microorganisms on to humans. Chlamydia are a large group of bacteria-like organisms that have become an alarmingly common cause of sexually transmitted disease.

Fungi are another group of pathogenic, or infection-causing, microorganisms. Fungi such as yeasts and molds can enter the body and wreak havoc, especially in those with weakened immune systems. There are about 100,000 known fungi, but relatively few cause human disease.

Finally, parasites such as protozoa (single-celled) and worms comprise another type of foreign invader. In these infections—or, more correctly, infestations—the parasite spends part of its life cycle in the human body, usually creating tissue damage or symptoms that cause the infected individual discomfort or pain.

Infectious diseases are transmitted in several ways. Most often, we experience infection after direct contact with the infectious agent. For example, if a person with a cold coughs into his or her hand and then picks up a public telephone, the people who use that phone shortly afterward will likely pick up the microorganism. All it takes at that point is for those people to rub their eyes or noses, and the invasion begins. Fortunately, not all infectious agents can survive on your hand or on a telephone receiver. Some infectious agents, however, are particularly hardy. Bacteria that cause tuberculosis can be transmitted in airborne particles, which is why the disease is so contagious.

THE BODY'S DEFENSE

The body has many and complex lines of defense against infectious agents (see chapter 15). When these systems are activated, they may produce signs of infection that can be detected using diagnostic tests. For instance, in the bloodstream and other tissue fluids, white blood cells fight infection on the cellular level. Their number may increase dramatically when infection is present.

Another detectable disease fighter that circulates in blood and other tissue fluids is the antibody. Antibodies are proteins that attach themselves to specific proteins, called antigens, found in the invading organisms. The antibody-antigen complex is extremely important in the diagnosis of some infectious diseases. In many cases, we know which antibodies link to particular antigens and thus can test for them. Antibodies render antigens ineffective by attracting certain cells that destroy the antigen; by causing the antigens to clump together (agglutinate), making them larger targets for elimination; and by enhancing the destructive abilities of white blood cells. Each disabling method produces signs that can be detected or duplicated with diagnostic tests.

While it is attacking foreign invaders, the body also "memorizes" each antigen. Thus, if a specific antigen returns—if you are exposed to the same virus or bacteria, for example—some white blood cells "remember" it and respond more readily to it the second time around. Signs of this memory may be detected in the blood.

HOW YOUR DOCTOR DIAGNOSES AN INFECTIOUS DISEASE

Doctors who diagnose and treat infectious diseases are considered some of the best detectives of medicine, and with good reason: Infectious diseases can affect any body system, be acute (short-acting) or chronic (long-acting), occur with or without fever, strike any age group, and overlap each other.

The patient history takes on major importance in these cases. Your doctor may begin by asking you to describe the symptoms you are experiencing—fever, pain, rashes, stomach upset, and so on. He or she may also inquire about factors, some of them very personal, that may not seem at all related to your health, including the following:

- What have you been immunized against, and when?
- Do you have any pets?
- Do you work in a job in which you are frequently exposed to young children or sick people?

- Do you travel a great deal? If so, where?
- Have you used intravenous drugs?
- What is the nature of your sexual activity?

These questions help in diagnosis because each disease has a description, called an epidemiology, that sums up all the factors that contribute to the likelihood of infection. These elements include how the disease is transmitted, where it is most prevalent, and what groups of people are most likely to be susceptible to it.

Knowing about your home and work environments, habits, and lifestyle can help your doctor determine if you are at risk for a particular infectious disease. For example, toxoplasmosis is an infectious disease caused by the protozoan *Toxoplasma gondii,* and cats are the definitive host. When people handle a cat's litter box or garden in areas that might contain cat feces, it is possible for them to contract the disease. Your eating habits also provide clues. If you regularly eat sushi or other raw or undercooked meat, you are at increased risk for several protozoal infections. Perhaps the most critical disclosure concerns your sexual activity. If you are not in a mutually monogamous relationship, you may be considered a candidate for sexually transmitted disease.

Clues from your history may lead to more pointed questions about your condition. The doctor may also have an idea of what to look for during a physical examination. For example, if you live in or recently visited the mid-Atlantic states, and you have fever and joint aches, one possibility your doctor might investigate is Rocky Mountain spotted fever, which is carried by ticks that are found in large numbers in that area. During the physical examination, he or she may come closer to this diagnosis by spotting its characteristic red rash.

Your doctor will then analyze these factors—your history, your symptoms, and the epidemiology of different infectious diseases—for any overlapping areas. In most cases, especially for commonly

PATIENT TIPS

You can help control the proliferation of infectious organisms that are resistant to treatment if you do the following:

- Do not insist that your doctor give you an antibiotic when there is no clear indication that you have a bacterial infection. The antibiotic won't help you if you have a viral or fungal infection; in fact, it may make it worse. At the same time, it may alter a type of bacteria living harmlessly in your body so that it becomes resistant to the antibiotic. This resistance can then be passed on to disease-causing bacteria.
- Always finish your full prescription of antibiotics, even if your symptoms disappear before you have taken all your pills. If you don't, you may simply weaken, not kill, the bacteria, which may then become resistant to the drug and may cause repeat infection.
- Never refill your prescription to use on another illness without checking with your doctor.

encountered infections, your doctor will use this information to make an educated guess about the infection and prescribe a standard treatment. However, there is great concern about the overuse of antibiotics; a number of drugs are now ineffective against today's more resistant infectious organisms. In addition, antibiotics are of little use if a virus or fungus is responsible for your infection.

For these reasons, many doctors are not so quick to pull out the prescription pad. If your doctor prefers to be conservative about prescribing antibiotics, he or she may suggest some diagnostic testing.

General Tests Used in Diagnosing Infectious Diseases

Most tests for infectious disease involve laboratory analysis of body fluids—blood, urine, cerebrospinal fluid, genital secretions, sputum, and others. Basic procedures in obtaining these specimens are described in chapter 4. How they apply to the diagnosis of infectious diseases is described below.

Smears

A small portion of the sample is looked at under a microscope for identification of the cells present. It is a quick way to see some microorganisms or detect abnormal cell activity such as white blood cell response to an invader.

Cultures

The best way to make a diagnosis involving an infectious agent is to isolate and identify the microorganism itself. A culture is often the best method of accomplishing this task. The culture can be performed using fluids such as blood, cerebrospinal fluid (CSF), or joint fluid to screen for a wide variety of bacteria. Or it can be used to look for specific organisms, such as salmonella or shigella (common causes of gastrointestinal infection), in stool samples. The sample is placed in an environment, or medium, that is designed to encourage specific organisms to reproduce. This medium is usually a jellylike substance that provides nutrients for the microorganisms. If the organism is present, it may multiply rapidly or it may take several weeks to grow.

Sometimes a culture is used to determine which drug will best treat your infection, a procedure called *antibiotic susceptibility testing.* The drug is added to the cultured sample directly to see if it kills the offending organism. This procedure may help determine further drug therapy when standard treatments fail or when a particularly unusual or virulent organism is responsible for illness.

Antigen and Antibody Tests

Tests to identify antibodies or antigens are usually performed on blood serum, the liquid product that is left when blood clots and the clot is then removed. Tests performed using blood serum are called serologic tests or serology. Some of these tests are designed simply to identify a particular substance in the serum. Others, called titers, measure the concentration of that substance.

In *antigen* tests, a known antibody is used to test a blood specimen for antigens with which it might associate in response to different infections. This mimics the immune system's antigen-antibody reaction. In *antibody tests,* the process is done in reverse: a known antigen is used in an attempt to identify the antibodies that might be attracted to it. There are several techniques used for both kinds of tests. These include the following:

The problem is that some infectious agents are difficult to detect or isolate, and test results may not be available for days or weeks. Meanwhile, the infection can grow and cause more difficulty. Thus, the doctor's conclusion takes all these factors into consideration. If your doctor prescribes a treatment that does not take care of the infection in a reasonable amount of time, he or she may then turn to one or more of the diagnostic tests listed on the following pages to determine a new course of treatment (see table 22.1, the box on general tests used in diagnosing infectious diseases, and the specific tests described below).

- Observing for a *precipitation reaction.* A substance may separate or "precipitate out" of a mixture once the antigen-antibody reaction has taken place. This occurs because the substance cannot dissolve in its environment. Rain and snow are called precipitation because they result when the skies cannot "contain" any more moisture and some of it must precipitate out of the atmosphere. These conditions can be produced in a beaker in a laboratory. If some component of a human sample reacts with something added to it, then the product may be observed; it may separate and settle on the bottom of the beaker if the test is run in a solution that cannot dissolve or contain that product.
- Observing for an *agglutination reaction,* a clumping of antigen or antibody cells that occurs when they come into contact with their corresponding antibody or antigen. This is the same thing that happens in the body when antibodies cause agglutination of antigens so the offending microorganisms can be eliminated more easily.
- Initiating a *complement fixation,* or CF, in which an antigen binds with an antibody and this combination allows the complement (a unique set of proteins) to become fixed at the same location. This fixation reaction can be detected indirectly, thereby identifying the original antigen.
- *Tagging* specific antibodies with special dye, so that the antigens they attract can be seen. They show up as green, glowing particles under a fluorescent microscope. This test is sometimes called the *fluorescent antibody test,* or *immunofluorescence.*
- *Enzyme-linked immunosorbent assay (ELISA)* or *radioimmunoassay (RIA)* are two other techniques that rely on tagging and identification. In ELISA, the antibodies are tagged with certain enzymes, which are proteins the body uses to speed up a variety of bodily functions. In RIA, the antibodies are tagged with radioactive material.

Other Tests

Other tests described elsewhere in this book also help the doctor determine a diagnosis. In fact, the diagnosis of infectious disease often occurs when these tests are done for other reasons.

- *Imaging tests* (see chapter 3) include X-rays, computed tomography (CT) scans, and bone and other radionuclide scans. These are often useful in diagnosing infection because of their ability to show inflammation of inner organs or fluid buildup that may not be obvious from simple observation.
- *Invasive tests* are accomplished by introducing a fiber-optic scope or fine needle into the body to visualize internal structures or obtain a biopsy—a sample of tissues or fluid. Examples include bronchoscopy (for examining the bronchial tubes; see chapter 7), coloscopy (for examining the large intestine; see chapter 8), and thoracocentesis (for withdrawing fluid present in the chest cavity; see chapter 7).

TABLE 22.1 Selected Infectious Diseases, Their Symptoms, and Appropriate Diagnostic Tests

Viral Infections

Diagnostic tests for viral infections generally involve the search for antibodies that are produced to fight a particular virus. Often no diagnostic tests are necessary because many viruses, such as measles or chicken pox, require no treatment in otherwise healthy children except to relieve symptoms. They run a limited course, and usually result in lifelong immunity. In certain situations, your doctor may run tests to see if you have an immunity to a particular virus. This is frequently the case when a woman decides to become pregnant. Her doctor may assess her immunity to viruses such as rubella, which causes an otherwise mild disease but could be dangerous to her developing fetus if the mother contracted it during pregnancy.

Disease	Symptoms	Diagnostic Tests
AIDS (acquired immunodeficiency syndrome)	Weakened immune system causes numerous symptoms such as fatigue, swollen glands, fever, and increased susceptibility to other infections.	HIV antibody by ELISA, HIV, p24 antigen, and Western blot (a more specific antibody-detection test). (Also see chapter 21.)
Chicken pox/shingles (*Varicella zoster* virus—VZV)	Painful skin blisters.	*Varicella zoster* virus (VZV) culture, VZV titer, and VZV antigen from tissue samples.
Encephalitis	Inflammation of the brain, high fever, headache, delirium, nausea, and vomiting.	Titers for the different viruses that can cause encephalitis: California, Eastern equine, and Western equine viruses; and CSF culture.
Flu (influenza)	Fever, chills, sore throat, cough, aches and pains, and fatigue.	Influenza A and B titer, influenza virus culture, and influenza virus direct antigen detection.
Hepatitis	Swollen, painful liver, nausea/vomiting, and diarrhea.	Hepatitis A, B, and C antigen and antibody tests.
Herpes simplex (genital herpes)	Painful, recurrent blisterlike sores in genital area.	Herpes simplex virus 2 (HSV2) culture, HSV direct antigen detection, and HSV2 antibody.
Herpes simplex (oral herpes)	Painful blisterlike sores around the mouth and nose.	Herpes simplex virus 1 (HSV1) culture, HSV direct antigen detection, and HSV1 antibody.
Infectious mononucleosis (caused by Epstein-Barr virus)	Constant fatigue, persistent fever, swollen glands, and sore throat.	Epstein-Barr virus (EBV) antibody titer, and heterophil antibody (an antibody toward EBV) agglutination test.
Measles	Fever followed by red spots inside cheeks followed by pink rash.	Measles virus antibody titer.
Rabies	Range from fever and headache to severe brain inflammation and death.	Rabies virus direct antibody detection, and rabies virus antigen detection in tissues.
Rubella (German measles)	High fever, skin rash, joint pain, and swollen lymph nodes.	Rubella virus culture and rubella antibody test.
Viral meningitis	Severe headache, stiffness in neck and back, high fever, and skin rash.	Titers for viruses that cause meningitis such as Coxsackie A or B virus, poliovirus, echoviruses, mumps virus, and antibody titers.

Bacterial Infections

In diagnosing bacterial infections, cultures are the most commonly used tools. Treatment may be concurrent or may precede any diagnostic tests. For example, the signs of an infection such as gonorrhea or pneumonia may be so obvious that your doctor may deem it unimportant to determine the specific bacterium responsible; prompt treatment with an antibiotic that kills a wide variety of organisms may be the best course

Diseases	Symptoms	Diagnostic Tests
Bacterial gastroenteritis	Stomach pain, diarrhea, nausea/vomiting, and appetite loss.	Cultures of bacteria that commonly cause gastroenteritis: salmonella, shigella, campylobacter, E. coli, and yersinia.
Bacterial meningitis	Severe headache, stiffness in neck and back, high fever, and skin rash.	Cultures of CSF and blood for meningitis-causing bacteria, and test for bacterial antigens in CSF.
Gonorrhea	Pain and burning upon urination, itching, and genital pus discharge.	Gonorrhea culture or smear.
Legionnaires' disease (type of pneumonia)	Flulike symptoms with coughing and diarrhea.	Tests for Legionnaires' disease antibodies, and *Legionella pneumophila* culture.
Leptospirosis	Fever, chills, muscular aches, headache, and jaundice.	Leptospira urine, urinary legionella antigen, and CSF culture.
Lyme disease	Joint pain, fever, chills, and fatigue.	Blood and/or CSF serology for antibody against *Borrelia burgdorferi.*
Pertussis (whooping cough)	A barking-type cough, fever, sneezing, and runny nose.	*Bordetella pertussis* nasopharyngeal culture.
Pharyngitis	Sore throat and fever.	Throat culture for Group A streptococcus and *Corynebacterium diphtheriae.*
Pneumonia (bacterial)	Severe cough producing thick, off-colored sputum, high fever, fatigue, and chills.	Cultures of sputum for pneumonia-causing microorganisms including *Streptococcus pneumoniae, Mycoplasma pneumoniae, Chlamydia pneumoniae, Klebsiella pseudomonas,* and *Staphylococcus aureus*; and chest X-ray.
Sinusitis	Swelling and/or blockage of sinus passages causing difficulty breathing and pressure headache.	Culture of sinus samples.
Staphylococcus aureus infection	Vary according to disease produced.	*Staphylococcus aureus* culture.
Streptococcal (strep) infection	Vary according to disease produced.	Streptococcal culture.
Syphilis (caused by a spirochete microorganism, *Treponema pallidum*)	Sores called chancres, fever, joint pain, headache, and fatigue.	*Treponema pallidum* dark-field examination, Veneral Disease Research Laboratory (VDRL) test (antibody test named for the laboratory that developed it), FTA-ABS (fluorescent treponemal antibody absorption test), and MHA-TP (microhemagglutination assay for *Treponema pallidum*).
Tuberculosis (TB)	Fever, cough, chest pain, and difficulty breathing; also weight loss and fatigue.	Tuberculin skin test, chest X-ray, and sputum culture for TB.

(continued next page)

TABLE 22.1 (continued)

Chlamydial Infections

Chlamydia microorganisms can cause a variety of illnesses. For instance, chlamydial infection is the leading sexually transmitted disease in the United States. In the past, it has often been overlooked or misdiagnosed. If untreated in women, it can progress to pelvic inflammatory disease (PID), a leading cause of infertility. Because of this and the fact that it is difficult to culture, doctors usually begin treatment as soon as they suspect chlamydial infection.

Disease	Symptoms	Diagnostic Tests
Chlamydia trachomatis infection (conjunctivitis or pink eye, and sexually transmitted chlamydia)	For conjunctivitis: Redness and inflammation of tissue around eyes, excessive eye discharge, and tearing. For sexually transmitted chlamydia: Burning sensation during and frequency of urination.	Chlamydia culture, *Chlamydia trachomatis* complement fixation test, and immunofluorescence tests for IgM.
Chlamydia pneumoniae infection (pneumonia)	Symptoms of pneumonia including fever and productive cough.	Chlamydia culture and serology.

Rickettsial Infections

Rickettsial diseases are spread through ticks, fleas, or lice. People become infected when they are bitten or come into contact with insect feces. Often these infections are spread by rodents carrying the ticks, fleas, or lice. Because of public health measures to limit rodent populations, many of these infections, such as typhus, are rare in the United States, and thus are not mentioned here. One exception is Rocky Mountain spotted fever, which is transmitted by the dog tick in the eastern United States and by the wood tick in the west. It is characterized by a red skin rash, fever, and joint pain and is tested for by *Rickettsia rickettsii* serology and Weil-Felix reaction (an agglutination test).

Fungal Infections

Fungal infections often occur because of the use of antibiotic drugs for other conditions. In addition to killing the offending microorganisms, the antibiotic may also kill off the "good" bacteria that normally keep fungi at bay. For example, women who take tetracycline to control acne may develop a vaginal yeast infection. Fungal infections are also a major problem for people with weakened immune systems, such as AIDS patients.

Disease	Symptoms	Diagnostic Tests
Aspergillosis	Vary according to the syndrome produced, such as bronchial infection, skin infection, or sinusitis.	Aspergillus serology (antigen and antibody), tissue biopsy, and sputum culture.

Candidiasis (oral thrush, thrush nipples, and vaginitis)	For oral thrush: White patches in mouth and mouth pain. For thrush nipples: Red spotted rash, peeling skin, and pain in nipples of breast-feeding women. For vaginitis: Thick, curdlike, vaginal discharge, and pelvic pain.	Cultures for *Candida albicans* on samples from affected areas.
Cryptococcosis	Symptoms of pneumonitis or meningitis.	Cryptococcus antigen titer, cryptococcus culture, and stain of tissue biopsy.
Histoplasmosis	Flulike symptoms such as fever, cough, headache, chest pain, and loss of appetite.	Fungal antibody screen, culture with stain of biopsy tissue, and urine antigen assay.

Parasitic Infections or Infestations

This category includes infections caused by protozoal microorganisms and worms (sometimes called helminthic infection). The latter set up shop in the intestines and can cause considerable gastrointestinal discomfort and diarrhea. Protozoal infections often occur during or after travel to a foreign country. A microorganism that the local people tolerate well may wreak havoc in a visitor's system. "Traveler's diarrhea" is a general term for this condition. The infections are highly contagious—the parasites can be ingested in food or water or passed by even casual contact—so usually the whole family must be diagnosed and treated. The same is true for parasitic worm infection. Diagnosis of parasitic infections relies on serology and stool examination for eggs (ova) or the microorganisms themselves.

Disease	**Symptoms**	**Diagnostic Tests**
Amebiasis	Diarrhea, abdominal cramps, and loss of appetite.	*Entamoeba histolytica* serologic tests, and ova and parasite exam of stool.
Ascariasis (worms)	Symptoms of lung infection including cough.	Stool exam for ova and parasites.
Giardiasis	Diarrhea and abdominal cramps.	Ova and parasite exam of stool.
Malaria	Fever, chills, headache, nausea, and anemia.	Malaria smear for plasmodium in blood.
Pinworms	Itching in and around the anus, especially at night; most common in children.	Stool exam for ova and parasites.
Tapeworms	Usually none, sometimes nausea, diarrhea, and abdominal pain.	Stool exam for ova and parasites.
Toxoplasmosis	Fever, headache, swollen glands, stiff neck, and sore throat.	Serology for *Toxoplasma gondii* antibodies (IgG and IgM), and biopsy of involved tissue.

TUBERCULIN SKIN TESTING

General information

Where It's Done	Who Does It	How Long It Takes	Discomfort/Pain
Doctor's office or hospital.	Nurse or doctor.	10 minutes for test; 2–3 days for reading.	Some discomfort upon injection.
Results Ready When	**Special Equipment**	**Risks/Complications**	**Average Cost**
2–3 days.	Tuberculin syringe.	None.	$

Other names PPD (purified protein derivative) test or Mantoux test. (Also see chapters 14 and 17.)

Purpose Tests for exposure to *Mycobacterium tuberculosis.*

How it works Tuberculin antigen is injected into the skin. If you have been exposed to tuberculosis, your body will have developed an immune response, which will travel to the injection site and cause a reaction, such as slight redness or swelling.

Preparation None.

Test procedure

- A small amount (0.1 mL) of material obtained from a culture of *Mycobacterium tuberculosis* (MTB) is injected just under the skin, usually on the forearm.
- The site is observed for any reaction immediately after the test and then two to three days later.

After the test

- You are free to leave and resume normal activities.
- You are asked to return to the testing site within two to three days so that the area of injection can be observed for any reaction.

Factors affecting results

- Recent vaccinations for measles, rubella, mumps, polio, or another infectious disease.
- Current therapy with steroids.
- Infection with nontuberculosis mycobacteria.

Interpretation Redness, raised skin, and hard lumps larger than 9 millimeters (about 1/3 of an inch) in diameter indicate a positive reaction. The larger the reaction, the more likely it is that you are infected with *Mycobacterium tuberculosis*. This means you have been exposed to or have had tuberculosis and may require medication.

Advantages

- It's quick.

- It's relatively painless.
- It's a sensitive test.

Disadvantages

- Some people have skin reactions that are borderline and therefore do not deny or confirm exposure.
- It does not distinguish between current disease and past infection.
- False-positive and false-negative results are possible.

The next step

- If the test is positive, treatment may be necessary.
- If test results are equivocal, the test will be repeated.
- If the test is negative but symptoms persist, additional tests may be performed.

STOOL EXAMINATION FOR PARASITES AND/OR THEIR EGGS (OVA)

General information

Where It's Done	Who Does It	How Long It Takes	Discomfort/Pain
Doctor's office or laboratory.	Doctor or technician.	A few minutes.	None.
Results Ready When	**Special Equipment**	**Risks/Complications**	**Average Cost**
Immediately.	Sterile collection cup.	None.	$

Other names Pinworm detection.

Purpose To diagnose parasitic infection.

How it works Direct and/or microscopic examination of a stool sample detects the presence of parasites or their ova (eggs).

Preparation None.

Test procedure

- You will receive one or more sterile containers in which to collect your stool sample at home.
- You defecate directly into the container and seal it. Your doctor will tell you if you must collect more than one sample. You do not need to handle the stool, and it need not be refrigerated.
- You deliver the stool sample to the doctor's office or laboratory within 12 hours.
- The sample is observed for evidence of parasites. A slide may be prepared for microscopic examination.

After the test

- You are free to resume normal activities.
- If your test is positive, your doctor will recommend that members of your household and other close contacts be tested as well.

Factors affecting results Delay in submitting sample.

Interpretation A positive test means that a particular parasite or its ova are present.

Advantages

- It's quick, painless, and inexpensive.
- It's simple but effective.

Disadvantages

- Some people find collecting and transporting the sample unpleasant.
- The parasite may be present but not show up in a particular sample.

The next step

- If the test is positive, treatment can begin immediately.
- If the test is negative but symptoms persist, the test may be repeated or a string test may be ordered.

Lawrence M. Brass, MD

23 The Nervous System

Tests Covered in This Chapter

The case of Henry R., a 58-year-old electrical engineer:

I had my first ministroke [transient ischemic attack, or TIA] without even knowing it. All of a sudden, my left leg became numb, almost causing me to fall. I sat down, and in a few minutes, sensation returned and I continued walking to my office.

Two days later, a more alarming episode occurred while I was reading a report. All of a sudden, the vision in my right eye became blurry, and it seemed that a shade was being slowly drawn, completely blocking my sight in that eye. About ten minutes later, my vision returned, but I put in a call to my doctor anyway. When he heard what had happened, he told me to take an aspirin and to have a colleague bring me to the hospital as soon as possible.

The Tests The doctor quickly detected a characteristic murmuring sound, or bruit, as he listened to blood flowing through the carotid artery in Henry's neck. He immediately ordered a Doppler ultrasound study of Henry's carotid arteries, which showed a severe narrowing on one side and a lesser one on the other. Henry was put on heparin, a drug that prevents blood clots, and was scheduled for arteriography to get a better picture of the carotid obstruction.

The Outcome The tests, coupled with a history of two TIAs, indicated that Henry was at a high risk of having a stroke. His doctor advised prompt surgery to remove the fatty plaque that was severely blocking a 2-inch segment of the right carotid artery. The operation was successful, and after recovery, Henry was put on low-dose aspirin therapy as a preventive measure. He was also instructed to have annual Doppler ultrasound studies, both to monitor the smaller obstruction on the left side and to make sure circulation on the right side was still normal.

INTRODUCTION

The nervous system is a complex network of nerve cells and fibers that receives information from inside and outside the body and sends instructions to various organs. These signals regulate all mental and physical processes in the body, from thought and speech to movement, heartbeat, and perspiration.

The core of the nervous system is the central nervous system, or CNS, which consists of the brain and the spinal cord. The human brain comprises about 100 billion nerve cells, called neurons. It can be

Lobes of the Brain and Their Functions

Frontal lobe: Motor function, planning, and expression of language.

Temporal lobe: Hearing, memory, and behavior.

Parietal lobe: Interpretation of sensation and understanding of language.

Occipital lobe: Perception and interpretation of visual information.

divided into the brain stem, which controls many of the body's basic functions, including breathing, swallowing, and eye movement; the cerebellum, which coordinates movements and balance; and the cerebrum, the thinking part of the brain. The cerebrum, also known as the cerebral cortex, has two hemispheres, each further divided into four lobes (see the accompanying box). In most people, the ability to perform language functions is largely concentrated in the left brain, while the right side of the brain controls musical ability and the capacity to understand spatial relations, recognize faces, and focus attention.

The spinal cord is a long structure extending from the brain stem to the lower back, that consists of neural fibers and is protected by skeletal vertebrae. Both the brain and the spinal cord are covered with three layers of membranes called meninges and bathed in cerebrospinal fluid, which cushion them against the encasing bones.

The brain and the spinal cord are connected to the rest of the body by the peripheral nerve system, or PNS, which has three parts and controls the sensory organs (eyes, ears, nose, taste buds, and those controlling touch), the voluntary muscles (such as those used to walk), and the autonomic or involuntary nervous system, which in turn controls unconscious body processes, such as the heartbeat, breathing, salivation, digestion, and constriction and enlargement of blood vessels.

COMMON NERVOUS SYSTEM DISORDERS

Neurological disorders are extremely varied and can affect the entire nervous system or its parts. The major causes of these disorders are blood flow disruption in the brain, infection, tumors, trauma, and abnormalities that may be present from birth. Some of the most common disorders of the nervous system are described below.

Migraine. This disorder is characterized by recurrent attacks of severe headache that can last several hours or even days and may be accompanied by visual disturbances, nausea, vomiting, and intolerance of light.

Stroke. Stroke affects nearly 500,000 Americans annually and can be divided into two major types: (1) ischemic stroke, caused by interrupted blood flow to the brain, and (2) hemorrhagic stroke, in which blood leaks into brain or adjacent tissues.

Trauma to the brain and spinal cord. Injuries to the central nervous system may be direct, such as gunshot wounds, which account for about one-fourth of brain and spinal cord injuries, or indirect, such as, for example, when brain structures are shaken and pulled inside the skull during a car accident.

Peripheral neuropathies. Compression of a nerve due to injury and such factors as vitamin deficiencies may cause a localized loss (due to weakness) of function or abnormal sensation, such as the dropping of a wrist or the sensation of pins and needles in the hand. More rarely, such disorders may affect the entire peripheral nervous system, causing generalized weakness.

Multiple sclerosis. In this autoimmune disease, the body's natural defenses turn against it and attack myelin, a fatty substance found in the cells covering nerves within the brain. This results in either brain signals being incorrectly conducted or not conducted at all. The recurrent "attacks" of multiple sclerosis may lead to severe disability.

SIGNS AND SYMPTOMS OF NERVOUS SYSTEM DISORDERS

Damage to the brain, depending on its location, can lead to thousands of different mental and physical symptoms, including difficulties with thought, vision, speech, memory, and movement. The following are the major symptoms that may occur if the nervous system is diseased. It should be noted, however, that most of these symptoms can have other causes and may not be serious. Therefore, this list also specifies those conditions under which these symptoms may indicate neurological problems that require immediate evaluation. (See also the accompanying box, which lists those neurological symptoms requiring emergency medical care.)

Headache—when extremely severe and unexpected, or when there is a change in the usual headache pattern.

Back pain—when the pain radiates to the feet, toes, or other parts of the body, or is accompanied by weakness or shooting pain in the legs, disruption of bowel or bladder function, and impotence.

Dizziness and vertigo—when vertigo (a sensation that the room is spinning) can't be attributed to allergy or inner ear problems, when light-headedness is persistent, or when the dizziness is associated with unsteadiness or a lack of coordination.

Numbness and loss of sensation (paresthesias)—when there is a persistent numbness or a tingling or crawling sensation under the skin of the affected part of the body, or a complete loss of sensation to pain, heat, and cold.

Impaired mental ability and memory problems—when short-term memory loss is regular and persistent, when there is difficulty thinking clearly, or when poor judgment in simple activities of daily living comes on suddenly.

Disruption of movement—when movement is either abnormally slow or abnormally fast.

Tremors and seizures—when tremors are chronic, severe, and accompanied by slowed movement, lack of coordination, or impaired mental ability. Seizures are neurological in origin and require evaluation.

Muscle weakness—when the weakness is not simple fatigue from strenuous activity, persists even with rest and worsens with time, or is accompanied by numbness.

Fainting (syncope)—when not an isolated incident related to dehydration, fatigue, excess alcohol consumption, or an extreme emotional upheaval; when accompanied by weakness on one side of the body, difficulty speaking or swallowing, double vision, or shaking; or when it lasts for more than a minute.

Sleep problems—when the cause is not obvious (stress, illness, medications, drug or alcohol use, chronic lack of sleep, or a disrupted sleep-and-wake cycle); when excessive daytime sleepiness is involved; or when there are sudden attacks of sleep during the day (narcolepsy).

HOW YOUR DOCTOR DIAGNOSES NEUROLOGICAL DISORDERS

The vast number and variety of symptoms makes identifying neurological disorders one of the most challenging diagnostic tasks in medicine. In 90% of cases, however, a careful history and complete physical exam can suggest a diagnosis. Tests may then be ordered to confirm the diagnosis or locate the abnormality. For example, subtle clues obtained during an exam may allow a doctor to distinguish between dementia due to Alzheimer's disease and those due to stroke, both of which cause confusion, but a CT scan may be ordered to help verify the doctor's conclusions.

Your doctor will focus on different parts of the nervous system, usually beginning with the brain. You may be asked to follow simple commands, like pointing to an exit, or to perform more complex tasks, like making calculations or interpreting a proverb. The doctor may also ask about memory problems and your ability to recognize objects. Different parts of the brain perform highly specialized tasks, and an abnormality may affect a very narrow aspect of your neural functioning. For example, some people with stroke lose the ability to speak but retain the ability to sing.

The doctor will observe the movements of your eyes and tongue and ask about taste, smell, and hearing. This is usually followed by an examination of the spinal cord, the peripheral nervous system, and the muscles. An important element of this exam is testing the reflexes. Any muscle can have this involuntary response, but generally the reflexes are tested by tapping the knees, ankles, biceps, and triceps. When a doctor briskly taps your knee, the pressure stretches the knee tendon and sends a signal to the spinal cord that is interpreted as a sudden shift in body position. In real life—as, say, when you trip over a curb—your brain would respond by stretching the leg outward to keep you from falling. Since in this case the brain cannot distinguish between real life and an exam, it responds with the familiar knee jerk. Normally, the response is relatively mild. A weak signal, however, may mean that the impulse traveling up the spinal cord is blocked, or that the nerves or muscles of the leg are affected by disease. In contrast, a very strong response may indicate an abnormality in the upper part of the spinal cord or in the brain.

Next, using a wisp of cotton, a pin or other sharp object, or test tubes of hot and cold water, the doctor may test and compare sensation in your peripheral nerves on both sides of the body. Finally, to evaluate muscle strength and coordination, you will be asked to flex and extend your arms or legs and hold them in the air, and to perform several maneuvers, such as touching your nose with a finger. The doctor will also observe your walk, which may reveal problems of movement and coordination.

Various tests may be ordered, depending on your symptoms and the suspected problem. Since the nervous system may be damaged by disorders that start elsewhere in the body, the doctor may first prescribe tests the are not geared specifically toward the nervous system, such as a routine blood test for infection or an endocrine test for hormonal abnormalities. Blood sugar concentration may be measured to rule out low glucose levels, and an electrocardiogram may be performed to rule out a heart attack.

The tests geared specifically toward the nervous system can be grouped into three major categories. First, there are imaging tests, such as X-rays, CT scans, and MRI, which provide the physician with a picture of the brain and spinal cord. In ordering these tests, the doctor seeks to detect or rule out not the most common disorders, but those that are most life-threatening. For example, the most common diagnosis for a severe headache is a migraine, but imaging tests may be ordered to rule out a brain tumor. Certain imaging tests can also provide information about movement within the tissues of the nervous system, such as the flow of blood in the blood vessels leading to the brain.

The second category encompasses tests that focus on the function of the nervous system. It includes tests like nerve conduction velocity, which examines the ability of the nerves to transmit signals. These tests may reveal abnormalities in structures that appear normal in imaging examinations, but are unlikely to establish the location of the abnormalities or their cause. Further tests are usually required to make the diagnosis more specific.

The third category includes chemical tests of body fluids. They detect abnormalities or imbalances in substances in the blood or cerebrospinal fluid that may affect the functioning of the brain and other parts of the nervous system. While imaging tests are effective in revealing abnormalities confined to one area, chemical tests are useful in diagnosing disorders that affect the entire nervous system.

Symptoms Requiring Emergency Medical Care

- Sudden loss of function, including weakness or numbness on one side of the body, vision loss or double vision, or loss of ability to speak or understand speech.
- Back pain after an accident or trauma that is severe and lasts for more than a few hours. Also severe upper back pain that does not appear to be caused by strenuous physical activity.
- Sudden onset of a severe headache.
- Impaired memory or mental ability that begins after taking a new medication.
- Fainting accompanied by weakness on one side of the body, difficulty speaking or swallowing, double vision, abnormal movements such as shaking, or unconsciousness that lasts for more than a minute, or if these symptoms persist beyond the fainting episode.
- Vertigo (the sensation that the room is rotating or spinning) that is severe and comes on suddenly.
- Seizures, in which case you should try to protect the person from self-harm by moving furniture and sharp objects out of the way rather than by trying to confine the person's movement, which during a seizure is impossible.

ELECTROENCEPHALOGRAPHY (EEG)

General information

Where It's Done	Who Does It	How Long It Takes	Discomfort/Pain
Hospital, doctor's office, or commercial laboratory.	Doctor, nurse, or EEG technician.	2 hours; longer in special circumstances.	Possible itchiness from the glue used to affix electrodes to scalp. If test is done for seizures, you may have to go without sleep the previous night.

Results Ready When	Special Equipment	Risks/Complications	Average Cost
Immediately.	EEG recorder, and electrodes.	Low risk, although seizures may occur as a result of underlying disease.	$$–$$$

Other names Electroencephalogram.

Purpose

- To assess brain electrical activity in order to evaluate the nature or cause of seizures; diagnose coma; evaluate sleep disorders; establish the presence and location of brain tumors, abscesses, or brain injuries; diagnose and evaluate the severity of stroke; and identify certain brain or spinal cord infections.
- To monitor brain activity during surgery or assess the depth of anesthesia.

- To distinguish psychiatric conditions from neurological diseases affecting mental status.
- To predict whether a person is likely to develop seizures after head trauma.
- To determine brain death.

> **PATIENT TIPS**
>
> If you are being evaluated for seizures, you will be told to do the following to increase the likelihood that the EEG will detect a seizure or seizure-related electrical activity:
>
> - Taper down your dose of anti-seizure medication.
> - Stay up as long as possible the night before the test—a variation called a sleep-deprived EEG.

How it works Electrical signals produced by the brain neurons are picked up by the electrodes and transmitted to a polygraph, where they produce separate graphs on moving paper using an ink writing pen or on a computer screen.

Preparation

- Avoid taking sedative drugs, such as benzodiazepines and barbiturates, before the test.
- Unless you are having a sleep-deprived EEG, come to the test well rested to avoid distorted results.
- Wash your hair the night before the test. Do not use hair cream, oils, or spray afterward.

Test procedure

- You lie down on the examining table or bed while eight to 20 electrodes are attached to your scalp.
- You are asked to relax and lie first with your eyes open, then closed.
- You may be asked to breathe deeply and rapidly or to stare at a flashing light both of which produce changes in the brain-wave patterns.
- If you are prone to seizures, you may experience one during the test.
- If you are being evaluated for a sleep disorder, EEG may be performed continuously during the night while you are asleep. Such a recording, which may involve an evaluation of other body functions during sleep, is referred to as polysomnography.

After the test

- The electrodes are removed and the glue that held them in place is washed away with acetone. You may have to use additional acetone at home to completely remove the glue.
- Unless you are actively having seizures or are restricted by your physician, you may drive home.
- If the EEG was performed overnight, you should arrange to have someone drive you home.
- If you stopped taking anticonvulsant drugs for the EEG, you can usually start taking them again.

Factors affecting results

- Lack of sleep before the test can distort some of the brain waves.
- Movements of the eyes, tongue, head, or body during the recording.
- Low blood sugar that may be caused by fasting.
- Medications that affect the brain.

Interpretation A neurologist examines the EEG recording for abnormalities in the brain-wave pattern, which may reflect diseases of the nervous system. In most psychiatric disorders, multiple sclerosis, and Alzheimer's disease, the EEG is generally normal or shows only minor abnormalities.

Advantages

- It's noninvasive.
- It's highly informative.

Disadvantages

- Results may be slightly abnormal in healthy people and normal in people with disease.
- It's less helpful than imaging techniques in determining the location of injuries or their precise nature for some diseases such as stroke.

The next step Other imaging studies of the brain, possibly including CT scans and MRI.

SINGLE-PHOTON EMISSION COMPUTED TOMOGRAPHY (SPECT)

Other names None.

For a full description of this test, see chapter 3.

Purpose

- To evaluate the flow and volume of blood in the brain.
- To detect bleeding and blockage of blood vessels in the brain.
- To diagnose epilepsy and evaluate its severity.

Interpretation The doctor examines the brain map and looks for signs of abnormalities. The map reveals areas with changes in blood flow. Abnormal patterns on the map correspond to different diseases. For example, blood flow increases during a seizure, decreases during a stroke, or may show characteristic changes in conditions such as Alzheimer's disease.

POSITRON-EMISSION TOMOGRAPHY (PET)

Other names None.

For a full description of this test, see chapter 3.

Purpose

- To evaluate the brain blood flow and use of oxygen or glucose (blood sugar) by the brain.
- To diagnose brain disorders, particularly dementia, epilepsy, brain tumors, and movement disorders.
- In research, to identify the areas of the brain that are involved in various mental and physical tasks.

Interpretation The doctor examines the brain map for abnormalities. For example, the map usually reveals areas with interrupted blood flow and reduced oxygen consumption. Abnormal patterns on the map correspond to different diseases.

SKULL AND SPINAL X-RAYS

General information

Where It's Done	Who Does It	How Long It Takes	Discomfort/Pain
Hospital, commercial X-ray facility, or doctor's office.	X-ray technician.	Minutes.	Generally none.

Results Ready When	Special Equipment	Risks/Complications	Average Cost
A few hours.	X-ray machine (portable or stationary).	Risks associated with radiation, particularly during pregnancy.	$$

Other names Skull and spinal films, radiography, or roentgenography.

Purpose

- To check quickly for injuries or abnormalities after trauma, especially of the cervical (upper) spine.
- To detect skull fracture and bone abnormalities.

How it works X-rays (electromagnetic energy emitted by an X-ray tube) are absorbed differently by various body tissue. When the tissue is exposed using special photographic film, various types of tissue show up as shadows, as dark gray areas, or as white opaque areas.

Preparation

- For a skull X-ray, remove all hair accessories and jewelry from your head. For a spinal X-ray, remove all clothing and jewelry and wear a hospital gown.
- For a spinal X-ray, pin up hair if it is long so that no locks hang over the chest or shoulders.

Test procedure

- The technician positions you against the X-ray machine and tells you to remain still while X-rays are taken.

- For the skull, X-rays are usually taken from the front, side, and back. Depending on the suspected problem, additional X-rays may be taken at different angles.

After the test

- You get dressed and are free to leave if testing is elective.
- The film is processed in a developing machine, and X-ray pictures are produced.

Factors affecting results

- Metal jewelry may obstruct the view.
- Movement during the test may distort the image.

Interpretation The doctor studies the X-ray pictures for abnormalities in the skull and spinal column.

Advantages

- It's simple, quick, and noninvasive.
- It's relatively inexpensive.
- It's also highly informative and widely available.

Disadvantages

- It involves a small amount of radiation exposure.
- It often detects the existence of an abnormality but does not establish a specific diagnosis.

The next step

- More definitive imaging studies, including CT scans or MRI.

CRANIAL AND SPINAL COMPUTED TOMOGRAPHY (CT) SCAN

Other names Computed axial tomography (CAT) scan or computed transaxial tomography.

For a full description of this test, see chapter 3.

Purpose

- To determine the type and location of brain injury (eg, ischemic versus hemorrhagic stroke).
- To establish the cause of certain symptoms, such as severe headache or back pain.
- To determine the anatomy of all the brain and spinal cord structures prior to surgery.
- To obtain a better view of brain abnormalities revealed by a regular X-ray study.

Interpretation The doctor studies the images for abnormalities that may be caused by disorders of the brain or spine.

The next step Treatment according to diagnosis; for some findings (eg, tumor) or some locations (eg, spinal cord) subsequent MRI may provide additional diagnostic information.

MAGNETIC RESONANCE IMAGING (MRI) OF THE BRAIN AND SPINAL CORD

Other names Magnetic resonance scan of the brain and spinal cord.

For a full description of this test, see chapter 3.

Purpose

- To scan the brain for the presence of stroke, tumors, bleeding, abnormal blood vessels, infectious and inflammatory conditions, seizures, and disorders characterized by abnormal accumulation of iron.
- To look for changes in brain structure associated with degenerative brain diseases (eg, Huntington's disease).
- To detect tumors, blood vessel abnormalities, herniated disks, degenerative diseases of the spinal column or spinal cord, multiple sclerosis, traumatic injury, infectious and inflammatory diseases, and other problems of the spinal cord.
- A recent variant of MRI technology called magnetic resonance spectroscopy (MRS) measures specific brain chemicals and may be used in the diagnosis of stroke, tumors, and multiple sclerosis.
- To assess oxygen levels and blood flow to the brain.

Interpretation The doctor studies the views of your brain and spinal cord on a monitor or on film for abnormalities.

The next step Treatment according to diagnosis; for some abnormalities (eg, changes in the bones of the skull), a subsequent CT scan may provide additional diagnostic information.

BRAIN ULTRASOUND

Other names Transcranial Doppler sonology (TCD).

For a full description of this test, see chapter 3; also see chapter 5.

Purpose

- To evaluate blood flow in the brain.
- To detect abnormal narrowing or malformations of the brain arteries.

Interpretation The doctor studies the image, called a brain ultrasonogram, and assesses the shape, and flow of blood within, the brain arteries.

The next step Possibly other imaging studies, including CT scans, MRI, or angiography.

BRAIN ANGIOGRAPHY

Other names Cerebral angiography or arteriography, or digital subtraction angiography (DSA).

For a full description of this test, see chapter 3.

Purpose

- To detect blood vessel abnormalities, including blockages and malformations, in the brain, especially when the patient is having or at risk of having a stroke.
- To detect bleeding in the brain when the patient has headaches or generalized visual problems that can't otherwise be explained.
- To evaluate a patient for surgery to remove a brain tumor.

Interpretation The doctor examines the image obtained, called a cerebral angiogram, for the presence of malformations, narrowing, bulging, bleeding, tumors, or a blood clot.

The next step Treatment.

MYELOGRAPHY

General information

Where It's Done	Who Does It	How Long It Takes	Discomfort/Pain
Hospital imaging suite or radiology laboratory.	Doctor.	45–60 minutes.	Some discomfort during lumbar puncture and as table is tilted.

When Results Ready	Special Equipment	Risks/Complications	Average Cost
A few hours to a few days.	Fluoroscope and X-ray equipment with a tilting table, contrast dye, spinal needle, and local anesthetic.	Risks associated with radiation, particularly during pregnancy; seizures; stroke; bleeding; infection and inflammation; headaches; nausea and vomiting; allergic reaction from the contrast dye.	$$

Other names Cervical, lumbar, or thoracic myelography.

Purpose

- To detect herniated discs, tumors, injuries, enlarged blood vessels, and other abnormalities, especially compression of the spinal cord.
- To evaluate problems in the spinal cord before surgery.
- To detect injuries to the nerve roots branching off the spinal cord.
- To detect tumors in the lower part of the brain.

How it works Contrast dye injected into the cerebrospinal fluid (which surrounds the brain and spinal cord) makes it possible to view internal structures with the help of fluoroscopy, a type of moving X-ray.

PATIENT TIP

Tell the doctor if you have bleeding problems or if you are taking anticoagulant drugs.

Preparation

- Avoid eating or drinking for eight hours before the test.
- You remove your clothing and don a hospital gown.
- A lumbar puncture is usually performed before myelography to inject the dye.

Test procedure

- Local anesthesia is administered at the site where the spinal needle will be inserted.
- A long needle is inserted into the spinal canal, with the help of a fluoroscope, and guided to the subarachnoid space, between the layers of membrane that surround the spinal cord.
- Once the needle is in place, a contrast dye is injected and X-ray pictures are taken.
- To move the dye to structures of interest, you may be slowly tilted head down during parts of the test. Care will be taken to prevent the contrast dye from entering the brain.

After the test

- You are free to leave but you must rest in bed for 12 hours with your head elevated.
- Drink a great deal of fluids.

Factors affecting results

- Failure to observe dietary restrictions before the test.
- Amount of contrast dye injected.

Interpretation The doctor examines the X-ray images, called a myelogram, for signs of abnormalities. Abnormalities can also be detected by observing the flow of the contrast dye under a fluoroscope. If the spinal canal is blocked or narrowed, the dye will not spread evenly or will be blocked, and the contour of the spinal cord will also be distorted.

Advantages Obstruction and abnormalities are easily seen and well defined on X-rays.

Disadvantages

- Additional diagnostic information may be obtained from the spinal fluid (see LP testing).
- It's invasive.
- It involves exposure to radiation.
- It cannot be performed in people with severe curvature of the spine or increased intracranial pressure.

The next step Treatment.

LUMBAR PUNCTURE (LP)

General information

Where It's Done	Who Does It	How Long It Takes	Discomfort/Pain
Doctor's office or hospital outpatient suite.	Doctor and possibly a nurse or technician.	20–30 minutes.	Position patient must assume may be uncomfortable. Some discomfort when needle is inserted.

Results Ready When	Special Equipment	Risks/Complications	Average Cost
A few hours to a few days.	Syringe, lumbar-puncture needle, and manometer.	Headache, backache, or bleeding from the puncture site; dangerous if there is infection on the lower back, such as an infected pressure sore.	\$–\$\$

Other names Cerebrospinal fluid (CSF) analysis, spinal fluid analysis, and spinal tap.

Purpose

- To detect infection, inflammation, or bleeding in the brain or spinal cord.
- To diagnose or rule out leukemia and lymphoma or other cancers involving the brain or central nervous system.
- To diagnose central nervous system disorders that are characterized by tissue destruction, such as multiple sclerosis, and neuropathies (nerve diseases).
- To diagnose some forms of hydrocephalus (water on the brain), for example, normal pressure hydrocephalus.
- As treatment, to lower the pressure of the spinal fluid or to administer drugs to the spinal canal.

How it works By measuring the pressure and withdrawing cerebrospinal fluid and analyzing it for such substances as antibodies, blood, bacteria, cancer cells, and excess protein or white blood cells, diagnoses of various disorders can be made.

Preparation

- You will have a CT scan (see chapter 3) first to see if there is an increase in pressure within the skull, possibly from a brain tumor or an abscess.
- You remove all clothing and wear a surgical gown.
- The site of the needle puncture on your back is cleaned, and local anesthesia is administered to the site.

Test procedure

- You lie on your side with your back to the person performing the test, your knees drawn up to the abdomen, and your forehead bent toward the knees. (Less commonly, the test may be performed while you are sitting.) This opens up the spaces between the vertebrae, making it easier to insert the needle. (See also Variations below.)

- The needle is inserted through your lower back into the spinal canal.
- A sample of cerebrospinal fluid (CSF) is withdrawn (which takes about five minutes) and sent to the laboratory for analysis. Some tests may need to be sent to specialized regional laboratories.

> **DID YOU KNOW?**
>
> Twenty years ago, needles used for spinal taps were dull and crudely made, making the procedure painful. Today's needles are so thin and flexible that you could wrap them around your fingers and they wouldn't break. This has reduced the discomfort of the procedure considerably.

- If you experience discomfort during the procedure, the needle can be repositioned.
- Pressure of the CSF is measured by attaching a manometer to the lumbar-puncture needle.

Variations If you have a problem with the lower back, such as a fused spine, that precludes assuming the curled position necessary for the spinal tap, the fluid sample may be drawn at the top of the spine at the back of the neck. In this case, the procedure is known as a *cisternal puncture.*

After the test

- A small adhesive bandage is placed over the puncture site.
- You lie down for ten to 15 minutes, which helps distribute the CSF to the brain. (The amount removed will be replaced by the body in about one hour.)
- Unless you are among the less than 1% of patients who experience a severe headache, you are free to leave. Otherwise you will remain in the facility until the headache subsides.
- You should drink extra fluids for the next 24 hours.
- If headache occurs, it is usually relieved by bed rest. If severe, you should call your doctor.

Factors affecting results A punctured blood vessel may lead to blood in the cerebrospinal fluid sample.

Interpretation The doctor receives an immediate impression about the CSF from its appearance. Normal CSF is clear and contains no blood. The presence of blood or a yellowish color may indicate spinal cord obstruction or bleeding in the brain or spinal cord. High pressure of the CSF may indicate the presence of a tumor, swelling, or bleeding. In addition, the CSF will be analyzed in a laboratory for the presence of various substances (see above).

Advantages It can quickly identify the presence of infection and other abnormalities in cerebrospinal fluid.

Disadvantages It's invasive.

The next step Other imaging studies, which may include CT scan or MRI.

ELECTROMYOGRAPHY (EMG) AND NERVE CONDUCTION VELOCITY (NCV)

General information

Where It's Done	Who Does It	How Long It Takes	Discomfort/Pain
Hospital outpatient department.	Doctor or technician.	Less than 1 hour for both tests.	Discomfort at site of needle insertion; possible anxiety over insertion of needle electrodes.

Results Ready When	Special Equipment	Risks/Complications	Average Cost
Within 24 hours.	Needle and surface electrodes, nerve stimulator, amplifier with filters, oscilloscope, and device to store data, such as a magnetic tape recorder.	Very rare possibilty of short-lived bacterial infection.	$$

Other names Electrodiagnostic study (needle exam) or latency studies.

Purpose

- To determine the severity and exact site of nerve entrapment (in such disorders as carpal tunnel syndrome or a herniated disk).
- To confirm diagnosis and measure the severity of peripheral nervous system disorders, such as polyneuropathies.
- To diagnose or evaluate disorders of the muscles and motor neurons, such as amyotrophic lateral sclerosis and myasthenia gravis.

How it works As they contract, the muscles give off a weak electrical signal that can be detected, amplified, and tracked, giving information about how well they are working. Electrical signals traveling along nerves can be measured. By measures at two points, the velocity of conduction can be measured.

Preparation

- Avoid taking aspirin and other nonsteroidal anti-inflammatory drugs for five to seven days before the test.
- If you take Mestinon for myasthenia gravis, stop taking it 24 hours before the test under the discretion of your physician.

- Wear loose-fitting clothes that will allow you to expose the necessary muscles and nerves during the test. You may have to disrobe and wear a hospital gown if your hip or shoulder muscles are being tested.
- Do not use hand cream or skin lotion before the test (so that the electrodes adhere properly).

> **PATIENT TIP**
>
> If you take an anticoagulant (blood-thinning) medication such as Coumadin, be sure to tell your neurologist. If this is the case, it may not be necessary to have the electromyography part of the exam.

Test procedure You sit or lie on the examination table and expose the muscles and nerves that need to be tested. One or both of the following studies are performed.

Electromyography:

- The appropriate area is cleaned with alcohol, and the needle electrode (a very thin, solid needle that is similar to a pin) is inserted into the muscle.
- The electrical activity of the muscle during relaxation, slight contraction, and forceful contraction is picked up via the electrodes, amplified, recorded on the oscilloscope, and converted to auditory signals via a speaker.
- Several muscles or areas of muscle may be tested one by one in this manner.

Nerve conduction studies:

- Recording and stimulating electrodes are placed on the skin overlying a nerve supplying a muscle or muscle group.
- A mild and brief electrical stimulus is delivered to the stimulating electrodes.
- The response of the muscle is picked up by the recording electrodes, amplified, and displayed. The speed with which the signal generated by the muscle travels through the nerves, called nerve conduction velocity, is measured. The amplitude (strength) of the signal is also measured.
- The maneuver is repeated on different nerves.

After the test You are free to return to previous activities, although you should try not to strenuously exert yourself for the rest of the day. If you feel any pain, it will be a mild muscle ache, no stronger than if you had bumped yourself.

Factors affecting results

- The position of the electrodes.
- Muscle-relaxing and anticholinergic medications.
- Skin temperature.

Interpretation

- *Electromyography*. Normally, there is no electrical activity in the muscle when it is relaxed, only when it contracts. If the muscle is diseased, it may have electrical activity in the relaxed state; when it contracts, its electrical activity may produce abnormal patterns. By examining these abnormalities, the doctor may determine the nature of the disease and identify the nerves and muscles affected.
- *Nerve conduction studies*. Nerve conduction velocity reflects the speed with which electrical impulses travel along the nerve. Various diseases can cause the impulses to slow down, or to be slower on one side of the body than on the other. The magnitude of the response to stimulation also gives clues to diagnosis and the extent of the injury.

Advantages

- It's only mildly invasive.
- It can help quantitate subjective symptoms.

Disadvantages It usually provides no definitive diagnosis although it adds clues to the physical examination.

The next step

- Treatment.
- There may be additional laboratory testing to look for the underlying cause of a neuropathy (eg, diabetes or hypothyroidism).

EVOKED POTENTIALS

General information

Where It's Done	Who Does It	How Long It Takes	Discomfort/Pain
Doctor's office or hospital.	Neurologist.	1 hour.	Moderate.
Results Ready When	**Special Equipment**	**Risks/Complications**	**Average Cost**
Immediately.	Scalp electrodes, signal amplifier and filter, and a computer for signal processing.	None.	$$

Other names Evoked responses.

Purpose

- To confirm the diagnosis of multiple sclerosis.
- To assess hearing, especially in children.
- To assess eyesight in infants and children.
- To diagnose disorders of the optic nerve.
- To detect tumors and other abnormalities affecting the brain and spinal cord.
- To assess brain stem function in coma.

- To monitor brain activity and signals from the nerves during surgery on the brain or spine, or during general anesthesia.
- To determine whether loss of sensation in an arm or leg is due to injury in the brain or spinal cord.
- To assist in the determination of brain death.

How it works Stimuli delivered through sight, hearing, or touch evoke minute electrical signals which travel along nerves and through the spinal cord to specific regions of the brain. These signals can be recorded via electrodes, amplified, and displayed.

Preparation

- Wash your hair the night before the test, but do not use hair cream, oils, spray, or lacquer afterward.
- Remove all jewelry and other metal objects from your body.
- Same preparation as for EEG (see above).

Test procedure

- Electrodes are placed on your scalp, as in electroencephalography. Three types of testing may be performed.

Visual evoked response (VER):

- You are seated in a specially equipped room, about 3 feet away from a screen.
- Electrodes are placed on your scalp over the regions responsible for vision.
- You are asked to focus your gaze on the center of the screen.
- You close one eye at a time while a shifting checkerboard pattern is presented on the screen (the squares reverse color once or twice a second).
- Electrical activity in the optical nerve and its branches is recorded.

Brain stem auditory evoked response (BAER):

- You sit in a soundproof room and put on earphones.
- Electrodes are placed on the top of your head and on the earlobe of first one ear and then the other.
- Clicking sounds are delivered through the earphones to the tested ear. Signals produced by the brain in response to clicks are recorded.

Somatosensory evoked response (SSER):

- Recording electrodes are placed on your scalp and neck.
- Electrodes delivering stimuli may be placed on the lower back, wrist, knee, or ankle over peripheral nerves that are known to function properly.
- Minute electrical shocks are delivered to the peripheral nerves.
- Signals produced by the brain in response to every shock are recorded.

After the test You are free to return to previous activities.

Factors affecting results

- Severe nearsightedness.
- Muscle spasms in the head or neck.
- Severe hearing impairment or sensory loss (neuropathy).
- Earwax or severe inflammation of the middle ear.

Interpretation Evoked signals are faint compared with the brain's background electrical activity. In the test, the signals are amplified, separated from the background, and presented as a wave. The doctor examines the waves and detects abnormalities that are characteristic of various disorders.

Advantages

- It's noninvasive and safe.
- It picks up small abnormalities.

Disadvantages It detects abnormalities but does not produce a specific diagnosis.

The next step Other diagnostic tests to determine underlying cause of abnormalities that may be found.

OCULOPLETHYSMOGRAPHY (OPG)

General information

Where It's Done	Who Does It	How Long It Takes	Discomfort/Pain
Hospital or office.	Doctor or nurse.	30 minutes.	None.
Results Ready When	**Special Equipment**	**Risks/Complications**	**Average Cost**
Immediately.	Oculoplethysmograph, corneal and earlobe pulse sensors, and anesthetic eyedrops.	Cannot be performed in people who had eye surgery in the preceding 6 months; may be dangerous if you had recent detachment of the retina or eye infection.	$$

Other names Carotid patency evaluation and ocular pneumoplethysmography.

Purpose To detect narrowing or blockage of the carotid arteries that run on both sides of the neck. Their narrowing can interrupt blood supply to the brain and cause transient ischemic attacks or stroke.

How it works It provides an indirect measurement of blood flow in the opthalmic artery, which reflects the blood flow to the brain through the carotid arteries.

Preparation You remove contact lenses if you wear them, and anesthetic eyedrops are placed into your eyes.

Test procedure

- Eye pressure is measured through small suction cups placed over the eyes.
- Eyecups that look like contact lenses are attached to the corneas of the eyes, and probes are attached to the earlobes. Both have sensors that allow them to detect the pulse rates in the vessels supplying the eyes and ears.
- As a vacuum is applied to the eyecups, they may be used to measure the blood pressure in the eye artery.

After the test

- You are free to resume normal activities.
- Avoid rubbing your eyes for 30 minutes.
- After 30 minutes, you can reinsert your contact lenses.
- You may experience blurred vision for a short while.

Factors affecting results

- Blinking and eye movements.
- High blood pressure.
- Abnormal heart rhythm.

Interpretation The pulse rates in the eye and earlobe are compared. Normally, the pulse should occur simultaneously in the two locations. If there is a delay between the pulses, a carotid artery may be narrowed or blocked.

Advantages It's quick and noninvasive.

Disadvantages

- It detects only severe narrowing or blockage.
- Other tests (ultrasound or angiography) are required to confirm the diagnosis and have largely replaced this technique.

The next step Angiography.

ELECTRONYSTAGMOGRAPHY (ENG)

General information

Where It's Done	Who Does It	How Long It Takes	Discomfort/Pain
Doctor's office or diagnostic clinic.	Physician.	1 hour.	Nausea can be severe.
Results Ready When	**Special Equipment**	**Risks/Complications**	**Average Cost**
Immediately.	Electrodes and recording devices.	Nausea, vomiting, and dizziness.	$$

Other names Calorics or vestibular test.

Purpose To measure involuntary eye movements, called nystagmus, in order to evaluate the function of the vestibular system and associated brain areas.

How it works The electrical charge in the retina is slightly negative, while that in the cornea is positive. Electrodes placed on either side of the eye can measure the eye movements by picking up the displacement of the charges. Patterns in the movements can help detect disorders.

Preparation

- Avoid eating for four hours before the test.
- Avoid taking sedatives and tranquilizers for two to three days before the test; abstain from consuming caffeine and alcohol for 24 to 48 hours before the test.
- Bring your eyeglasses and hearing aid with you if you use them.
- Clean your ears of excessive earwax.
- The person performing the test will examine your ears for the presence of wax, inflammation, or other problems in the ear canal.

Test procedure

- You will be instructed to look up, down, and to the sides and to follow a slowly moving target with your eyes as your eye movements are recorded.
- Involuntary eye movements in the dark may be recorded behind closed eyelids.
- If you have symptoms only when your head assumes a certain position, you will be asked to move your head, and any involuntary eye movements will be recorded.
- In a part of the test known as caloric testing, your eye movements will be recorded as warm and cool air or water are placed into the external ear canal.

After the test Same as after oculoplethysmography (see above).

Factors affecting results

- Earwax or irritation of the ear canal.
- Ruptured eardrum.
- Impaired vision.
- Nausea and vomiting.
- Blinking.
- Medications.

Interpretation Involuntary eye movements can be used to detect abnormalities in the vestibular system or in the nerves that connect the vestibular system to the brain and the muscles of the eye.

Advantages

- It's noninvasive.
- It can quantitative subtle eye movement abnormalities.

Disadvantages The patient may become very nauseated.

The next step X-ray studies or CT of the skull and brain, MRI, or treatment.

THE TENSILON (EDROPHONIUM) TEST

General information

Where It's Done	Who Does It	How Long It Takes	Discomfort/Pain
Doctor's office or hospital.	Doctor, nurse, or lab technician.	15 minutes.	None.
Results Ready When	**Special Equipment**	**Risks/Complications**	**Average Cost**
Immediately.	Syringe and needles, edrophonium, and catheter.	Nausea, dizziness, slow heartbeat, and blurred vision.	$$

Other names Neuromuscular junction test.

Purpose To diagnose myasthenia gravis or other disorders in which the muscles grow weak because they have lost the ability to pick up signals from the nerves.

How it works The test serves to promote the neurotransmitter (acetychlorine) that activates muscle, by reducing its breakdown (blocked by edrophonium).

Preparation You should not have taken any medication within four hours of the procedure.

Test procedure

- A small needle or catheter is placed in your vein.
- You receive an injection of a small dose of the drug edrophonium through the catheter.
- If the drug does not restore power to the muscles within a minute or two, the dose is increased. The maneuver is usually repeated three to four times.
- If muscle is restored, the effect lasts only a few minutes.

After the test If the test is positive, you experience a dramatic increase in muscle strength—but then this strength dissipates very rapidly.

Factors affecting results The dose of edrophonium.

Interpretation If the muscle power is temporarily restored, you have myasthenia gravis or a related disorder of the connection between the nerve and muscle. However, if the injections produce no effect, the disorder cannot be ruled out. Some people, particularly the elderly in whom the myasthenia affects only the muscles that control the movements of the eyes, may have no chemical abnormalities characteristic of the disorder and may therefore fail to respond to the test even though they do have the disease.

Advantages

- It's rapidly performed and analyzed.
- It's remarkably specific for myasthenia gravis.

Disadvantages

- It's invasive.
- Edrophonium produces side effects such as abdominal discomfort.

The next step Treatment.

BRAIN BIOPSY

General information

Where It's Done	Who Does It	How Long It Takes	Discomfort/Pain
Hospital.	Doctor (neurosurgeon or neurologist), in the presence of a pathologist.	1 hour.	Discomfort associated with general anesthesia.

Results Ready When	Special Equipment	Risks/Complications	Average Cost
1–3 days.	Surgical instruments.	Possible increased risk of seizures.	$$$

Other names None.

Purpose To diagnose or confirm the diagnosis of Alzheimer's disease, tumors, infection, inflammation, and other brain disorders. Used rarely, often as a measure of last resort, when other tests have failed to provide a diagnosis.

How it works A tiny sample of brain tissue is obtained with a long needle and examined under the microscope for damage or abnormalities.

Preparation You are placed under general anesthesia.

Test procedure

- A small burr hole is drilled in the skull, and a needle is then inserted into the brain.

- A pathologist, who is usually present during the operation, promptly prepares the removed sample of brain tissue for analysis. The sample is studied under a microscope with available laboratory tests. If sufficient tissue has been removed, it may be frozen for further analysis.

After the test The patient is taken to the recovery room and monitored for several hours.

Interpretation The removed tissue sample provides information about various brain abnormalities. For example, in Alzheimer's disease the cortex contains plaques, abnormal collectons within brain cells. If the brain is affected by infection, the infectious organism can be cultured from the sample and identified. If a tumor is removed, it can be classified as cancerous or benign.

Advantages It provides an opportunity to examine brain tissue directly.

Disadvantages

- It's invasive and includes the risks of surgery and anesthesia.
- It leads to removal of brain tissue and may be associated with brain injury.
- It leaves a scar on the brain that can potentially trigger seizures.

The next step Treatment.

MUSCLE AND NERVE BIOPSY

General information

Where It's Done	Who Does It	How Long It Takes	Discomfort/Pain
Hospital.	Doctor.	1 hour.	Moderate.
Results Ready When	**Special Equipment**	**Risks/Complications**	**Average Cost**
2–4 days.	Surgical instruments.	Local pain.	$$

Other names None.

Purpose

- To diagnose muscle disease, such as muscular dystrophy.
- To diagnose nerve disease, such as neuropathy.
- To establish whether a neurological disorder originates in the nerve or muscle.

How it works A tiny sample of nerve or muscle tissue is obtained with a long needle and examined under the microscope for damage or abnormalities.

Preparation A local anesthetic is injected into the area from which the biopsy sample will be removed. General anesthesia may be used in children.

Test procedure

- A clamp is placed on the muscle to prevent it from contracting.
- A sample of muscle and/or nerve is removed and sent to a laboratory for analysis.

After the test Local suturing is done and a sterile dressing applied.

Factors affecting results

- The site from which the tissue was removed.
- If the removed sample is too damaged by disease, it may be impossible to make a diagnosis.

Interpretation Various abnormalities can be identified by testing the tissue samples and studying them under a microscope.

Advantages It provides an opportunity to examine muscle and nerve tissue directly.

Disadvantages

- It's invasive and associated with some discomfort.
- There is usually a small area of sensory loss beyond the area of the biopsy.

The next step Treatment of underlying disease.

Maurice J. Mahoney, MD, JD

24 Genetic Diseases

Tests Covered in This Chapter

The case of Donna M., 28, and her 5-month-old son, Billy:

> *Because I'm relatively young and neither my family nor my husband's had any history of genetic disease, I had no reason to have prenatal testing. So I was really distressed when Billy was born with a cleft palate, a defect of the eye called coloboma, and poor muscle tone. The doctors did some tests and diagnosed a chromosomal disorder.*
>
> *Billy spent three weeks in the hospital. His oxygen level needed constant monitoring and he required tube feeding. But then we took him home and gradually he grew stronger and healthier until we were able to take him off the monitor and begin bottle-feeding him.*

The Tests Doctors analyzed the chromosomes in samples of blood from Billy and his parents. Chromosomes are collections of genes—strings of chemicals that program every trait and function in the body. Once in a while a chromosome breaks. While machinery in the cell usually repairs the break, in rare instances two broken chromosomes exchange pieces before the repair is made and form what is called a translocation. The tests showed that Billy and Donna both have translocations. Donna's is called a balanced translocation because the exchanged chromosomes have not lost or damaged any genes crucial to health, body form, or structure. Because its overall effect is benign, she was never aware of it.

Billy, however, has what is called an unbalanced translocation, because genetic material is either missing, damaged, or overabundant. This usually occurs when one parent, in handing down half of his or her 46 chromosomes, passes on only one of the two or more rearranged chromosomes. The health effects caused by such an imbalance depend on which genes are involved.

The Outcome Although it's too early to predict, Billy may suffer profound retardation and his organs may not develop normally. Or his problems could be comparatively minor: learning disabilities, slight behavioral disorders, and mild physical deformities that would not be considered handicaps. The appearance of his ears, eyes, or the creases around his mouth or eyes may be a little abnormal, or his fingers may be longer or shorter than normal. So far, the muscle tone in his upper body is still weak, and his development is a little slow, but doctors won't be able to measure his mental function until he is about 2 years old. They will also monitor him for any physical defects that can be corrected surgically.

INTRODUCTION

Every cell in the human body contains about 100,000 genes, the units of hereditary material that determine the regulation of body processes and a person's physical characteristics, such as hair color or height (see figure 24.1). Except for eggs and sperm, each cell possesses an identical

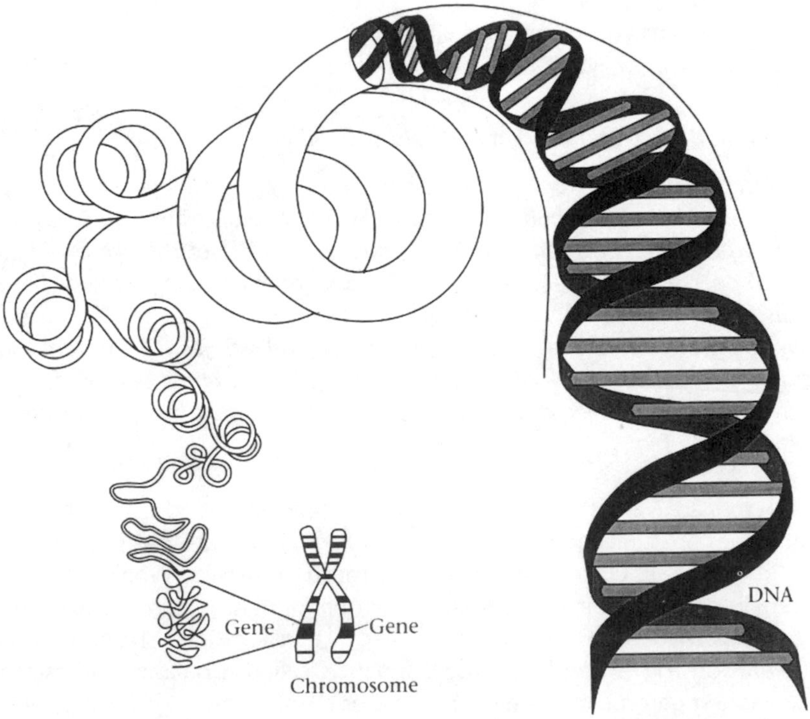

FIGURE 24.1 Blueprints of Life

The tightly coiled strands of DNA that make up each of the body's millions of genes carry that individual's unique genetic code. Genes are responsible for individual characteristics; myriad hereditary or genetic diseases also may be carried by these genes.

gene set. These genes are arranged in 23 pairs of tiny strings, called chromosomes. A person's entire set is inherited: In every pair, one chromosome comes from the mother and one from the father.

Of these 23 sets, 22 are arranged in matching pairs, called autosomal chromosomes. The 23rd pair, the sex chromosomes, are matching in women but not in men. The female sex chromosomes consist of two strings, known as XX, while the male chromosomes are known as XY. Since the mother can only contribute an X chromosome, it is always the father who determines the sex of a child, depending on whether he contributes an X or a Y.

GENETIC DISORDERS

Genetic disorders may be influenced by several factors. When a disease runs in a family, faulty genes are passed from parent to child. Or a change in the genetic material—a mutation—may occur during formation of an egg or sperm cell, as happened in the cases of Donna M. and her son, Billy. Mutations may also appear during fetal development. In these cases, children with genetic abnormalities may be born to parents without genetic disorders.

The major types of genetic disorders are described below.

Chromosomal disorders are abnormalities in the number or structure of the chromosomes. These disorders are often severe and include mental retardation and a variety of physical deformities. Examples include Down syndrome, Turner syndrome, and Klinefelter syndrome.

Single-gene (or Mendelian) disorders are caused by a defect in a single gene or pair of genes. Most of these are rare, but together they cause significant illness. They may vary greatly in severity and may not produce symptoms until late in life. These conditions include the following:

Autosomal dominant disorders, such as Marfan syndrome and Huntington disease, which occur when one gene is abnormal and the corresponding one is normal.

Autosomal recessive disorders, such as cystic fibrosis, sickle-cell anemia, and Tay-Sachs disease, which usually occur only when both genes in a pair are defective. While children in these cases may suffer genetic disease, both parents will be healthy because their defective genes are paired with normal copies.

X-linked disorders, such as hemophilia, color blindness, and some muscular dystrophies, which are caused by genes located on the X chromosome. Women are less prone to X-linked disorders because if they have an abnormal X chromosome, they usually have a normal one to compensate for it. However, a man who inherits an abnormal X chromosome with a defective gene will develop the disease even if the gene is recessive, since his Y chromosome can't compensate for it.

Multifactorial (or polygenic) genetic diseases are the most common but the least understood of all genetic diseases. Although a person inheriting one or more of these genes has an increased risk of a particular disorder, environmental factors will determine whether the disease manifests itself. This category includes such common chronic disorders as coronary heart disease, diabetes mellitus, schizophrenia, and cleft palate.

Somatic gene disorders are conditions in which gene abnormalities develop only in certain cells. Genetic defects responsible for these disorders are not inherited; rather, they occur in the developing fetus or at some time after birth. For example, cancer is usually a somatic gene disorder in which only genes in the diseased tissue are aberrant.

HOW YOUR DOCTOR DIAGNOSES GENETIC DISORDERS

Now that many more diseases are recognized as having a genetic component, genetic testing is playing an increasing role in diagnosing diseases of all the organ systems. Disease detection, however, is only one reason for genetic testing (see the accompanying box).

For most disorders, the doctor first orders tests to evaluate the diseased organ and only later to establish whether the disorder has

Why Genetic Tests Are Done

The main uses of genetic testing are as follows:

- To determine whether apparently healthy individuals carry genes that will cause disease later in life or predispose them to developing a particular disorder. The results may help determine if there is a need for periodic monitoring or measures to help prevent severe complications. For example, people who carry the genes for familial polyposis, a hereditary disorder that increases the risk of colon cancer, may undergo regular screening for the early detection of this malignancy.
- To screen fetuses for genetic disorders. While some disorders discovered this way may be treated in the womb, in most cases their detection offers the parents the option of terminating the pregnancy or being prepared for the birth of an affected child (see chapter 25).
- To screen newborns for about a dozen genetic diseases that can be treated or even prevented if treatment is begun early. These include sickle-cell anemia, galactosemia, hypothyroidism, and phenylketonuria (PKU).
- To screen people who may carry defective genes and are planning to have children, in order to evaluate their risk of passing on a genetic disease.
- To diagnose certain genetic conditions. Even when no treatment is available, a diagnosis may help predict the outcome of the disorder or put an end to unnecessary testing.
- To increase the success of organ transplantation. The closer the match between the genetic types of donor and recipient, the lower the risk of the donor organ being rejected by the recipient's immune system.

genetic origins. For example, if you have had a heart attack at a relatively young age, initial tests will evaluate the heart while further tests may be used to detect familial hypercholesterolemia (an inherited tendency to extremely high cholesterol levels), which may be an underlying cause.

There are cases, however, when doctors believe that disorders are largely or primarily due to a genetic defect. For example, if a newborn baby has recurrent pneumonia, cystic fibrosis may be suspected. In this case, tests aimed at clarifying the genetic origin of the disease are ordered immediately.

Family History

If you suffer what seems to be a genetic disorder, your doctor will want to know about your first-degree relatives (parents, siblings, and children), with whom you share certain genes. The doctor will ask about their age and health and, if they are deceased, what the cause of death was. Certain racial and ethnic groups are more susceptible to particular genetic diseases, so identifying your heritage is also crucial.

Genetic disorders may be diagnosed indirectly, by examining your signs and symptoms, or directly, by examining your genetic tissue (see table 24.1). In the indirect approach, the doctor studies your family history and orders tests that are not specifically genetic. For example, if you are diagnosed with a certain type of kidney disease, the doctor may establish its hereditary origin by simply drawing your family tree and indicating the disorder's distribution among family members.

TABLE 24.1 Some Genetic Disorders and Their Diagnosis

Disorder	Diagnostic Tests
Basal-cell nevus syndrome	X-rays of skull and skeleton.
Cystic fibrosis	Sweat test, direct gene analysis.
Familial hypercholesterolemia	Cholesterol in blood.
Familial hyperparathyroidism	Calcium in blood, parathyroid hormone.
Familial polyposis of the colon	X-ray of colon, colonoscopy, gene linkage.
Fragile X syndrome	Chromosome analysis, direct gene analysis.
Gilbert disease	Bilirubin in blood.
Hemophilia	Clotting factors in blood, linkage, direct gene analysis.
Hereditary hemorrhagic telangiectasia	X-ray of lungs.
Huntington disease	Direct gene analysis.
Muscular dystrophies	Electromyography (EMG), muscle biopsy, creatine phosphokinase (CPK), electrocardiogram (ECG), direct gene analysis when available.
Osteogenesis imperfecta	X-rays of bones. Collagen analysis using cultured skin cells.
Polycystic kidney disease	Urinalysis, ultrasound, renal arteriogram, blood pressure measurement, direct gene analysis.
Tay-Sachs disease	Enzyme analysis (hexosaminidase A), direct gene analysis.

Genetic Tests

When doctors know what function the problematic gene performs in the cell and what proteins it makes, the disorder can be diagnosed by measuring these proteins or enzymes, known as gene products, with standard tests used to analyze blood, urine, or other body fluids. If the genetic material contains an error, the gene product may be abnormal or present in unusual amounts. For example, Tay-Sachs disease is linked to decreased levels of the enzyme hexosaminidase A. In children and adults, the disease can be diagnosed by measuring the concentration of the enzyme in blood, and in fetuses, by measuring levels in amniotic fluid.

> **DID YOU KNOW?**
>
> Gene analysis has become more widely available thanks to a method of testing called polymerase chain reaction, or PCR. This swift, automated technique helps expand minute amounts of DNA thousands to hundreds of thousands of times. The technique is particularly useful when material available for analysis is scarce, because it allows gene analysis to be performed on genetic material extracted from a single cell. Some forensic medicine specialists now use it to analyze bits of evidence found at crime scenes.

The tests described in this chapter examine either chromosomes or individual genes. But while chromosome analysis is performed in numerous medical centers, direct gene analysis is expensive and only beginning to reach the public. The advantage of gene analysis is that it can sometimes lead to a more definitive diagnosis. For example, chromosomal abnormalities are detected in only a small percentage of all mentally retarded people; in a larger percentage, the retardation is probably caused by a single gene. (Other significant factors are environmental—fetal alcohol syndrome, lead poisoning, birth trauma, and so on.)

The cost of gene analysis is expected to drop soon as the tests become routinely available in hospitals and commercial laboratories throughout the country.

CHROMOSOME ANALYSIS

General information

Where It's Done	Who Does It	How Long It Takes	Discomfort/Pain
Doctor's office, hospital, or commercial laboratory.	Doctor, nurse, or technician.	Usually less than 5 minutes.	Slight (from drawing blood or obtaining tissue sample).
Results Ready When	**Special Equipment**	**Risks/Complications**	**Average Cost**
3 days to 2 weeks.	Supplies for drawing blood, possibly a biopsy tool, possibly an aspiration needle (for amniocentesis).	Negligible for drawing blood; other risks depend on which tissue cells are extracted for analysis.	$$

Other names Chromosome karyotype or cytogenetics.

Purpose

- To look for the cause of birth defects, mental retardation, or retarded growth.
- To detect chromosomal disorders in the fetus.
- To reveal the cause of infertility or repeated miscarriages.
- To evaluate couples with chromosomally abnormal children.
- To evaluate women who aren't menstruating.
- To examine abnormal sexual development, particularly when there is doubt about true gender.
- To diagnose certain cancers or evaluate their course and the effectiveness of treatment.

How it works Chromosomes isolated from cells are examined, and their number and structure are evaluated.

Preparation None for analysis of blood, skin, or bone marrow samples. See chapter 25 for pregnancy related tests.

Test procedure

- Cells are removed to examine their chromosomes. These cells can be from the blood, skin, or bone marrow or, in a pregnant woman, from the placenta, amniotic fluid, or chorionic villi.
- The cells are cultured, and a karyotype (a picture of the chromosomes) is created.

After the test

- The care you receive depends on the procedure used to obtain a tissue sample for chromosome analysis. (See other chapters for individual tests.)
- The slides with chromosomes are preserved for several years until they fade and can no longer be used. Photographs will last much longer.

Factors affecting results

- Chromosomes that are too condensed or stretched out may be difficult or impossible to evaluate in number or structure.
- Samples may contain insufficient cells or ones that divide infrequently.
- Fetal cells may be mixed with the mother's cells.

Interpretation

- A doctor or lab technician examines the chromosomes for abnormalities in structure or number.
- Some chromosomes can be analyzed by *fluorescent in situ hybridization (FISH)*, a new procedure that uses a DNA probe and is being rapidly added to the traditional ways of analyzing chromosomes.

- In *mosaicism*, in which abnormal chromosomes are interspersed with normal ones, the ratio of the two types is used to predict the severity of the genetic disorder. This is difficult in prenatal diagnosis.

Advantages The test is completely accurate for most chromosomal disorders.

Disadvantages

- It's expensive.
- It detects abnormalities only in chromosomes and not in single genes, so it often fails to produce a diagnosis.
- It requires a high level of technical expertise and specialized equipment.

The next step A positive diagnosis is considered definitive. This may lead to further counseling, treatment, and, if appropriate, reproductive decisions. If the result is negative, further tests (eg, MRI, enzyme tests, and urine biochemistry) may be ordered.

GENE ANALYSIS

General information

Where It's Done	Who Does It	How Long It Takes	Discomfort/Pain
Doctor's office, hospital, or commercial laboratory.	Doctor, nurse, or lab technician.	Usually less than 5 minutes.	Slight (from drawing blood or obtaining tissue sample).
Results Ready When	**Special Equipment**	**Risks/Complications**	**Average Cost**
2–4 weeks.	Supplies for drawing blood or a cheek brush (for removing cheek cells); rarely, a biopsy tool.	Almost negligible risk associated with obtaining tissue cells.	$$–$$$

Other names DNA analysis or direct gene analysis.

Purpose

- To diagnose diseases caused by defective genes (see table 24.1). In some cancers, to predict the course of the disease.
- To detect genes that may cause or increase the risk of disease later in life or be passed on to offspring.
- To detect a severe genetic disorder in a fetus when there is a family history.

How it works Blood or other tissue is analyzed for a known disease-causing gene by using specific chemicals that bind to defective genes.

Preparation None for blood test. For tests on fetal tissue, see chapter 25.

Test procedure Tissue or blood is taken for genetic analysis.

After the test If blood has been taken, follow the normal procedure for drawing blood (see chapter 4). Otherwise, care depends on the procedure used to obtain a tissue sample.

DID YOU KNOW?

A relatively new technique, *fluorescent in situ hybridization (FISH)*, allows chromosomes and genes to be analyzed simultaneously. Scientists apply a fluorescent dye, called a genetic probe, that attaches itself only to its exact copy. So a probe containing a colon-cancer gene will attach to and light up another colon-cancer gene. More than 50 different colors can be used to identify genes or sets of chromosomes.

Factors affecting results Samples are sometimes contaminated with someone else's DNA.

Interpretation

- Genetic material is examined for alterations, rearrangements, or deletions in genes that cannot be seen under a microscope.
- In such cancers as acute lymphoblastic leukemia and non-Hodgkin's lymphoma, identifying specific genetic changes helps establish the diagnosis and, in some cases, prognosis.

Advantages It provides a definitive diagnosis of disorders caused by known genetic defects.

Disadvantages

- It's expensive.
- It's limited to disorders for which specific genes have been identified.
- It's not widely available for many genes, although this is changing rapidly.

The next step Both positive (abnormal gene present) and negative (abnormal gene not present) findings are considered definitive. A positive test result may lead to further counseling, treatment, and, if appropriate, reproductive decisions. If the result is negative, further tests may be ordered to investigate the problem. They will vary with the symptoms.

LINKAGE ANALYSIS

General information

Where It's Done	Who Does It	How Long It Takes	Discomfort/Pain
Doctor's office, hospital, or commercial laboratory.	Doctor, nurse, or lab technician.	Less than 5 minutes.	Slight (from drawing blood or obtaining tissue sample).
Results Ready When	**Special Equipment**	**Risks/Complications**	**Average Cost**
2–4 weeks.	Supplies for drawing blood or a or cheek brush (for removing cheek cells); rarely, a biopsy tool.	Almost negligible risk associated with obtaining tissue cells.	\$–\$\$

Other names None.

Purpose

- To detect genes that may cause or increase the risk of disease later in life or be passed on to offspring.
- To detect a severe genetic disorder in a fetus when there is a family history of it.

How it works DNA "markers" linked to the problem genes are identified in your chromosomes and those of your close relatives.

Preparation None.

Test procedure

- Blood is usually drawn (although other tissue samples may be taken) from the patient and several of his or her relatives.
- The DNA of affected and unaffected relatives is extracted and analyzed to determine which DNA structures are most likely to represent markers of the disease-causing gene.
- The patient's DNA is examined for the presence of the markers.

After the test If blood has been taken, follow the normal procedure for drawing blood (see chapter 4). Otherwise, the care you receive depends on the procedure used to obtain a tissue sample.

Factors affecting results

- Correctly identifying how people in a particular family are related to each other is crucial to accurate results.
- The test will have limited value if close relatives crucial to establishing linkage relationships are not available.
- Occasionally, DNA segments may have changed places when the subjects' eggs and sperm were formed, causing the markers to move from their usual locations.

Interpretation

- The presence of DNA markers can help predict whether a fetus or a person with no symptoms carries the defective genes that run in the family.
- If the markers are not found, the presence of abnormal genes cannot be ruled out because DNA structures in the vicinity of the gene may have been rearranged when inherited.
- A small number of disorders have gene markers that are found in most people with the disease (and in few people without the disease), but in most cases the markers are specific to a particular family, and will differ from family to family.
- In an experimental approach with limited availability, results can be used to make cancer treatment decisions or take preventive measures.

Advantages

The test makes it possible to diagnose genetic abnormalities when the gene causing the disorder has not yet been identified.

Disadvantages

- It's expensive.
- It's available in only a few medical centers and for a limited number of disorders.
- Close relatives must be available for testing.
- It's laborious, more time-consuming, and less reliable than direct gene analysis.

The next step

Both positive (abnormal gene present) and negative (abnormal gene not present) findings are considered highly informative. Either result may lead to further counseling, treatment, and, if appropriate, reproductive decisions. Direct gene analysis may be suggested in the future if it becomes available for the gene in question.

Joshua A. Copel, MD

25 Pregnancy

Tests Covered in This Chapter

The case of Fiona P., a 31-year-old mother and PR executive (and, at the time, 36 weeks pregnant):

> *I had a wonderful first pregnancy three years ago. During that pregnancy, I had an alpha-fetoprotein test [which tests the mother's blood for levels of a protein produced by the fetus]. I didn't have any anxieties about having AFP, but this time, I went through a bit more soul searching. My first baby was fine, so why should I get tested now? But then I started to wonder: "What am I going to do if the results indicate a problem?" I ended up choosing AFP again, and it was fine.*

Then around my eighth month, I had a bit of a scare. My obstetrician thought I was measuring very small and recommended that I have ultrasound to check the size of my baby. I was apprehensive about whether they might have to perform an early delivery.

The Tests Fiona's ultrasound showed that the baby's limbs and abdomen were a healthy size, the weight was average, and the surrounding amniotic fluid was plentiful (lack of fluid may be a sign of inadequate growth). The baby's movement was normal, as was fetal breathing, which may be restricted if the baby's brain isn't receiving sufficient oxygen.

The Outcome The ultrasound assured the doctor that Fiona's baby was growing normally, much to Fiona's relief. She was amazed that he could measure the baby's limbs and point out the four operating chambers of the heart. Just one week later, Fiona gave birth to a healthy baby boy.

INTRODUCTION

Pregnancy begins with conception, when a woman's egg is fertilized by a sperm. The chromosomes of the egg and sperm unite, forming a new set of chromosomes containing the genetic material of the future child. The fertilized egg begins dividing almost immediately so that by the third day after conception it contains four to eight cells. By the end of the 12th week, the limbs and internal organs of the fetus are fully formed and assume a distinctly human shape. The fetus is surrounded by a membrane, called the amnion or amniotic sac, which is filled with amniotic fluid, and which is in turn enveloped by another membranous sac, the chorion. The umbilical cord connects the fetus to the placenta, which mediates an exchange of nutrients and oxygen between the mother and child.

Dating a Pregnancy

Since the exact time of conception is generally unknown, pregnancy is, by convention, dated from the woman's last period. An average pregnancy lasts about 40 weeks from the last period, but since conception is most likely to have occurred at the time of ovulation, or about two weeks *after* the last period, the actual duration of an average pregnancy is about 38 weeks from conception.

Early Signs of Pregnancy

Missing a period is not a foolproof sign of pregnancy. Weight loss, strenuous exercise, emotional stress, or illness may suppress menstruation in women who aren't pregnant. Conversely, some pregnant women experience minor bleeding (spotting) during the first three months, which they may mistake for a period. In particular, spotting may occur about ten to 14 days after conception, when the cells forming the future embryo attach themselves to the wall of the uterus.

Common symptoms in early pregnancy include fatigue, dizziness, nausea, and vomiting. Many pregnant women also experience enlarged and tender breasts, a frequent desire to urinate, and changes in appetite. Symptoms vary, however, and some women experience nothing unusual in the early months of pregnancy except missed periods. Women usually begin to show, or have noticeable abdominal swelling, around the 14th or 16th week of pregnancy.

HOW YOUR DOCTOR DIAGNOSES PREGNANCY

Pregnancy tests used today are sophisticated enough to detect a pregnancy as early as four days after a missed period, although they are most accurate if they are done at least ten days past the normal time of menstruation. Urine tests are most commonly used, but a blood test may be more accurate, can detect pregnancy earlier, and can detect an ectopic pregnancy (one that develops outside the uterus—an emergency situation). A blood test may also help establish the age of the fetus if there is a doubt about the time of conception. By the time your period is about two weeks late, your doctor can determine pregnancy by a simple pelvic exam, although the results of the exam will be confirmed by a blood or urine test.

> **PATIENT TIP**
>
> Home pregnancy tests are generally reliable in detecting pregnancy when they are used precisely according to directions. Inexperienced users, however, are less likely to get accurate results. The chances of accuracy are increased if you wait at least ten days after a missed period and if you test your first urine of the day.
>
> Always confirm a positive result with your doctor. You should also consult your doctor if the result is negative but you are experiencing symptoms of pregnancy.

TESTS ORDERED AT FIRST PRENATAL VISIT

Ideally, a woman should have a medical checkup before conception to discuss special care during pregnancy and the need for genetic screening. If you think you are already pregnant, you should schedule the first prenatal visit with your doctor as soon as pregnancy is confirmed.

During the visit your doctor will ask you about past illnesses, pregnancies, miscarriages, and abortions. The doctor will also record a history of diseases in your family and your partner's family. If there is a possibility that either of you carries a genetic disease that may be transmitted to the offspring, you may be referred for genetic counseling (see below).

Your doctor or other health care provider will check your weight and blood pressure and conduct a pelvic examination to evaluate the size and structure of your uterus, confirm the age of the fetus, and evaluate your pubic bone size. He or she may do a Pap smear for cervical cancer (see chapter 26), particularly if you do not have this test done regularly. A cervical culture for gonorrhea is also performed (see chapter 22).

A number of tests are routinely ordered during the first prenatal visit (see table 25.1). Your blood type and Rhesus (Rh) factor are established, and a complete blood count is performed to check for anemia and establish the dose of supplemental iron you will need to take during your pregnancy. Your blood will also be tested for various abnormal antibodies and signs of infection, including rubella, hepatitis B, and syphilis (a syphilis test is required by law in most states). Pregnant women at risk of infection with the human immunodeficiency virus (HIV), which causes AIDS, will be offered an HIV test (see chapter 21).

A urinalysis is ordered to check for such conditions as kidney disorders and urinary tract infection. Pregnancy relaxes the pelvic muscles, and thus the bladder cannot be emptied as completely, increasing susceptibility to these infections, which are more likely to occur without symptoms during pregnancy than at other times.

Additional tests may be ordered, depending on your ethnic origin. African-American women as well as those of Italian, Greek, or Southeast Asian descent may be screened to see if they carry the hereditary blood disorders sickle-cell anemia or thalassemia. Ashkenazi Jews may be screened to see if they carry the genes for Tay-Sachs disease, an inherited disorder that causes blind-

DID YOU KNOW?

If you have a chronic disease, you should consult your doctor before you conceive. If you need diagnostic tests for your condition, they are best performed before you become pregnant; some tests, such as a radioactive scan for thyroid disease, may be harmful to the baby.

Medications used to treat some diseases, such as phenytoin (Dilantin) for epilepsy, may also pose a risk for the baby and may have to be discontinued or reduced.

Sometimes the disease itself may affect the pregnancy, and special measures must be taken to protect the baby. For example, severe asthma attacks may disrupt oxygen supply to the fetus. Conversely, pregnancy may affect the course of the disease, calling for an adjustment in treatment.

TABLE 25.1 Screening Tests for Pregnant Women

Stage of Pregnancy	Appropriate Tests (When Indicated)
First prenatal visit	Blood type, Rh type, antibody screen, hemoglobin and hematocrit, rubella antibodies, syphilis, hepatitis B, gonorrhea culture, Pap Smear, and urinalysis.
8–18 weeks	Ultrasound, alpha-fetoprotein, and amniocentesis or chorionic villi sampling.
24–28 weeks	Hemoglobin and hematocrit, glucose challenge test for diabetes, and Rh antibody screening (if Rh negative).
32–36 weeks	Ultrasound, syphilis, gonorrhea culture, and hemoglobin and hematocrit.
Optional additional tests	HIV, sickle-cell anemia or thalassemia, and chlamydia.

ness, mental retardation, and paralysis. (Preferably, women should have the screening test before conceiving because pregnancy can alter the test results.) A test performed on amniotic fluid can determine whether the baby carries the genes for the disorder.

Depending on your and your partner's medical histories, you may be tested for genital herpes or chlamydia, which can damage the baby. If you have an active herpes infection at the end of your pregnancy, you should deliver by cesarean section to protect the baby from contracting the virus during delivery.

If your due date falls after your 35th birthday, you will usually be offered amniocentesis or chorionic villi sampling to check for Down syndrome (see below).

TESTS ORDERED AT FOLLOW-UP PRENATAL VISITS

After the initial examination, your doctor will probably want to see you about once a month until your seventh month, every two to three weeks in the eighth month, and every week during the last month, unless you have a high-risk pregnancy that requires more frequent visits. During these follow-up visits your doctor will measure your blood pressure, record your weight and the growth of your uterus, and perform a dipstick urine test to screen for abnormal levels of proteins and glucose. The baby's heartbeat, which can usually be heard by the 12th week of pregnancy, will also be monitored. Your doctor will usually ask about the baby's movements and, if they appear to slow down, may order an ultrasound exam or electronic fetal heart monitoring.

Between the 14th and 17th weeks of pregnancy, you should be offered a test that measures alpha-fetoprotein (AFP), which can help detect spina bifida and poor fetal growth. In women who do not undergo amniocentesis, AFP can help identify women at risk of having a baby with Down syndrome. An enhanced version of this test, called triple screening, measures two hormones in addition to AFP. Triple screening helps identify more fetuses with Down syndrome than AFP alone, and many doctors recommend that all women undergo this test. If results of the AFP test or triple screening suggest a problem, ultrasound or amniocentesis may be performed to confirm the diagnosis.

At 24 to 28 weeks, the glucose challenge test for diabetes is usually performed. Some doctors recommend that all pregnant women have this test, which involves having your blood sugar levels measured after you have swallowed 5 ounces of a very sweet liquid (see chapter 19). The American College of Obstetricians and Gynecologists recommends that the test be performed in pregnant women who are 30 or older and in those who have a family history of diabetes or have previously had a stillborn baby or a baby that weighed close to 9 pounds or more, as well as in pregnant women who are obese or have glucose in their urine.

GENETIC COUNSELING AND PRENATAL DIAGNOSIS OF GENETIC DISORDERS

Your doctor may recommend genetic counseling and testing (see chapter 24) if there is a concern that your baby may have a genetic abnormality. Birth defects caused by these abnormalities are rare, accounting for only about 3% of all births. And about 95% of prenatal tests are negative, indicating no identifiable fetal abnormalities. Detecting an abnormality before delivery allows you time to consider an abortion or prepare for a baby who may have special needs. However, a negative test provides no absolute guarantee of a normal baby, as these tests are able to screen for only certain birth defects.

You may be concerned about your baby's genes if you or your partner has a genetic disease in the family, if you already have a child with an inherited disorder or birth defect, or if you are in your late 30s or 40s. Genetic testing may also be advised if you and your mate are blood relatives, such as first cousins, or if either of you has been exposed to radiation, medication, chemicals, or infection that may pose a risk to the fetus.

Tests are now available for detecting hundreds of genetic diseases, including cystic fibrosis, Tay-Sachs disease, sickle-cell anemia, beta thalassemia, Gaucher disease, Huntington disease, hemophilia, Duchenne muscular dystrophy, and fragile X syndrome. Of course, most of these disorders are rare. A particular test may be ordered only when the disorder is severe and there is a significant risk that the baby carries the genes for this disease. Thus, the risk of Down syndrome occurring in babies born to women under age 35 is not sufficiently high to warrant amniocentesis, a test that itself carries certain risks.

Genetic tests may be performed on future parents to check whether they carry recessive, or hidden, genes for a disease. Generally, there is a risk to the baby only if both parents are found to be carriers of the abnormal gene. Tests involving the fetus may consist of evaluating the fetal chromosomes, measuring enzymes or other products produced by genes, or evaluating the genes themselves (see chapter 24). If a suspected disorder affects only babies of one sex, determining the gender of the fetus may serve as an initial screening method.

There are several ways to obtain fetal genetic material. Most often, fetal cells are extracted from the amniotic fluid that surrounds the fetus (a process known as amniocentesis). In chorionic villi sampling (CVS), genetic analysis is performed on cells obtained from a portion of the amniotic sac because the genes in these cells are identical to those found in the fetus. In a relatively new technique known as fetal blood sampling, or cordocentesis, fetal blood cells are withdrawn for analysis via a needle inserted into the umbilical cord.

In the past, fetal blood and tissues for biopsy were removed with the help of fetoscopy, which involves inserting a rigid viewing tube into the uterus in order to obtain blood and tissue samples. However, because this technique results in miscarriages in up to 7% of cases, it has now been largely replaced by cordocentesis when a fetal blood sample is required and by ultrasound when there is a need to check for structural abnormalities.

PREGNANCY TEST

General information

Where It's Done	Who Does It	How Long It Takes	Discomfort/Pain
Commercial laboratory or hospital.	Doctor, nurse, or lab technician.	5 minutes or less to draw blood; less for urine sample.	Minor, from drawing blood.
Results Ready When	**Special Equipment**	**Risks/Complications**	**Average Cost**
A few minutes for urine test; 24 hours for precise blood test.	Supplies for drawing blood or container for collecting urine.	Negligible for drawing blood; none for urine test.	$

Other names Blood or urine pregnancy test and human chorionic gonadotropin (hCG).

Purpose

- To determine whether a woman is pregnant.
- To establish the stage of pregnancy (blood test only).

How it works The blood or urine is analyzed for the pregnancy hormone, human chorionic gonadotropin (hCG), which is released by the chorion (the membrane that becomes the placenta) within six days of conception. hCG levels peak between the eighth and 12th weeks of pregnancy.

Preparation Urine collection is best done first thing in the morning when hCG concentrations are highest. Avoid drinking or urinating during the previous night.

Test procedure Various testing techniques are used. The newest tests add blood or urine to monoclonal antibodies that recognize hCG (see chapter 15). In the urine test, color changes signify the presence of hCG.

After the test You may resume normal activities.

Factors affecting results

- hCG may be present in blood up to four weeks after an abortion or miscarriage.
- hCG may be released by trophoblastic tumors (molar pregnancies)—uncommon, benign tumors that usually develop in the placenta but may also occur when a piece of the placenta is left behind in the uterus after delivery, miscarriage, or abortion.

Interpretation

- The presence of hCG in blood or urine signals pregnancy.
- The simplest urine test is quick and inexpensive but is not accurate until at least two weeks after a missed period. (A more complex, more accurate urine test takes two hours but can be used about a week after a missed period.)
- A blood test is generally more reliable than a urine test in very early pregnancy; it is almost always accurate by the tenth day after conception.
- A blood test detecting hCG can establish the stage of pregnancy, but ultrasound is more accurate and can reveal an ectopic (tubal) pregnancy.

Advantages

- It highly reliable. By the sixth week of pregnancy, tests are virtually 100% accurate.
- Blood tests are generally positive one to two weeks before urine tests.
- Blood tests can detect hCG levels.
- Urine tests are quick, inexpensive, and noninvasive.

Disadvantages

- Urine tests may produce false-negative results a few days after conception.
- Urine tests only reveal presence of hCG.

The next step If result is positive, you should be scheduled for regular prenatal care.

ALPHA-FETOPROTEIN (AFP)

General information

Where It's Done	Who Does It	How Long It Takes	Discomfort/Pain
Commercial laboratory or hospital.	Doctor, nurse, or lab technician.	Less than 5 minutes.	Minor, from drawing blood.
Results Ready When	**Special Equipment**	**Risks/Complications**	**Average Cost**
Less than a week.	Syringe, needle, and blood collecting tube.	Negligible.	$

Other names Fetal alpha globulin.

Purpose

- To detect spina bifida and other abnormalities in the fetus.
- To evaluate the risk of Down syndrome in younger women.

How it works AFP, released by the baby's liver, is present in the mother's blood. Abnormally high AFP levels may signal abnormalities including neural tube defects (such as spina bifida), kidney problems, malformations of the digestive tract, threatened miscarriage, or death of the fetus. Abnormally low AFP levels may indicate Down syndrome, but this diagnosis must be confirmed by other tests.

Preparation The test is usually performed between the 15th and 18th weeks of pregnancy.

Test procedure Blood is drawn from a vein.

Variations *Triple screening*: In addition to alpha-fetoprotein, the blood sample is analyzed for human chorionic gonadotropin (hCG) and unconjugated estriol. All three substances, which are produced by the fetus or the placenta and enter the mother's bloodstream, can provide an estimated risk of the baby's having Down syndrome, spina bifida, and other significant birth defects, and of premature labor and other third-trimester complications. Although these tests can't be used to diagnose these conditions, this information can help determine if more definitive testing, such as amniocentesis or chorionic villi sampling, is necessary.

Because pregnancy after age 35 greatly increases the odds of chromosomal abnormalities such as Down syndrome, women in that age group are routinely offered either amniocentesis or chorionic villi sampling. These tests are not normally recommended for younger women, whose odds of having a miscarriage as a result of the tests are higher than their odds of having a Down syndrome baby. However, eight in ten Down syndrome babies are born to women under 35. Triple screening helps identify fetuses of younger women at risk, who can then be offered these tests.

DID YOU KNOW?

In nonpregnant women and in men, high blood levels of AFP (manufactured by the liver) may indicate cancer of the liver, pancreas, stomach, and gallbladder. AFP levels may also be raised in noncancerous conditions, including certain forms of hepatitis and cirrhosis of the liver.

After the test You may resume normal activities.

Factors affecting results

- Age of the fetus.
- Number of fetuses.
- Obesity, diabetes, and race.

Interpretation The doctor analyzes the levels, which vary with the age of the fetus and other factors.

Advantages It's noninvasive.

Disadvantages It produces a relatively high rate of false-positive and false-negative results, which are somewhat offset by the more sensitive "triple screening" (see Variations).

The next step

- If a high level is found, ultrasound is usually performed to check the age of the fetus and the number of fetuses.
- A low-level result may be followed by amniocentesis to check for Down syndrome.

PREGNANCY ULTRASOUND

General information

Where It's Done	Who Does It	How Long It Takes	Discomfort/Pain
Hospital, doctor's office, or commercial lab.	Doctor or sonographer.	15 minutes to 1 hour.	Mild when full bladder is required for imaging during early pregnancy.
Results Ready When	**Special Equipment**	**Risks/Complications**	**Average Cost**
Preliminary results, immediately; full report, 1–2 days.	Ultrasound monitor and transducer.	None.	$$

Other names Pelvic ultrasound scanning or sonography.

Purpose

- To establish the age and number of fetuses, evaluate their size and well-being, determine the location of the placenta, establish the amount of amniotic fluid, and detect abnormalities in the fetus and mother's pelvis.
- To reveal fetal malformations and severe disorders such as spina bifida.
- If the baby is at risk of inheriting a sex-linked disease, to determine the sex of the baby.
- May be performed to monitor fetal growth in late pregnancy.
- To assist in other procedures, such as amniocentesis, CVS, and fetal blood testing, that require placement of a needle in the uterus.

How it works High-frequency sound waves (see chapter 3) provide an image similar to an X-ray. The image, called a sonogram, shows the baby's entire body, organs, and the surrounding tissues.

Preparation

- If the test is performed during the first trimester, you will be asked to drink a great deal of fluids beforehand (a full bladder descends, allowing a better view of the uterus, and the fluid is a good medium for transmission of sound waves).

- Later in pregnancy, this is not necessary because the amniotic fluid provides the medium, and the enlarged uterus not only pushes the bladder down but extends so that it lies directly against the abdomen.
- You can remain dressed but you will be asked to expose your abdomen.

Test procedure

- Gel is applied to your abdomen, and an ultrasound transducer is swept across the area.
- The tester observes the image displayed on the screen.
- The sonogram, printed on film, videotape, or paper, may later be examined more carefully (although the doctor may analyze the scan immediately during the procedure).

Variations

Transvaginal ultrasound: This technique uses a small ultrasound transducer (about the size of a tampon) that is inserted directly into the vagina rather than pressed against the abdomen. This eliminates the need for women to fill up on fluids beforehand. For this test you disrobe from the waist down and lie on your back on a pelvic-exam table. A sterile condom is slipped over the transducer, or probe, which is then covered with lubricating gel and placed in the vagina. (If you find this uncomfortable, which few women do, you can ask to insert it yourself.) The probe rests up against the cervix (see figure 25.1). This produces a much sharper image, not only because of the close proximity to the uterus, but also because the transducer's crystal can vibrate at a higher frequency. The rest of the test proceeds the same way as transabdominal ultrasound. (For other uses of transvaginal ultrasound, see chapter 11.)

After the test

You are free to empty your bladder and return to previous activities.

Factors affecting results

- Obesity.
- Scars from abdominal surgery.
- In early pregnancy, a less-than-full bladder may obscure the results.

Interpretation

- A doctor examines the sonogram for structural abnormalities in the fetus, including congenital heart defects and bone deformities.
- The well-being of the fetus is evaluated by its movements and heartbeat.
- The doctor looks for problems in the mother, such as an incompetent cervix, which is prone to become dilated in pregnancy, leading to miscarriage.
- The sex of the fetus can be established around the 16th to 18th week of pregnancy.

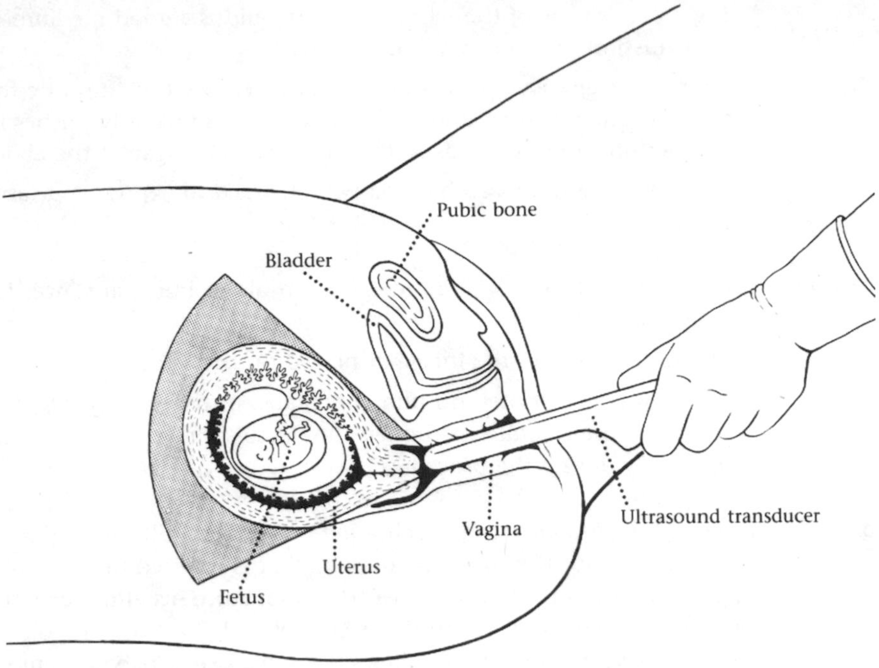

FIGURE 25.1 Transvaginal Ultrasound

As an alternative to an ultrasound examination through the abdominal wall, a doctor may insert a small transducer into the vagina. This method produces a better image of the fetus than can be obtained through the abdominal wall.

Advantages

- It entails no exposure to X-ray radiation.
- It's noninvasive.
- It produces quick results.
- It creates a moving image.

Disadvantages

- It's less reliable than amniocentesis or CVS in diagnosing certain disorders, such as Down syndrome.
- False-positive and false-negative results are possible.

The next step Suspected abnormalities should be confirmed at facilities with extensive experience at diagnosing fetal abnormalities.

AMNIOCENTESIS

General information

Where It's Done	Who Does It	How Long It Takes	Discomfort/Pain
Hospital, clinic or doctor's office.	Doctor with sonographer.	20–45 minutes.	Some discomfort when needle enters the skin and then the uterus.

Results Ready When	Special Equipment	Risks/Complications	Average Cost
1–2 weeks.	Syringe with needle, collecting tubes, and ultrasound guidance equipment.	Miscarriage rate of 0.5%–2%, injury to the fetus or placenta (rare), bleeding, and infection. Risk lowest when performed at 14–16 weeks.	$$$

Other names Amniotic fluid analysis.

Purpose

- To detect abnormalities in the fetus.
- To reveal chromosomal abnormalities, diseases caused by defective genes, and certain metabolic problems when one is suspected.
- To detect Down syndrome when the mother will be over age 35 at due date, has a family history of severe birth defects or metabolic disorders, or has had a low alpha-fetoprotein test result.
- To determine whether a baby expected to be delivered prematurely can survive outside the womb.
- In Rh-negative mothers carrying Rh-positive babies, to help evaluate the condition of the fetus and the need for an early delivery or fetal blood transfusion.

How it works A sample of fluid that fills the amniotic sac surrounding the baby is drawn (see figure 25.2), and cells shed from the baby's skin and digestive tract are cultured (grown in the laboratory), allowing analysis of genes and chromosomes and measurement of other substances in the fluid.

Preparation

- The test is performed between the 15th and 20th weeks of pregnancy.
- Your abdomen is cleansed with alcohol or iodine.

PATIENT TIP

One of the main concerns women have about amniocentesis is whether it will hurt. You *will* feel some discomfort when the needle enters the skin, and more when it penetrates the uterus, but most women find the test quite tolerable. If you are offered a local anesthetic, keep in mind that it will require an extra needle stick, which also adds time to the procedure and causes a slight burning sensation at first. Also remember that it numbs only the skin, not the uterine wall.

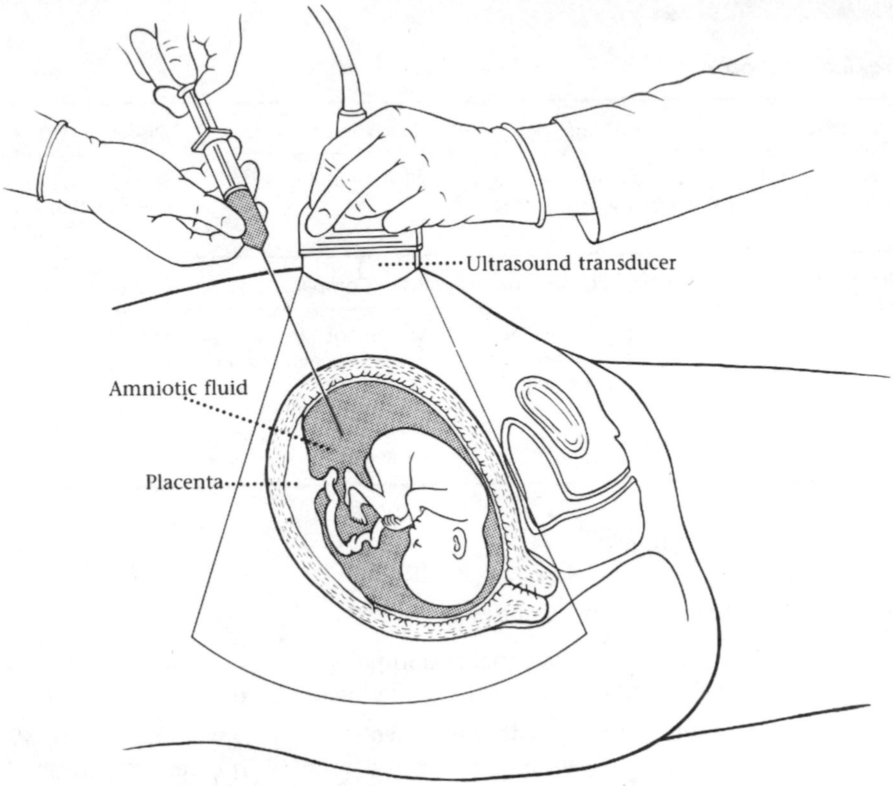

FIGURE 25.2 Amniocentesis

Using ultrasound as a guide, a doctor uses a hollow needle to withdraw some of the amniotic fluid surrounding the fetus. Fetal cells in this fluid are then analyzed for various chromosomal abnormalities.

Test procedure

- Ultrasound is often used to locate the placenta and make sure that there is sufficient amniotic fluid.
- A local anesthetic may be applied to your stomach.
- You lie on your back with your hands folded behind your head.
- A thin needle is inserted through the abdominal wall, and about a tablespoon of fluid is removed.

After the test

- Avoid strenuous activities for about 24 hours.
- Call your doctor immediately if you experience abdominal cramps, vaginal bleeding, leakage of clear fluid from your vagina, unusual behavior of the fetus, or anything else unusual.

Factors affecting results

- If the placenta is penetrated by the needle, some blood may enter the fluid and influence tests such as those for fetal lung maturity or spinal defects.
- Previous vaginal bleeding may discolor the fluid but does not affect chromosome analysis.

Interpretation

- The general appearance and content of the amniotic fluid is evaluated.
- Blood may signal damage to the fetus, placenta, or umbilical cord; the presence of feces in the third trimester may indicate fetal distress, or it may be normal.
- Chromosomes may be analyzed for Down syndrome, and the levels of alpha-fetoprotein may be measured to check for spina bifida (see above).
- Chromosome analysis also reveals the sex of the fetus and the risk of sex-linked disorders such as hemophilia.
- Other genes may be analyzed, as well as substances related to metabolic and developmental disorders.

DID YOU KNOW?

Many women worry about the needle accidentally pricking the baby. This is extremely uncommon, especially with direct ultrasound visualization. But it may put your mind at ease to know that for certain tests needles are deliberately put into fetuses, and they actually tolerate this quite well.

Advantages

- It detects numerous disorders before birth.
- It is virtually 100% reliable in revealing Down syndrome and spina bifida.

Disadvantages It cannot be performed as early in pregnancy as CVS, and takes longer for results.

The next step If an abnormality is detected, you will be referred to a genetic counselor, who can explain the implications of the test results.

CHORIONIC VILLI SAMPLING (CVS)

General information

Where It's Done	Who Does It	How Long It Takes	Discomfort/Pain
Hospital, clinic, or doctor's office.	Doctor and sonographer.	5–7 minutes.	Minor discomfort; cramping when the needle or catheter is inserted into the uterus.

Results Ready When	Special Equipment	Risks/Complications	Average Cost
2–5 days.	Catheter, syringe, collecting tubes, and ultrasound equipment.	Risk of miscarriage (about 1%–2% greater than amniocentesis), injury to the placenta and amniotic sac, bleeding, infection, and fetal damage when performed at less than 9½ weeks.	$$

Other names Chorionic villus sampling.

Purpose

- To detect suspected genetic abnormalities in the fetus.
- To identify chromosome disorders—most commonly, Down syndrome in women over 35.

How it works A thin tube, inserted either through the vagina and cervix or a needle inserted through the uterine wall, takes cells from the placenta (see figure 25.3).

Preparation If the test is done in the first trimester, you will be asked to drink enough to fill your bladder, since the fluid enhances the view of the uterus.

> **DID YOU KNOW?**
>
> *Villi* is the medical term for the tissue in the placenta, which contains genetic material identical to that of the fetus. With CVS, doctors can diagnose hundreds of birth defects. To be practical, however, they look at the parents' medical histories and then test only for the most likely defects.

Test procedure

- You disrobe and lie on your back on a pelvic-exam table.
- The sonographer uses ultrasound (see above) to observe the position of the uterus and placenta. The position helps determine whether a catheter will be inserted through the vagina and cervix or a needle inserted through the abdomen and uterine wall.
- If the sample is taken through the uterine wall, a local anesthetic may be applied first.
- For the needle method, an ultrasound transducer is placed on the abdomen as for amniocentesis.

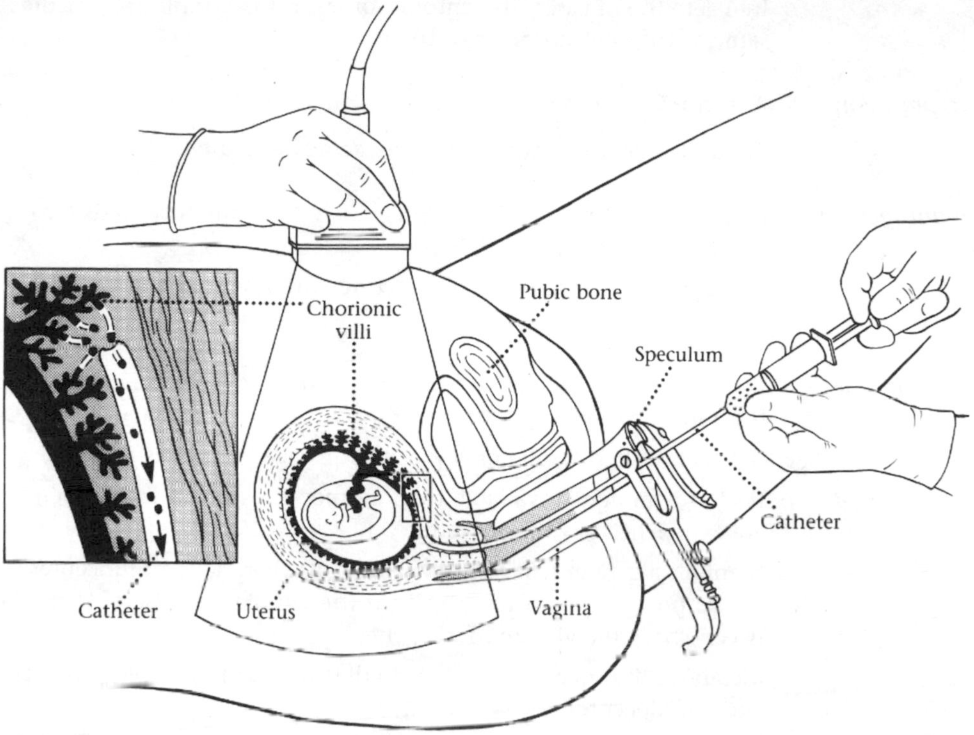

FIGURE 25.3 Chorionic Villi Sampling

In order to obtain cells from the placenta surface, a thin catheter is inserted into the cervix and uterus and a sampling of cells is suctioned into the tube. Ultrasound is used to guide placement of the catheter.

- For the catheter method, a thin metal rod is inserted into the cervix to help identify it on the ultrasound scan and show how best to insert the catheter into the uterus.

After the test

- Avoid strenuous activities for about 24 hours.
- You may experience mild cramping for a few hours, especially if needle withdrawal was used.
- If the transvaginal method was used, you may have some light spotting. Because iodine is used to prep the vagina, you may also leak iodine, which looks like dried blood.
- Contact your doctor immediately if you experience severe abdominal cramps, vaginal bleeding that is more than spotting, fluid leakage, fever, or anything else that feels abnormal.

Factors affecting results

- Presence of the mother's cells in the sample may distort measurements.

- In 1% to 3% of cases, the chromosomes in the sample are not the same as the chromosomes of the fetus.

Interpretation

- A doctor evaluates the fetal chromosomes for disorders.
- The cells may be cultured for more accurate results.

Advantages

- It can be performed earlier in pregnancy than amniocentesis (at around ten weeks).
- It is almost 100% reliable in detecting chromosomal and genetic defects.

Disadvantages

- It does not measure alpha-fetoprotein (AFP), so a supplemental blood test must be used.
- It entails a slightly higher risk of miscarriage than does amniocentesis.
- It's less commonly available than amniocentesis, and fewer doctors are experienced in the procedure.
- It entails a greater risk of distorted results than does amniocentesis due to presence of mother's cells in the sample and discrepancies between chorionic villi and fetal genes.
- Metabolic disorders are difficult to diagnose and must be confirmed with amniocentesis.
- Because of the early gestational age at which the test is performed, fetal anatomy cannot be seen as well as it can at the time amniocentesis is performed.

The next step If an abnormality is detected, you will be referred to a genetic counselor, who can explain the implications of the test results.

FETAL BLOOD TEST

General information

Where It's Done	Who Does It	How Long It Takes	Discomfort/Pain
Hospital or doctor's office.	Doctor and sonographer.	5 minutes to 1 hour.	Similar to having blood drawn.
Results Ready When	**Special Equipment**	**Risks/Complications**	**Average Cost**
A few minutes to a few days, depending on the extent of testing.	Spinal needle and ultrasound equipment.	Risk of miscarriage about comparable to amniocentesis (1%–2%), infection, and temporary slowing of fetal heartbeat.	$$$

Other names Cordocentesis, fetal blood sampling, umbilical cord blood testing, and percutaneous umbilical blood sampling (PUBS).

Purpose

- To rapidly verify the presence of Down syndrome or another fetal chromosomal abnormality.
- To evaluate the presence of chromosomal abnormalities when CVS results are ambiguous.
- To detect the presence of infectious disease such as toxoplasmosis, rubella, or cytomegalovirus in the fetus, so that it can be treated.
- To perform a blood count and check for anemia or low platelet levels in the fetus.

How it works

A sample of the baby's blood is withdrawn from the umbilical cord and analyzed (see figure 25.4).

Preparation

- If you are in the third trimester you may have to fast overnight in case an emergency cesarean delivery is required.
- Your abdomen is cleansed with an antiseptic solution.

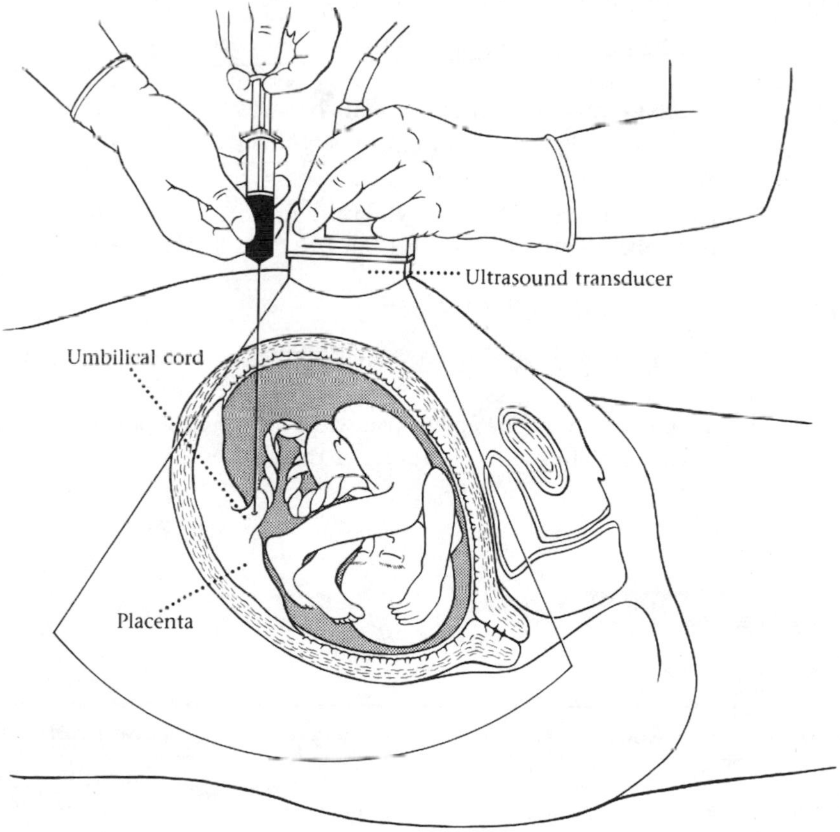

FIGURE 25.4 Fetal Blood Test

Guided by ultrasound, the doctor inserts a thin hollow needle through the abdominal wall and into the uterus to withdraw a sample of blood from the umbilical cord.

Test procedure

- Guided by an ultrasound image, the doctor introduces a long, thin needle through the abdomen and uterus into the umbilical cord.
- About a teaspoon of blood is drawn and checked to be sure it is fetal blood; a second sample may be taken.
- The baby's heartbeat is monitored during the procedure.

After the test

- Your breathing and pulse and the baby's heartbeat are monitored for about an hour, after which you are free to leave.
- Avoid strenuous activities for 24 hours.
- Contact your doctor immediately if you experience abdominal cramps, vaginal bleeding, leakage of amniotic fluid into your vagina, unusual behavior of the fetus, or anything else that feels abnormal.

Factors affecting results

The presence of maternal blood or amniotic fluid in the sample distorts results.

Interpretation

- The blood is analyzed for the same conditions as in CVS.
- The blood may be examined for the presence of antibodies.

Advantages

- It allows rapid evaluation of fetal chromosomes when quick decisions must be made about ending the pregnancy or delivering by cesarean section.
- It can help avoid abortion when the mother has an infection potentially threatening to the fetus but the fetus is not infected.

Disadvantages

- It has limited availability.
- The test is new, and its risks have not been firmly established.

The next step

If an abnormality is detected, you will be referred to a genetic counselor, who can explain the implications of the test results.

FETAL MONITORING

General information

Where It's Done	Who Does It	How Long It Takes	Discomfort/Pain
Hospital, birthing center, doctor's office, or at home with trained personnel.	Doctor, nurse, attendant, or midwife.	20–90 minutes, or intermittently.	Internal monitoring restricts movement.

Results Ready When	Special Equipment	Risks/Complications	Average Cost
Immediately for some results; interpretation by perinatologist may be done later.	Ultrasound device, tocodynamometer, straps to keep the devices in place, and fetal-scalp electrodes (for internal monitoring).	Risk of infection with internal monitoring.	$–$$

Other names External or internal fetal monitoring.

Purpose

- To monitor the baby's heart rate and other functions during late pregnancy and labor.
- To help assess fetal well-being, especially if the baby suddenly becomes less active than usual.
- To monitor for signs of early contractions or other indications that the mother may not carry to term, especially in cases of multiple babies, or if the mother has diabetes, high blood pressure, thyroid problems, or a history of stillbirths.

How it works

- Uterine contractions and the fetal heart rate, a major indication of fetal well-being, are measured with the help of ultrasound and recorded.
- Sometimes ultrasound imaging is used to assess the baby's breathing, muscle tone, and movements. During labor, a fetal blood sample may be taken to make sure the baby receives adequate oxygen.
- If you have high blood pressure, diabetes, or other factors that increase the risk of complications, monitoring may begin in the last stages of pregnancy.

Preparation

- If the test is performed before labor, you should eat to increase fetal movement.
- During labor, avoid eating or drinking.

PATIENT TIPS

- Be sure to eat before the test. If your blood sugar is low, your baby may respond by sleeping or being inactive, which will prolong the test. But avoid ingesting caffeine—in coffee, cola, or chocolate—which can accelerate the baby's heart rate and therefore prolong the test.
- If you have small children, try to leave them with a baby-sitter, bring someone along to watch them, or if that isn't possible, pack plenty of activities to entertain them. You'll be immobile during the test, but your toddler won't be!
- If you're uncomfortable lying on your back, ask to have your head elevated slightly. If you're really uncomfortable, once the baby's position and the amount of amniotic fluid surrounding the baby have been assessed, ask if you can lie on your side for the rest of the test.

Test procedure

- In the simplest test, a stethoscope is attached to your abdomen to listen to the baby's heartbeat.
- For typical external electronic monitoring, you sit in a recliner (unless you are in the delivery room) and a monitor is attached with straps to your abdomen. A tablespoon of gel is applied to your abdomen as a medium for the ultrasound transducer. The transducer transmits the fetal heartbeat to a recorder, which charts the beats. The heartbeat may be amplified and heard as a beeping sound.
- Ultrasound may be used to observe the baby for about 30 minutes. During this time, the rhythmic movements of the chest are monitored and movements are counted to evaluate fetal well-being.
- If you are having contractions, an external tocodynamometer records their pattern.
- In high-risk situations, fetal monitoring may be performed internally via electrodes inserted through the dilated cervix and attached to the scalp of the fetus (see figure 25.5).
- During labor, fetal blood may be drawn from the baby's scalp and checked for acidity.

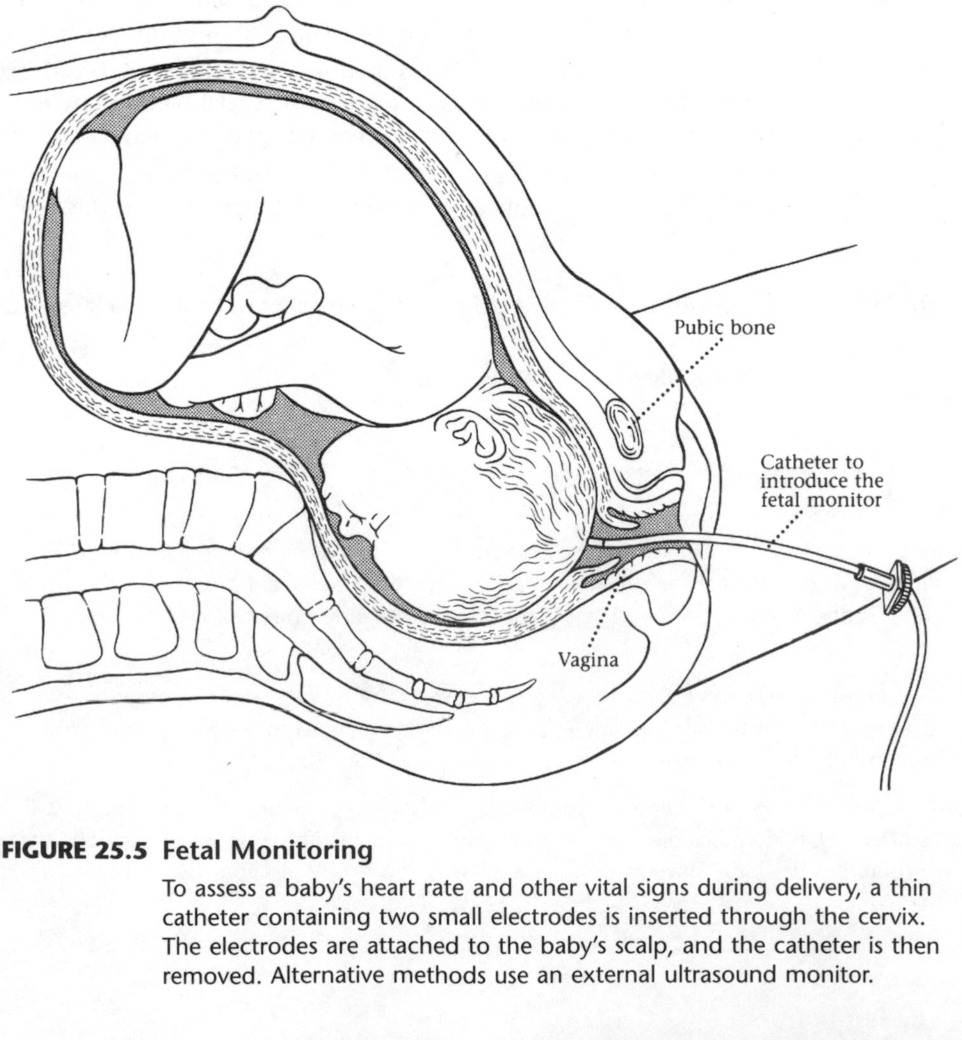

FIGURE 25.5 Fetal Monitoring

To assess a baby's heart rate and other vital signs during delivery, a thin catheter containing two small electrodes is inserted through the cervix. The electrodes are attached to the baby's scalp, and the catheter is then removed. Alternative methods use an external ultrasound monitor.

After the test No special aftercare is required.

Factors affecting results

- Certain drugs, including painkillers, anesthetics, and tranquilizers.
- Position at which external fetal monitor is placed.
- Body position and obesity.

Interpretation Fetal heart rate should accelerate periodically and should not drop with uterine contractions. Otherwise, the baby may not be receiving sufficient oxygen.

Advantages It allows for early detection of birthing complications.

Disadvantages

- It restricts mobility.
- False-positive results may occur, particularly in low-risk pregnancies, and lead to an unnecessary cesarean section.

The next step A result suggesting fetal distress in a near-term pregnancy may indicate the need for an emergency cesarean section.

KLEIHAUER-BETKE (K-B)

General information

Where It's Done	Who Does It	How Long It Takes	Discomfort/Pain
Hospital or commercial lab.	Doctor, nurse, or technician.	5 minutes.	Minor, from drawing blood.
Results Ready When	**Special Equipment**	**Risks/Complications**	**Average Cost**
Same day.	Syringe and needle, and equipment for analyzing blood sample.	Negligible.	$

Other names Acid elution for fetal hemoglobin.

Purpose To determine the amount of Rh immune globulin an Rh-negative woman must receive to prevent her from developing antibodies, or abnormal proteins, against her fetus.

How it works Blood is drawn and tested for the presence of fetal cells.

Preparation None.

Test procedure Blood is drawn from your vein and analyzed for the presence of fetal cells with a special staining technique known as the Kleihauer-Betke method.

After the test You may resume normal activities.

Factors affecting results Blood diseases in the mother that produce fetal types of hemoglobin.

Interpretation The greater the fetal blood leakage into the mother's circulation, the greater the amount of Rh immune globulin the mother must receive.

Advantages There is no risk to the mother or fetus.

Disadvantages None.

The next step The appropriate amount of Rh immune globulin is prescribed for the mother.

Janet B. Henrich, MD ■ *Florence Comite, MD*

26 Testing in Women

Tests Covered in This Chapter

The case of Marsha W., a 42-year-old attorney:

It had been two years since my last mammogram when my doctor suggested that I have a comprehensive evaluation at a specialized women's health clinic. It included such tests as a mammogram, a bone-density scan, electrocardiogram, and blood tests, and assessments by various health professionals.

After I had my mammogram, the technologist told me they needed a second set of my right breast. I didn't think anything was unusual. I perform breast self-exams fairly regularly, and I hadn't felt anything out of the ordinary. Of course, it's difficult to tell, because my breasts always feel very lumpy.

I was then asked to come back for a special type of mammogram called a spot compression. That's when I began to realize something was very wrong. Six years before, I'd had a benign fibroadenoma tumor the size of a walnut surgically removed from my other breast.

The Tests The spot on Marsha's mammogram was so tiny that it might have been an enlarged blood vessel or merely a speck of lint on the camera lens. None of the three physicians who examined her breast manually could feel a lump. Although some women with larger tumors might go directly from mammogram to biopsy, Marsha's case required additional tests. Spot compression applies pressure to a specific area of the breast, spreading out the tissues to enable a better view. When this test could not rule out a tumor, a breast ultrasound was performed. Cancer was ultimately diagnosed on the basis of a stereotatic biopsy, a sophisticated type of needle biopsy that uses mammography to help the doctor locate a mass that cannot be felt.

The Outcome Marsha's tumor was very small—less than 1 centimeter (about ⅖ of an inch) in diameter. She underwent a lumpectomy, the least invasive surgical procedure for breast cancer, followed by radiation therapy, and her prognosis is excellent. Had she waited another year to have a mammogram, the tumor might have doubled in size, at which point the average five-year survival rate would have dropped from 85% to 66%. Ironically, the same day that 42-year-old Marsha's initial mammogram showed a suspicious mass, the National Cancer Institute dropped its recommendation that women under 50 have regular mammograms (other experts continue to recommend them, however; see chapter 2).

INTRODUCTION

Because women live longer than men, they constitute the majority of the population that is most susceptible to disease. The same three diseases that kill most American men—heart disease, stroke, and cancer—are also the three leading causes of death in American women. Yet women have often been excluded from research into these diseases, leading some experts to wonder whether the information gleaned from research on men has been applied inappropriately to women, resulting in less than optimal care.

These concerns are now being met. An awakening to the importance of women's health has ushered in unprecedented efforts to provide better care for women in the United States. This means that you can expect much better access to information about the conditions that are most likely to affect you now and in the future, as results from newly implemented wide-scale research become available. You can take advantage of this awareness in the medical community by paying close attention to medical advice on disease prevention and early diagnosis. Screening and diagnostic tests are an important part of this process.

If you want to take control of your health, you must not only be informed but must also assume responsibility for your care, recognizing that it is your right to participate in decisions about your treatment. You should begin by scheduling timely appointments with an internist or family practitioner who can provide continuity to and oversee your general medical and routine gynecological care. If you are in your childbearing years or have gynecological problems, you may also want to find a gynecologist/obstetrician who will work well with your regular doctor.

Some health problems are unique to women, some express themselves differently in women, and others are simply more common in women. This chapter covers some of the diagnostic procedures most common in women. Chapter 11, The Female Reproductive System, covers other tests and procedures for diseases that involve the reproductive organs; breast self-examination is illustrated in chapter 2. Diagnostic tests for diseases that affect both men and women are found in various other chapters throughout this book.

HOW YOUR DOCTOR DIAGNOSES ILLNESSES COMMON TO WOMEN

Before a physical exam, your doctor or other health care professional will review your medical history, including information about your menstrual and reproductive history and what medications you are taking. Your doctor will want to know about the health of other members of your family, especially sisters, mother, and grandmothers. This information helps determine your personal risks for disorders that may be more common in families. For instance, the incidence of breast cancer is linked to family history. If any of your close relatives have had breast cancer, your physician may recommend earlier mammography screenings for you. There is some evidence that osteoporosis also runs in families. If your mother or father has osteoporosis, you may be a candidate for bone-density measurement tests as you approach menopause and your menstrual cycles become irregular.

Your physician should also inquire about your diet, exercise habits, and any unhealthy behavior such as smoking or excessive drinking. Many diseases that affect women as they age have origins in earlier health behavior that can be prevented or mitigated. The doctor may also ask about recent life events. The answers may explain symptoms such as menstrual irregularity or sleeplessness.

The focus of routine physical exams is to uncover information that might indicate recommendations for screening and further diagnostic tests. Many disorders that affect women have few early symptoms, so regular screening is necessary. (For a schedule of such screening tests, see chapter 2.)

A complete routine physical should include a professional breast exam involving palpation of each breast (extended to the underarm) and, depending on your age and medical history, a pelvic exam and Pap smear. If appropriate, it may also include diagnostic exams for breast disease and osteoporosis, as detailed below.

Breast Disease

Most benign breast lumps and cysts occur in women aged 35 to 50. If you or your doctor finds a lump, a mammogram, needle aspiration, and/or breast ultrasound (see below) may be recommended, depending on your age, to determine if the lump is a solid mass or a fluid-filled sac (a cyst). A biopsy, in which a tissue sample is removed for pathological study, may be necessary to determine if the lump is cancerous. The biopsy may be either percutaneous (nonsurgical) or surgical.

If a cancerous tumor is detected, it will usually be removed surgically and assessed for size and the factors that might cause it to grow, such as whether its growth is influenced by estrogen. Also, tests to determine if it has metastasized (spread to other parts of the body) will be performed immediately. Benign lumps are usually removed during a biopsy. In the case of cysts, the fluid may be withdrawn (aspirated) with a needle, or the entire cyst may be removed surgically.

Osteoporosis

Although loss of bone mass is part of the aging process for both men and women, it occurs earlier and progresses more rapidly in women, possibly leading to more severe consequences. Loss of up to several inches in body height, back pain, and deformity of the spine ("dowager's hump") are common manifestations of this disorder.

Osteoporosis affects most women to some degree. Bone loss starts at about 40 years of age and increases about twofold in the decade following menopause. Although widespread screening is not recommended, some women at risk because of a strong family history of osteoporosis, primary or secondary amenorrhea, use of steroid medication for such conditions as Crohn's disease, asthma, or thyroid disorders, and/or poor dietary calcium intake may benefit from earlier measures of bone density. Early detection may show premature loss of bone mass and allow time to take measures to prevent the complications of this disorder.

It is unfortunate and tragically unnecessary that many women are not diagnosed until they break a bone and/or their decreased bone mass becomes apparent on X-rays. At least a 30% loss of calcium from the bone must occur before an X-ray can detect signs of osteoporosis. By this time, the risk of serious injury is high. There are several more sensitive methods used to assess bone density, including quantitative digital radiography (QDR). At present, QDR is considered the best method. It is difficult, if not impossible, to determine the cause of bone loss. However, a bone biopsy is sometimes used to help sort out potential causes. Timely therapy with replacement hormones or nonhormonal medications can help prevent bones from becoming so brittle that they fracture.

HOW DIAGNOSTIC TESTS MAY DIFFER IN WOMEN

In tests for diseases that are not unique to women, gender may affect the way a test is performed or the reliability of its results. Some tests are gender-dependent because they are related to the hormonal effects surrounding the menstrual cycle, pregnancy, or menopause. For example, some blood tests used to diagnose endocrine system disorders, especially thyroid function tests, require special interpretation in women.

Hormones, especially estrogen, and hormone-related conditions can sometimes alter results from blood and urine tests. Women generally have lower red blood cell counts, and thus a smaller store of iron, because of loss during menstruation and pregnancy. This is considered normal and, depending on the blood count, is not necessarily a sign of disease if anemia is not present.

Body structure can also cause difficulty in certain diagnostic procedures. Primary examples are the exercise stress tests and isotope tests for heart disease, which are more difficult to interpret in women because of the presence of breast tissue. Also, a blood test for creatine phosphokinase, an enzyme released by the muscles and useful in assessing heart attack damage, has different results for men and women because men have a greater muscle mass.

Sometimes tests are not used in the same way for women as for men. Perhaps the most striking example of this disparity is in the diagnosis and management of coronary artery disease. Despite the fact that coronary artery disease is the number-one cause of death among American women, studies have shown that women are referred less often than men for procedures such as cardiac catheterization (see chapter 5). In one 1987 study of a group of 390 people who had abnormal results from an exercise radionuclide scan, 40% of the men were referred for cardiac catheterization, compared to only 4% of the women. Whether this test is overused in men or underused in women is not clear.

DISORDERS AND SCREENING AT DIFFERENT AGES

Birth to Young Adulthood

The first two decades in a woman's life constitute the period of primary physical and emotional development and maturity. Most adolescents and young women remain relatively free of those conditions that are the leading causes of severe disability or death in older women, such as heart disease, breast cancer, and osteoporosis. Injuries, motor vehicle accidents, and risk-taking behavior such as drug and alcohol use, smoking, and unprotected sexual activity take a higher toll among this age group. About 10% of females in this age group have a serious disease or disability. Those conditions that are more common among girls or occur for the first time during or are worsened by puberty include autoimmune disorders such as lupus and juvenile rheumatoid arthritis, scoliosis, and thyroid disorders. Tests relating to these diseases are cross-referenced in table 26.1, Important Causes of Illness and Disability in Women.

Some screening tests are recommended for young women, but they may be fewer and farther between than for older women.

TABLE 26.1 Important Causes of Illness and Disability in Women

The following conditions are of concern to women at different ages. Tests and procedures that detect risk factors for and early signs of these diseases are found in the indicated chapters.

Disorder	Chapter Reference
	Adolescence to Age 44
Risk-taking behaviors	
Early sexual activity	Chapter 11, The Female Reproductive System, and chapter 25, Pregnancy.
Substance abuse	Chapter 29, Toxicology, Monitoring of Drug Therapy, and Testing for Substance Abuse.
Scoliosis	Chapter 13, Rheumatoid and Musculoskeletal Disorders.
Sexually transmitted diseases (including AIDS)	Chapter 11, The Female Reproductive System; chapter 21, Human Immunodeficiency Virus (HIV) and Acquired Immunodeficiency Syndrome (AIDS); and chapter 22, Infectious Diseases.
Infertility	Chapter 11, The Female Reproductive System.
Complications of pregnancy	Chapter 25, Pregnancy.
Endometriosis	Chapter 11, The Female Reproductive System.
Chronic pelvic pain	Chapter 11, The Female Reproductive System.
Premenstrual syndrome (PMS)	Chapter 11, The Female Reproductive System.
Autoimmune disorders	
Lupus erythematosus	Chapter 15, The Immune System.
Juvenile rheumatoid arthritis	Chapter 15, The Immune System.
Thyroid disorders	Chapter 9, The Endocrine System.
Depression	Not covered in this book.
Sexual and physical abuse	Not covered in this book.
	Ages 45 to 64
Arthritis	Chapter 13, Rheumatoid and Musculoskeletal Disorders.
Osteoporosis	Chapter 26, Testing in Women.
Diabetes	Chapter 19, Diabetes.
Menopausal symptoms	Chapter 11, The Female Reproductive System.
	Ages 65 and Older
Frailty	Not covered in this book.
Arthritis	Chapter 13, Rheumatoid and Musculoskeletal Disorders.
Bone fractures	Chapter 13, Rheumatoid and Musculoskeletal Disorders.
Dementia	Chapter 23, The Nervous System.
Movement disorders (Parkinson's disease, etc)	Chapter 23, The Nervous System.
Peripheral vascular disease	Chapter 6, The Vascular System.
Digestive disorders	Chapter 8, The Digestive System.
Bladder problems	Chapter 12, The Renal System.

Although recommendations vary according to different professional organizations, a routine physical exam every three years, a professional breast exam and pelvic exam annually with a Pap smear every one to three years, and a breast self-exam monthly usually suffice for healthy women between puberty and age 35. Of course, during those years, women must be aware of choices in lifestyle that can lower the likelihood of more serious diseases later in life. For instance, avoiding bad habits such as smoking and recreational drug use and opting for good habits such as a proper diet and exercise during the early years may significantly decrease the incidence of osteoporosis, lung and other cancers, and heart disease later in life.

Young Adulthood to Menopause

Your reproductive years are still relatively free of chronic diseases and disabilities. Injuries, less common forms of heart disease, cancer, and AIDS are the most common for this age group. Most important during this time are the conditions related to sexual function, conception control, and pregnancy. Prevention of sexually transmitted diseases, including AIDS, is critical.

In their 30s, many women experience breast changes that are usually benign. This irregularity or "lumpiness" is usually referred to as fibrocystic disease or benign breast disease and can lead to diagnostic breast procedures in some women in an attempt to distinguish between benign conditions and breast cancer. The benefits of screening mammography have not been proven in women under 50 who have no breast disease symptoms. Because of this uncertainty, screening recommendations vary for women between the ages of 40 and 50. It is generally recommended that any woman with a personal history of breast cancer should have a professional breast exam and mammogram annually regardless of her age, as should any woman 40 and over with a strong family history of breast cancer.

Menopause to the Mature Years

The average age at menopause, the period in which many chronic diseases first make their appearance in women, is 51. Heart disease, cancer (especially breast and colon cancer), arthritis, osteoporosis, depression, diabetes, and some disabilities and injuries are the leading causes of ill health and death for this age group.

You can make managing your health care a personal priority by undergoing annual physical exams, becoming well informed about signs and symptoms of troubling conditions, and seeking prompt medical attention when you notice problems. You may also choose to take replacement hormones after menopause. Studies show that estrogen eases symptoms and has a protective effect against heart disease and bone loss, but it may increase the risk for certain types of cancer. Cardiac studies, bone-density tests, and the assessment of other risk factors for these disorders will help you and your doctor come to an informed decision.

It is important not to ignore the benefits of technology. For instance, mammography is the most effective tool in finding cancerous tumors that are not detected during breast exams and in distinguishing between benign and malignant breast lumps. Breast cancer is the most common cancer among women in the United States, but despite the statistics, many women do not regularly undergo mammography screenings. Even though it is hard to find time, the fact that mammography combined with breast examinations decreases the incidence of death from breast cancer in women over 50 should be a highly motivating factor. Women 50 and over should have a professional breast exam annually and a mammogram every one or two years even if they have no symptoms of breast disease.

The Mature Years, After 65

In the United States, women account for 59% of the population in this age group. They live about four to ten years longer than men. Aging by itself does not necessarily have to result in a decline in function and health. In fact, there are often opportunities to intervene to enhance health for many older women. Regular physical exams, screening tests, and proper diagnostic responses to signs and symptoms can identify those windows for intervention.

The diseases and disabilities that affect women in this stage of life include arthritis, cancer, dementia (including Alzheimer's disease), heart disease, neurologic disorders, osteoporosis, and urinary incontinence.

MAMMOGRAPHY

General information

Where It's Done	Who Does It	How Long It Takes	Discomfort/Pain
Outpatient radiology office or radiology section of hospital.	Radiology technician.	About 30–45 minutes from the time you arrive.	Some discomfort when breast is compressed between the plastic plates.
Results Ready When	**Special Equipment**	**Risks/Complications**	**Average Cost**
A few minutes to a few days, depending on findings and urgency of results.	Dedicated X-ray equipment accredited by the American College of Radiology.	X-ray exposure is very low. However, pregnant women should discuss the risks to the fetus versus the importance of the test.	$–$$ (depends on facility).

Other names None.

Purpose

- To screen for breast cancer in healthy women with no breast problems.

- To diagnose breast disease in women with symptoms, previous breast surgery, or previous abnormal mammograms.

How it works X-ray technology is used to view internal structures of the breasts.

Preparation You disrobe from the waist up, remove all jewelry, and don a front-opening hospital gown.

Test procedure

- You stand next to a special X-ray unit.
- The technologist gently positions your breast on top of an X-ray film cassette and compresses it from the top with a plastic compression plate.
- At least two X-rays (from two positions) are taken of each breast.

PATIENT TIPS

On the day of the test:

- Wear a two-piece outfit so you need only remove the top.
- Avoid using powder or deodorant, which can produce shadows on the mammogram.
- Try to avoid having the exam during premenstrual days or during your period, when breasts are swollen and tender.

After the test You may be asked to wait while the X-ray film is developed. Then you may dress and resume normal activities.

Factors affecting results

- Using deodorant or wearing jewelry on your upper body.
- Having lumpy breasts, which are more common before age 40.
- Breast implants or other previous breast surgery.

Interpretation A radiologist who specializes in mammography examines your X-rays for abnormalities, which appear as opaque spots on the film (see figures 26.1 and 26.2a–b).

Advantages

- It's the best method for detecting breast cancer when it is still early enough to be curable.
- It's noninvasive.

Disadvantages

- A small amount of radiation is involved.
- For women with very dense breasts, some breast tumors may be difficult to detect.

The next step

- If the results are normal, you should have your next mammogram in one to two years, depending on your age.
- If any abnormalities are found, you may have to have another mammogram, an ultrasound, or a breast biopsy.

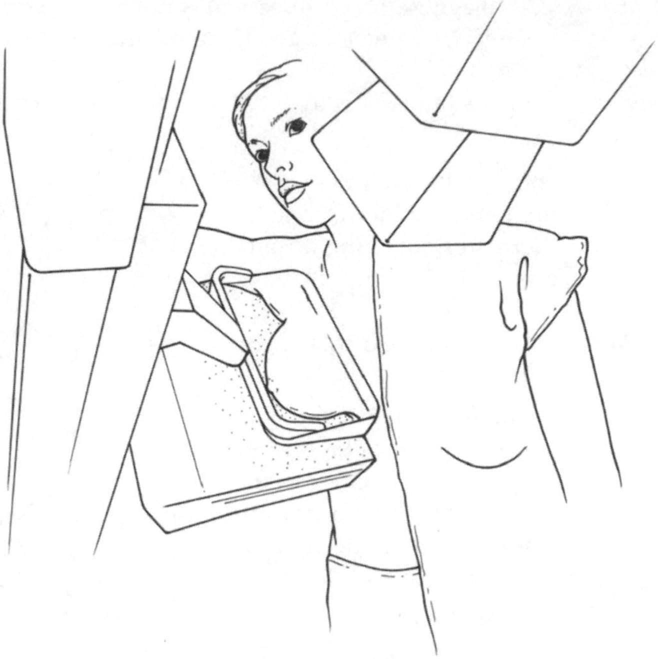

FIGURE 26.1 During mammography, a special low-dose X-ray machine is used to produce images of the breast. In many instances, these images can detect breast cancers in a very early stage when they are still too small to be felt during a physical examination.

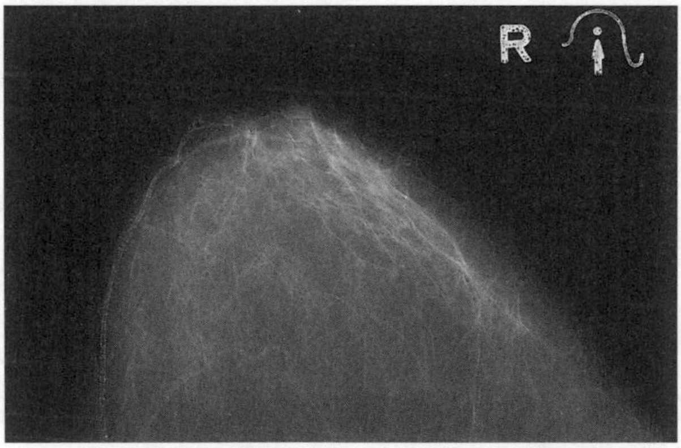

FIGURE 26.2a A mammogram of a normal breast.

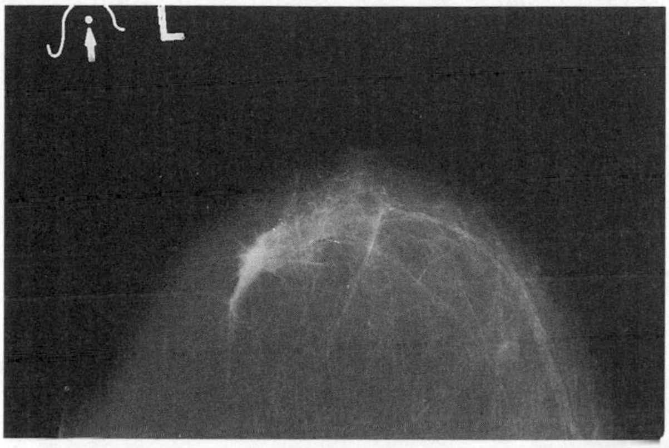

FIGURE 26.2b A mammogram showing an abnormal growth. A biopsy is needed to confirm whether this is indeed cancer.

BREAST ULTRASOUND

General information

Where It's Done	Who Does It	How Long It Takes	Discomfort/Pain
Outpatient radiology office or radiology section of a hospital.	Technician, usually female.	About 30–45 minutes.	None.
Results Ready When	**Special Equipment**	**Risks/Complications**	**Average Cost**
From a few minutes to a few days, depending on urgency of results.	Ultrasound equipment.	None.	$$

Other names None.

Purpose To determine whether a lump in the breast is a cyst (usually follows an abnormal mammogram).

How it works High-frequency sound waves (see chapter 3) are directed through the breast to provide an image of internal structures.

Preparation You disrobe from the waist up, remove all jewelry, and don a front-opening hospital gown.

Test procedure

- Gel is applied to your breast, and an ultrasound transducer is swept across the area.
- The technician observes the image displayed on the screen.
- The sonogram, printed on film, videotape, or paper, may later be examined more thoroughly (although the doctor may analyze the scan immediately during the procedure).

After the test You are free to leave and resume normal activities.

Factors affecting results A very large, dense breast makes it difficult to see small, deeply embedded lumps.

Interpretation A radiologist who specializes in ultrasound will examine the image for any abnormalities.

Advantages

- It's noninvasive.
- It can often distinguish between solid masses and benign cysts.

Disadvantages

- It may not be of use in women with large, dense breasts.
- It may miss small masses or solid tumors.

The next step

- If the results are normal, you should have your next mammogram in one to two years, depending on your age.
- If an abnormality is found, you may have to have a diagnostic mammogram, an ultrasound, or a breast biopsy.
- If a cyst is found, no additional tests are required, and treatment can proceed.

PERCUTANEOUS (NONSURGICAL) BREAST BIOPSY

General information

Where It's Done	Who Does It	How Long It Takes	Discomfort/Pain
Outpatient radiology office or radiology section of hospital.	Radiologist.	About 1 hour.	Slight discomfort when local anesthesia is administered.
Results Ready When	**Special Equipment**	**Risks/Complications**	**Average Cost**
Within 4 working days.	A special X-ray table and a computer that calculates the exact location of the breast lump.	Some bruising or pain may occur after the procedure.	$$

Other names Stereotatic-core needle.

Purpose To confirm or rule out malignancy.

How it works A tissue sample is physically withdrawn and sent to a pathology laboratory for examination and microscopic evaluation.

Preparation You disrobe from the waist up and don a front-opening hospital gown.

Test procedure

- You lie face down on a specially designed table with a hole in which the breast is positioned.
- Using ultrasound for guidance, the radiologist locates the lump or cyst.
- Within a fraction of a second, the large-core needle removes a sample (see figure 26.3).

After the test You dress and return to normal activities.

Factors affecting results Inadequate amount of tissue in the sample for diagnosis.

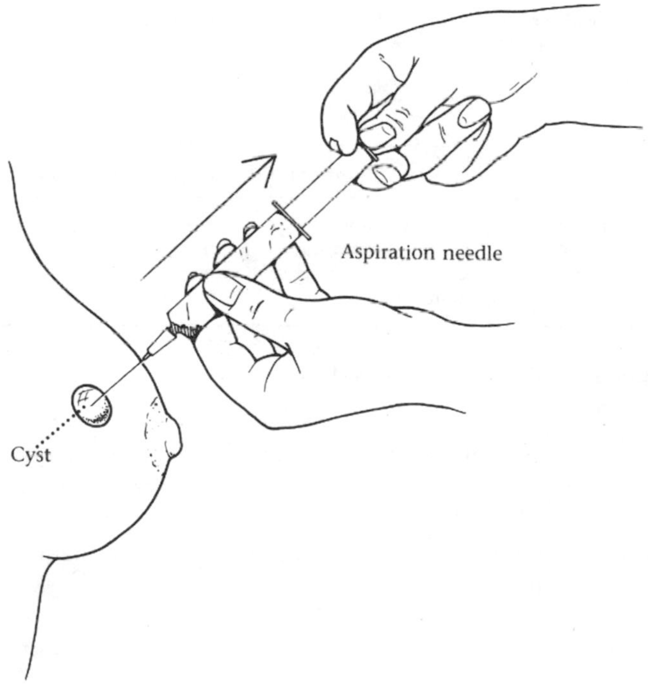

FIGURE 26.3 In a percutaneous breast biopsy, a thin, hollow needle is inserted into the suspicious growth and cells are withdrawn for laboratory analysis. In this instance, the growth is actually a benign fluid-filled cyst.

Interpretation The pathologist examines the tissue sample under a microscope for malignant cells.

Advantages

- It eliminates the need for surgical biopsy in women who have benign lumps or cysts.
- In most cases, it eliminates one surgical procedure for women who have malignant lumps.
- It requires one-third to one-half the cost of surgical biopsy.

Disadvantages Tissue sample may not be large enough to thoroughly check the site, requiring repeat procedure or surgical biopsy.

The next step

- If the tissue is benign, you may need follow-up exams at six-month intervals.
- If the tissue is malignant, biopsy results can help you discuss treatment options with a surgeon.

SURGICAL BREAST BIOPSY

General information

Where It's Done	Who Does It	How Long It Takes	Discomfort/Pain
Hospital, surgical center, or doctor's office.	Surgeon.	About 1 hour or less.	With local anesthesia, needle will cause mild pain; with general anesthesia, minor pain when IV is started.

Results Ready When	Special Equipment	Risks/Complications	Average Cost
Preliminary report available on day of biopsy; final report, in 3–4 days.	Mammography equipment or other method of locating lump.	Risks (infection, allergic reaction to anesthesia, etc) typically associated with surgery.	$$$

Other names Excisional biopsy.

Purpose To provide a tissue sample or the entire breast lump for microscopic examination to determine if it is cancerous or benign.

How it works Cancerous cells too small to be seen in mammography can be identified under a microscope.

Preparation

- If you are to receive sedation, you must not eat or drink for at least 12 hours before the procedure.
- You disrobe and don a hospital gown.
- You will be given a local anesthetic (often with intravenous sedation) or a general anesthetic (uncommon).

Test procedure

- The surgeon makes an incision over the lump and cuts it away from the surrounding tissue.
- After the bleeding is controlled, the incision is closed using clips or sutures, the site is bandaged, and the tissue sample is sent to the lab for examination.

Variations

Incisional biopsy: This procedure is the same as excisional biopsy except that only a part of the lump is removed. It is performed very rarely but may be done as a first step in cases in which the woman has a very large, abnormal breast mass.

After the test

- If the anesthetic was local, you may be able to dress and go home with some pain medication. If it was general, you will be observed in the recovery room while your vital signs are checked periodically.
- You can resume normal activities as soon as you are comfortable (within hours), avoiding heavy exertion for one to two weeks.
- If external sutures are placed, they will be removed in about a week.
- You should wear a supportive bra and change the wound dressing according to your doctor's orders.
- For minor pain, use acetaminophen (Tylenol) or the prescription medication provided. Some patients find an ice pack over the area helps as well.
- It is common to be slightly bruised after a breast biopsy. If the pain, swelling, or bleeding increases, or if there is any sign of infection, call your physician.

Factors affecting results

The tissue sample may not be adequate for analysis, requiring a repeat biopsy.

Interpretation

The pathologist examines the tissue sample under a microscope for malignant cells.

Advantages

The technique is definitive—the lump in question has been removed.

Disadvantages

- It's invasive.
- It leaves a scar, although it may be minimal and may fade over time.

The next step

- If the biopsy shows the lump to be cancerous, your doctor may perform other tests to see if the cancer has spread to other parts of the body.
- If the lump is benign, periodic monitoring may be recommended.

COMPUTED TRANSAXIAL TOMOGRAPHY, BONE-DENSITY STUDIES

General information

Where It's Done	Who Does It	How Long It Takes	Discomfort/Pain
Radiology section of hospital, doctor's office, or diagnostic center.	Radiologist or radiology technician.	10–20 minutes.	Occasional discomfort associated with having to remain motionless.

Results Ready When	Special Equipment	Risks/Complications	Average Cost
2–4 days.	Special X-ray equipment.	None.	$$

Other names Bone densitometry, single- and dual-energy photon absorptiometry, and QDR (quantitative digital radiography).

Purpose To study skeletal changes, such as bone loss that occurs with osteoporosis.

How it works Uses CT scan technology (see chapter 3), which allows visualization of the bones that is more sensitive than conventional X-rays.

Preparation You may be asked to disrobe and don a hospital gown, although some hospitals do not require this.

Test procedure You lie on a special table while the scanner is positioned over your spine, hip, and/or wrist.

After the test You resume normal activities immediately.

Factors affecting results

- Residual barium left in the gastrointestinal tract after barium studies.
- Calcium (such as in the blood vessels) overlying the area being scanned.
- An increase in bone sclerosis from conditions such as degenerative disease or compression fractures.
- Movement during the scan.

Interpretation A radiologist analyzes the images for bone mineral density.

Advantages

- It's noninvasive.
- It involves minimal radiation.
- It can discriminate between loss in different types of bone (cortical and trabecular).

Disadvantages If there are bone irregularities, results may not be accurate.

The next step Test results are considered definitive. If bone loss is indicated, preventive therapy can be started to help prevent futher loss.

27

Joseph B. Warshaw, MD

Testing in Infants and Children

Tests Covered in This Chapter

The case of Melanie M., age 4½, as recounted by her parents:

Melanie was born with a duplication of the upper part of the right kidney, which makes her prone to infections. Her left kidney functions perfectly. The doctors detected this before she was born when they did an ultrasound scan as part of amniocentesis. Another sonogram within hours after her birth confirmed it. So from the beginning, we knew that she would eventually need surgery. But she was so little, we wanted to wait and see if the condition caused any infections. If it didn't, we were hoping she might be able to avoid the operation.

For the first two and a half years, everything was normal. Then Melanie had her first infection. Antibiotics took care of it and she was fine for another two years. But the second infection caused her a lot of pain and she ended up in the hospital. That's when we decided to go through with the surgery.

The Tests In addition to the sonograms, which were not invasive and only required that she remain still, Melanie had an X-ray of her kidneys known as an intravenous pyelogram (see chapter 12). This involved injection of radioactive dye and was frightening for her, but her parents were able to hold and comfort her during the procedure. Together, these tests gave a clear picture of Melanie's problem: her right kidney resembled two kidneys on top of each other with an extra, malformed ureter (the tube that carries urine from the kidney to the bladder) that connected to the surface of the bladder but had no outlet. Because some of the urine could not drain properly from the kidney, there was a constant risk of infection. Without treatment, Melanie might have suffered inflammation and damage to the normal portion of the kidney and/or blood poisoning. To monitor her condition, Melanie's pediatrician and urologist did periodic urine cultures, watching for evidence of infection.

The Outcome The surgeon removed the upper half of Melanie's right kidney and the malformed ureter, leaving her with the bottom half of the kidney and its normal ureter. She was up and running around by the second day and able to go home by the fifth. Her doctors consider her completely cured.

INTRODUCTION

Children are not just small adults. Their physical and emotional needs are quite distinct. Some are too young to talk, and even when they can, they often cannot explain what is wrong, what hurts, or what feels different. Although almost all of the diagnostic tests that are available for adults can also be performed on infants and children, carrying out these tests is sometimes complicated by equipment that is too large and often by patients who are so frightened that they are unable to cooperate. All of these factors make diagnosing disorders in infants and children a challenge for doctors. When they perform tests and procedures, they must consider the risks and benefits, and the potential for both physical and emotional discomfort. All of this makes good communication between the practitioner and the family essential in arriving at an appropriate diagnosis and plan of treatment while maintaining the trust of the child and family.

The goal of this chapter is to describe how doctors are able to make diagnoses in infants and children—obtaining the necessary history, choosing the appropriate tests, and adapting them for pediatric patients without compromising the final outcome—and how parents and other caretakers play a key role in this process.

The most common tests used in the pediatric population are not diagnostic tests but screening tests. Screening tests are done on large numbers of people who have no symptoms of any particular disease but may be at risk for that disease. The objective is to detect disease before the onset of symptoms (see chapter 2). Diagnostic tests are performed when specific symptoms suggest an illness or condition but do not precisely define it.

SCREENING TESTS FOR INFANTS AND CHILDREN

Some of the most important screening tests for children are performed at the beginning of life and at regularly scheduled health maintenance visits. In most states, the law requires newborn blood screening for numerous conditions that show no symptoms at birth, but that if detected and treated as soon as possible, such detection and treatment may prevent serious disability later in life.

Among the diseases that are routinely tested for at birth are phenylketonuria, galactosemia, sickle-cell anemia, and thyroid deficiency. The blood is collected via a heel stick immediately after birth, and the test is repeated in two weeks, because some of the tests may not become positive until after the infant has been fed for at least 24 hours.

During subsequent so-called well-baby visits, your doctor will continue to do screening tests (see table 27.1), and will assess your child's vision, hearing, and developmental level.

Vision

Several tests are used to test vision. In the cover test, which checks for strabismus (cross-eyes), the doctor simply asks your child to stare at an object and then covers one eye with a hand, noting whether the other

TABLE 27.1 Schedule of Recommended Screening Tests

Age	Visits to Physician	Tests	Special Tests
Birth to 18 months	At 2, 4, 6, 12, 15, and 18 months.	Height and weight; and blood test for levels of hemoglobin (a protein in red blood cells that transports oxygen, needed by all cells in the body) and hematocrit (the ratio of the volume of red blood cells to whole blood) once during infancy (these can detect several kinds of anemia and other red blood abnormalities).	*Hearing:* At 18 months, or earlier if a child had an infection at birth, there were birth complications, or there is a family history of hearing impairment in childhood. *Erythrocyte protoporphyrin (lead poisoning test):* For infants exposed to lead or living near busy highways or hazardous waste sites (see chapter 29).
2–6 years	At least once for immunizations (measles, mumps, rubella, diphtheria, pertussis, tetanus, polio, hepatitis B, and *Haemophilus influenzae* type b).	Height and weight; blood pressure; eye exam for strabismus (crossed or wandering eye) and amblyopia (diminished vision in the affected eye), at ages 3–4; and urinalysis for bacteriuria (bacteria in the urine).	
7–12 years	As needed.	Height and weight, and blood pressure.	
13–18 years	At least once for immunizations (tetanus, possibly hepatitis).	Height and weight, and blood pressure.	

eye must move to focus on the object. If it does, strabismus may be a problem. Once your child is about 30 to 36 months of age or older, strabismus may be tested with a random-dot steriogram, in which the child is asked to identify a three-dimensional E among dots on a card.

When your child is 4 or 5, the doctor may use the standard eye chart to test his or her ability to read letters or indicate the direction of characters from a standard distance (see chapter 18). If the child seems to have difficulty, the physician may recommend a more comprehensive examination by an ophthalmologist.

Hearing

Your child's ability to hear sounds of varying frequency and volume is also assessed periodically. The doctor will use a simple, painless technique called tympanograhy to measure the eardrum's absorption of sound under different air pressures in the external ear canal. The result is a graphic printout called a tympanogram. Once the child is 4 to 5 years old, he or she will be tested using pure-tone audiometry, the delivery to each ear of the same tone over several different frequencies (see chapter 18). Many school systems also schedule this kind of hearing test to screen for potential educational difficulties.

Developmental Skills

Motor, speech, language, and interpersonal skills are assessed using standard indicators such as the Denver Developmental Screening Test. The doctor compares the child's ability to perform skills and respond to questions against that of other children of the same age. If the child does not function at the appropriate developmental level for his or her age, the doctor may suggest a referral for formal developmental testing. Parents are often involved in the assessment by means of a questionnaire regarding the child's motor, language, and interpersonal skills.

Laboratory Tests

Screening tests may require performing a blood test for hidden conditions such as lead poisoning. Iron-deficiency anemia is routinely screened for in the blood at 1 year. A skin test for tuberculosis is performed at 1 year and every two to three years after that, following the recommendation of the American Academy of Pediatrics (AAP). The AAP also recommends a screening urinalysis at 2 years and a urine culture for girls at 3, 5, and 8 years of age. These are all simple tests that are relatively inexpensive and do not cause a great deal of discomfort but can reveal underlying conditions that may be present but not producing symptoms.

HOW YOUR DOCTOR DIAGNOSES PEDIATRIC PROBLEMS

The observations of parents and caretakers are an integral part of the pediatric diagnostic process. Thus your pediatrician or family practitioner will rely on you for a thorough history of your child's symptoms before performing a physical examination. Your answers and the doctor's observations will help determine which, if any, tests are needed to confirm or rule out the doctor's preliminary diagnosis.

Some of the more common signs and symptoms that can easily be observed by a parent or caretaker include the following:

- Sunken or bulging soft spot on the head of an infant.
- Persistent irritability, lethargy, or lack of interest in activities.
- Increase in crying or change in nature of cry: high-pitched, hoarse, or louder.
- Unexplained chills, convulsions, body stiffness, or trembling.
- Prolonged, marked increase in appetite.
- Abnormally slow or fast heart rate.
- Unexplained increase in body temperature.
- Frequent or prolonged bouts of vomiting and/or diarrhea.
- Glassy, sunken eyes and/or dark circles under the eyes.
- Skin that is blue, pale, and cold or flushed, sweaty, and warm; unexplained rash; excessively dry skin.
- Difficulty breathing.
- Alteration in normal urination: marked increase or decrease in volume or frequency; painful urination; or urine that is bloody, coffee-colored, or has a strange odor.

If the problem can't be clearly defined and treatment suggested by your child's symptoms and the doctor's exams, one or more tests may be recommended. Here, too, good communication between the parent and practitioner is essential. The doctor or nurse should explain to you why the procedure is necessary, what the risks and benefits are, and what the alternatives are to performing the test. You are also entitled to hear, in language you can understand, exactly what the test will entail so that you can explain it to your child (see the accompanying box).

As your child's advocate, it is your role to ask questions: Is this test necessary? Will it be painful? Could a less invasive procedure yield the same information?

Tips for Parents

- If you want to remain with your child during test procedures, find out the hospital's policy in advance. Most hospitals now allow it. If yours doesn't, consider a change.
- Be sure that the test is fully explained to you ahead of time. If you understand what to expect, including how much pain or discomfort is involved, you can be calm and reassuring to your child.
- Your child will be greatly affected by your attitude toward the test. If you are overly anxious, your child will sense it immediately and become fearful.
- Know yourself. If you really can't control your anxiety, or if you faint at the sight of blood, your child may be better off if you wait outside.
- Know your child. Some children may interpret a parent's presence during a painful procedure as the utmost betrayal of their trust. Others may view a parent's leaving as abandonment during their time of need.
- If your child is old enough to understand, explain the procedure ahead of time. But don't do it too far in advance. Young children have a very different concept of time than adults do, and too much anticipation can stir up worry.
- Be honest with your child. If you say that inserting an IV needle isn't going to hurt and it does, you will end up losing the child's trust, and the child will be more fearful in the future. The best approach is matter-of-fact but sympathetic.
- Let your child know that it's okay to scream and cry. Say, "This is going to hurt a little, but I'm going to be there with you and it will be over soon."
- If your child has a comfort item such as a doll or blanket, bring it along.
- Remember that your role is not one of assistant or immobilizer for the procedure. Your most important duty, whether during or immediately after the procedure, is to comfort and console your child, to maintain your child's trust in you.
- If possible, plan a treat for afterward—a favorite activity you and your child can do together.

If the test is to be done in a hospital, your doctor should explain the hospital's policy about allowing parents to be present. Many hospitals no longer ask parents to leave the room when blood is drawn or other tests are performed. Parents can stay with their children during all diagnostic tests. They can hold the child while general anesthesia is administered so that the child falls asleep in Mommy's or Daddy's arms. They are allowed in the recovery area, and can even sleep over in their child's hospital room.

This enlightened attitude is reflected in test procedures as well. Special adaptations have been made for infants and children that allow tests to be performed quickly, painlessly, and compassionately without compromising sterility and accuracy. Accommodations have been made in test instruments—from child-sized blood pressure cuffs to dedicated pediatric cardiac catheterization laboratories—and almost as fast as new instruments are developed for adults, miniaturized ones appear in pediatric practices. The following section details some of the most common diagnostic tests and adaptations.

TESTS AND TECHNIQUES THAT DIFFER IN INFANTS AND CHILDREN

Most tests are performed for essentially the same reasons in both adults and children. Different methods have been developed, however, to replace standard adult techniques that are not practical for use with small children. These adaptations have been made to accommodate not only the differences in size but also in the emotional state of the child.

Immobilization

Manual restraint remains the standard method of immobilization for most procedures, especially with infants. Typically, an assistant holds the patient at the site at which the test is to be performed. Additional assistants may be necessary for bigger patients who are unable to hold still. When assistants are unavailable, means other than relying on parents are available. For blood specimens, a hospital sheet wrapped around the child is a simple and effective restraint that helps eliminate the element of struggle and allows the procedure to take place quickly and efficiently. For older children, an arm or leg can be immobilized by taping it to a small board. More elaborate restraints include papooses—boards with canvas covers and Velcro straps—in which an infant or toddler can be swaddled. In the case of certain diagnostic studies, simple plastic devices have been developed to help hold children in appropriate positions without compromising the final radiographic image.

Local Anesthetics

Anesthesia is not usually necessary for procedures such as venipuncture (drawing a blood sample from a vein), where the pain of injecting the local anesthetic equals that of the venipuncture itself. For procedures such as arterial puncture or lumbar puncture, however, local anesthetic can sometimes be helpful. A 1% solution of lidocaine is the agent most commonly used. Topical anesthetics have also been developed, but their use is limited because of the time it takes them to take effect.

Sedation

The need to provide generalized sedation varies from patient to patient. For most diagnostic procedures, manual restraint and a local anesthetic usually suffice. For imaging tests such as magnetic resonance imaging, where it is crucial that the patient be perfectly still, or bone marrow aspiration, when the size of the needle and the force with which it is inserted can be quite frightening, sedative medications given intravenously, or even general anesthesia, may be used.

Blood Tests

Numerous diagnostic tests can be performed on a blood sample. Obtaining the sample from an infant or child may involve one or more of the techniques described below. Since the arteries and veins of infants and children are proportionately smaller than those of adults, it is not uncommon to make more than one attempt or to change techniques midway in order to obtain the sample.

Skin-puncture sampling. In infants and children, skin-puncture sampling is a convenient and usually less distressing way of obtaining blood samples, especially when only a small sample is required. The sites used are usually the heel in infants and the second, third, and fourth fingers in older children.

To increase blood flow in the area, the sampling site is usually warmed with a cloth towel or disposable diaper soaked in warm water. The area is cleansed with alcohol and dried with a sterile gauze pad. A lancet is used to penetrate the skin, and after the first drop of blood is wiped away, the blood is collected using gentle massage to either the heel or finger.

Venipuncture. For obtaining blood samples for diagnostic tests, venipuncture is the quickest and most commonly used method. In older children, the veins in the hand or elbow crease are usually easily accessible. In infants and small children, however, these veins are proportionately smaller and are often not easily seen or felt beneath the subcutaneous fat. If this is the case, veins in the foot and neck—and in infants, in the scalp—will be used instead.

The child is immobilized using any of the methods described above. Then a tourniquet is applied to get the vein to distend, or bulge, making it more accessible. The tourniquet may be applied over clothing or some other cloth for comfort. For scalp veins, a rubber band may be placed circumferentially around the infant's head as a tourniquet. Other measures include warming the area when possible, tapping or flicking the vein with a finger, or swabbing the area repeatedly with alcohol. Once the vein is distended, the area is cleansed with alcohol and wiped dry with a sterile gauze. The doctor or technician then warns the child before sticking the needle into the vein. When collection is complete, the tourniquet is released, the needle is removed, and manual pressure with a gauze pad is used to control any further bleeding.

Arterial puncture. Certain tests require blood from an artery rather than from a vein. Such tests are usually investigating the balance of gases such as oxygen and carbon dioxide in the blood.

Arterial specimens are usually obtained from the radial artery, which is located on the thumb side of the wrist when the palm is facing up. Once again, this may be quite difficult in infants, in which case the arteries on the top of the feet can be used. No tourniquet is required for arterial puncture, as arteries are naturally distended and more easily located since they carry a pulse. The area is usually cleansed with both povidone-iodine and alcohol after the patient has been sufficiently restrained. Once the blood has been obtained, manual pressure is applied to the site for at least five minutes to control any further bleeding.

Urine Tests

For children who have the ability to urinate on command, urine testing is usually a straightforward procedure. For infants and toddlers who are not yet toilet trained, however, the techniques described below can be used.

Bagged urine specimens. When the specimen is not needed immediately—that is, when waiting for the next void will not compromise the patient or change management of the case—a bagged specimen is usually done, as it is the least invasive method. It requires a sterile plastic bag with an adhesive rim designed to stick to skin. The area around the genitals is cleansed thoroughly with iodine and allowed to dry before the bag is applied. When the patient voids, the bag is simply removed and the urine placed in the appropriate containers for analysis.

Bladder catheterization. When a sterile specimen is needed to check for infection or when rapid results are essential to treatment, bladder catheterization is a safe, quick method of obtaining a sterile urine specimen. The pubic area is cleansed with iodine and a well-lubricated catheter or feeding tube (used because of its small size) is inserted through the urethra into the bladder until urine flows. The infant or child may begin to urinate spontaneously before or during catheter insertion. If this happens, a midstream specimen may be "caught" in the sterile container.

Suprapubic bladder puncture. Withdrawing urine with a needle through the skin overlying the bladder, called suprapubic aspiration, is a common method of obtaining sterile urine specimens in babies under age 2. It can be easier than catheterization for tiny infants in whom even the smallest catheter is too big.

This procedure is performed at least 30 to 60 minutes after the infant's last void to ensure that the bladder is distended with urine. With the infant lying on his or her back in the frog-leg position, the lower abdomen is palpated to determine the position of the bladder. The area is cleansed with povidone-iodine and alcohol and the needle is inserted about 1 inch, or until urine starts to fill the syringe. Once the specimen is collected, the site is covered with an adhesive bandage. This procedure is no more painful than simple venipuncture. A small amount of blood in the urine after the procedure is normal and not cause for alarm.

Lumbar Puncture

Obtaining cerebrospinal fluid when infection, inflammation, or a malignancy is suspected requires a lumbar puncture. The key to doing it successfully is adequately restraining the patient. Infants and children are most commonly placed on their side with their back at the edge of the examining table. The child is then curled up, knees to chin, as much as possible. Alternatively, the child may be placed in a sitting position.

The area is cleansed with povidone-iodine and covered with a sterile drape. A local anesthetic such as 1% lidocaine may be injected. Once the exact location is identified, a special needle is inserted until spinal fluid begins to flow. The fluid is then allowed to drip into collecting tubes. Once the needle is removed, the site is covered with a small adhesive bandage. The child remains in position for a few minutes to be sure the flow has stopped.

COMMON DISORDERS AFFECTING INFANTS AND CHILDREN

Many common childhood problems are easily identified, self-limited, and have no specific treatment. Chicken pox is one example, although a recently approved vaccine should make this disease much less prevalent in the future. There are other disorders prevalent in childhood or limited to children that require one or more tests for definitive diagnosis. The most common ones and the tests used to diagnose them are listed in table 27.2. The tests themselves are described in other chapters in this book, according to the organ system they affect.

TABLE 27.2 Common Childhood Problems and the Tests Used to Diagnose Them

Disorder	Description/Symptoms	Diagnostic Tests
Acute appendicitis	Inflammation of the appendix that is the most common reason for emergency surgery in childhood. Symptoms include lack of appetite, immobility, irritability, fever, vomiting, keeping the legs flexed, and stomach pains that become constant.	Abdominal X-rays, ultrasound, and white blood cell count.
Anemia	A low red blood cell count that is usually a sign of an underlying disorder. Can be acute or chronic, inherited or acquired. Examples of underlying causes include malnutrition, iron deficiency, lead toxicity, sickle-cell anemia, or malignancy. Symptoms include fatigue, pallor, and dizziness.	Complete blood count, mean corpuscular volume, reticulocyte count, and peripheral smear (all done using a venipuncture sample). Depending on the results of these tests, further tests may be performed to identify the underlying cause.
Asthma	Recurrent, reversible obstruction of the airway (breathing passage), causing wheezing and difficulty breathing. Acute attacks are caused by numerous factors including irritants (such as smoke), viruses, changes in the weather, emotional stress, and exercise.	Peak flow and trial of airway relaxant medication.
Conjunctivitis ("pink eye")	Inflammation of the conjunctival layer of the eye. May be caused by viruses, bacteria, allergy, or irritants.	Eye culture if bacterial infection is suspected.
Croup	Inflammatory illness of the upper airway that occurs primarily in late fall and early winter. Characterized by a barking cough.	X-rays may be used to confirm clinical diagnosis.
Diabetes mellitus	Inability to process glucose normally. Initial symptoms may be increased urination and weight loss.	Blood glucose level.
Failure to thrive	A condition in which an infant does not grow or gain weight at the expected rate. This is a complex condition that is easier to diagnose than to find a cause for. Although severe birth defects or endocrine problems may be the cause, the most common one is malnutrition that may result from inadequate caloric intake, caloric losses from gastrointestinal disease, or an inborn error that prevents the proper utilization of nutrients. Environmental, social, or cultural forces may play a role in malnutrition.	Complete blood count, urinalysis, urine culture and sensitivity tests, serum electrolyte levels, BUN and creatinine levels, serum T_4 and thyroid-stimulating hormone levels, and erythrocyte sedimentation rate. Depending on the results of these tests, further tests may be performed to identify the underlying cause.
Fever in infants less than 8 weeks old	Infants in this age group do not have the same symptoms as older children when they have an infection. Usually reliable indicators such as alertness, playfulness, interaction with the environment, change in skin color, hydration status, and consolability may not be useful. Factors such as increased cry, irritability, lethargy, and poor feeding become important, but are not reliable indicators of the degree of illness.	Complete blood count, erythrocyte sedimentation rate, blood culture, urinalysis, urine culture, spinal fluid (for cell count, chemistries, and culture), and chest X-ray if indicated.

(continued next page)

TABLE 27.2 (continued)

Disorder	Description/Symptoms	Diagnostic Tests
Infectious mononucleosis	Self-limited disorder caused by the Epstein-Barr virus (EBV). Usually characterized by fever, sore throat, swollen lymph nodes, and fatigue.	Complete blood count with differential cell count, monospot or heterophile antibody test, and occasionally, EBV titers.
Jaundice	Yellow discoloration of the skin and mucous membranes as a result of increased bilirubin level in the blood. May be normal in the newborn or, if persistent or present in older infant or child, may represent underlying disease.	Bilirubin level (blood test), complete blood count with differential cell count, peripheral smear, reticulocyte count, Coombs' test, blood type, and urinalysis.
Lead toxicity	Usually results from chronic ingestion of lead in paint chips, gasoline fumes, and the like. Most patients have no symptoms. When severe, symptoms include irritability, decreased appetite, constipation, abdominal pain, and headache.	Lead level (blood test), complete blood count with peripheral smear, and free erythrocyte protoporphyrin.
Lyme disease	Caused by tick-borne organism. Symptoms include rash, fever, malaise, headache, and joint aches.	Lyme titers.
Meningitis	Infection of the lining of the brain. May be caused by virus, bacteria, or other inflammatory processes. Symptoms include high fever, headache, vomiting, stiff neck, and lethargy.	Complete blood count with differential cell count, blood culture, urinalysis and urine culture, and spinal fluid studies.
Pharyngitis	Sore throat that is most commonly caused by a virus. Some 20%–30% caused by Group A beta-hemolytic streptococcus (strep throat), requiring antibiotics to prevent rheumatic fever.	Throat culture.
Pneumonia	Lung infection that is usually viral, occasionally bacterial. Symptoms include rapid breathing, cough, and fever.	Complete blood count with differential cell count, blood culture, and chest X-ray.
Ringworm	Highly contagious fungal infection of the skin characterized by red, coin-shaped, crusty lesions.	Scrape culture of a lesion.
Sickle-cell disease	Hereditary disorder of red blood cells causing mild to severe anemia and painful crises.	Complete blood count with peripheral smear, and hemoglobin electrophoresis.
Urinary tract infection	Bacterial infection of the urinary tract. Symptoms vary with the age of the child. In newborns, symptoms include poor feeding, vomiting, diarrhea, irritability, and other nonspecific symptoms; in older infants, change in voiding pattern or foul odor to urine; in older children, pain on urination, urgency, and increased frequency.	Urinalysis and urine culture. In prepubescent children, initial studies are frequently followed weeks later by other studies to assess the anatomy of the urinary tract, including ultrasound, intravenous pyelography, or voiding cystourethrogram.

28

Peter Jokl, MD

Sports Medicine

Tests Covered in This Chapter

The case of Greg B., 36, owner of an express delivery service and sports enthusiast:

> *I love playing sports, especially hockey. But in March during a hockey game an opponent took my legs out from under me and sent me flying. Although I've been injured before, this was the worst, most uncontrollable pain I'd ever felt. I knew right away I had seriously damaged my knee—the same knee I had had surgery on before when I partially tore the anterior cruciate ligament.*

The Tests Conventional X-rays were the first step in determining the extent of Greg's injury. X-rays reveal bone chips and arthritic changes in the knee and often are sufficient to diagnose a knee problem. In Greg's case, magnetic resonance imaging (MRI), which uses a powerful magnet linked to a computer to produce cross-sectional pictures of the body, was also necessary. Unlike an X-ray, an MRI can clearly show soft tissues such as cartilage and ligaments. The MRI showed that Greg had torn his anterior cruciate ligament (ACL), the main ligament in the knee joint (see figure 28.1).

The Outcome The doctor first suggested Greg try compensating for the torn ligament by building up the surrounding leg muscles with exercise, but the knee kept buckling when he walked and he couldn't play any of the sports he loved. It became clear that playing competitively again would mean arthroscopic surgery—using a special instrument to probe and

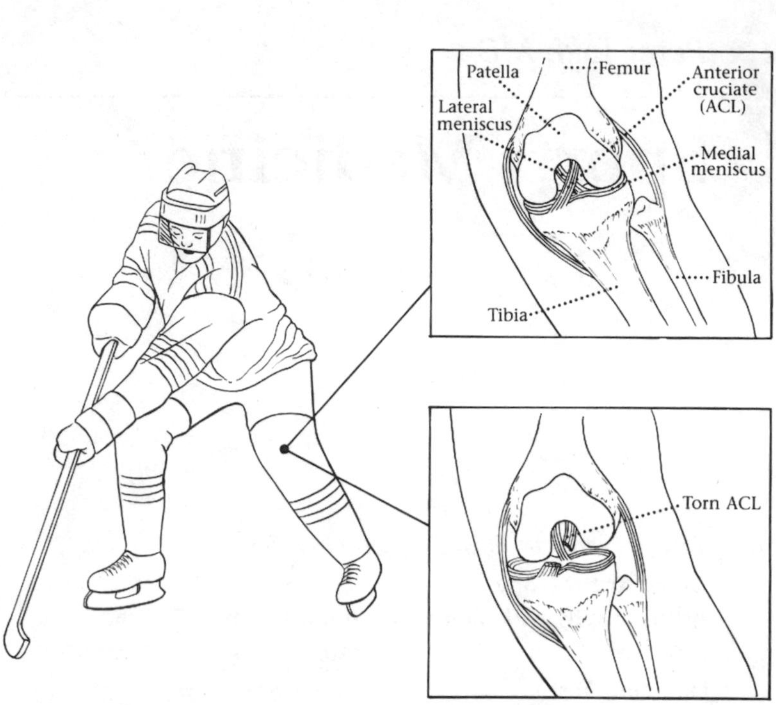

FIGURE 28.1 Anterior Cruciate Ligament

A rupture of the anterior cruciate ligament (ACL) is one of the most common of all sports injuries.

repair the inside of a joint. But this major surgery requires a conscientious follow-up program. The doctor made it clear that rehabilitating the repaired knee would take a big commitment on Greg's part—exercising the leg every day for four months to a year after the surgery.

Greg went ahead with the surgery and began a graduated physical therapy program to build stability, range of motion, and strength. By October he was able to reduce his therapy sessions to once every six weeks, but he continued to exercise on his own. In February, he returned to the ice for the first time since taking his spill nearly a year earlier. He wears a specially fitted brace to prevent hyperextending the knee.

INTRODUCTION

Many sports-related injuries would not occur if athletes—both professional and amateur—followed the prescriptions of their coaches and doctors:

- Condition yourself gradually and properly.
- Warm up before exercising by starting slowly.
- Prepare for environmental conditions such as cold or hot weather.
- Use equipment that is safe and in good condition.
- Be realistic when assessing your skill and ability to perform a sport.
- Know your limits so you don't overdo it.
- Cool down and do stretching exercises afterward.
- Go easy on your body when you suffer an injury, no matter how minor.
- Allow for adequate rehabilitation after being hurt.

Even if all sports and exercise enthusiasts followed these guidelines, there is still one major cause of such injuries for which no athlete can prepare—bad luck. In any cause, when you suspect an injury, you should stop immediately and use a first aid formula identified by the acronym RICE:

Rest: Stop exercising the injured area.

Ice: Apply cold packs to the area to prevent swelling.

Compression: Wrap the area with an elastic bandage to prevent fluid accumulation.

Elevation: Raise an injured extremity above chest level to prevent fluid accumulation.

If the pain does not begin to diminish and range of motion does not begin to return, however gradually, you should see a health care professional for further diagnosis or treatment. You may want to start with your family physician or visit one of the special centers devoted to sports medicine that have opened across the country. These facilities have special diagnostic equipment and many take a team approach, with physiatrists and other physicians specializing in sports medicine, orthopedic surgeons, and physical therapists working together to treat injuries and, equally important, to help you prevent them from recurring.

HOW YOUR DOCTOR DIAGNOSES A SPORTS-RELATED INJURY

When you visit your physician with a sports-related injury, you will be asked questions about your injury and medical history, and the doctor will physically examine the injured area. Initially the doctor will want to know the following:

- *What hurts?* To evaluate the injury and determine the parts of the body that need to be examined.
- *How did it happen?* To determine the mechanism of injury. Damage that results from contact with another person or object, for example, differs from an injury caused by a body part giving out spontaneously during activity.
- *What did it feel like at the time of the injury?* To indicate what structure gave way. For example, the buckling of a joint and a loud pop almost certainly signal a torn ligament.
- *What was new after the injury?* To determine the nature of the damage. A clicking knee points to torn cartilage or a kneecap problem. An inability to straighten a joint can indicate displaced torn cartilage or a dislocated kneecap.
- *Has it been injured previously?* To evaluate chronic weakness or problems.
- *How flexible are you?* To recognize the significance of your current flexibility during a physical exam. Having very flexible joints (often referred to in lay language by the misnomer "double-jointed") affords a normal flexibility that would indicate a severe injury in those who are less flexible.
- *Where did the injury occur?* To indicate likely causes. A particular geographic area may be associated with certain conditions. For instance, if you frequent wooded areas with ticks, Lyme disease may be the cause of soreness in your joints.

After analyzing some of your medical history, your doctor may be able to diagnose your injury based on a physical exam without the need for tests. The examination will focus on the injured area, as your doctor compares it to your uninjured joints and other parts of your body. He or she will evaluate visible signs of the injury such as broken, red, or discolored skin; swelling; and differences in joint mobility or appearance.

The doctor usually presses and squeezes the injured area, even if this produces pain, to feel for structural abnormalities. If the pain centers on a particular area, your doctor may be able to limit further examination and testing to the structures in that area. Manipulations test for the following:

- Localized tenderness.
- Sounds of grating or grinding.
- Restrictions in the range of motion of the injured area.
- Ability of the injured part to bear weight.

You may be asked to hop on one leg or go through other motions to reproduce the pain and give your physician further insight into your injury. Though the pain may be intense, this is the best way to help your doctor reach a diagnosis without further, more expensive tests.

Other questions the doctor may ask include the following:

- *Do you have other chronic conditions?* To indicate whether ailments like gout or high uric acid may be contributing to your problems.
- *Are you taking any medications?* To evaluate how drugs may be affecting your athletic activity. For example, insulin injections and beta blockers can hinder performance. Anabolic steroids taken to enhance performance can lead to ligament injuries.
- *Do you have any allergies?* To judge whether allergies are causing soreness.
- *Has previous surgery repaired the injured area?* To judge whether it has become necessary to repair previous surgical work. Screws used to repair broken bones may loosen, for example.
- *What is your family's medical history?* To decide if your problem is inherited. Bruising or bleeding problems, for instance, may run in your family.

From the physical exam and answers to these questions, your doctor will generally know if the injury has resulted in skeletal (bone) or soft-tissue (muscles, tendons, ligaments, or connective tissue) trauma. The choice of further tests will depend on this distinction.

Skeletal Trauma

X-ray analysis is the primary diagnostic procedure for spotting possible injuries such as fracture, infection, tumor, inborn anomaly of the bone, or, in some cases, a metabolic disorder such as osteoporosis. Several X-ray views are usually taken, depending on the location of the injury (see chapter 3 for more information on X-rays).

X-rays may miss small skeletal traumas such as stress fractures. In such cases, a bone scan of an area with a radioactive material called technetium, which displays the tiny breaks, may be needed (see chapters 3, 13, and 26 for more information on bone scans).

Tests providing three-dimensional images of skeletal trauma include computed tomography (CT) scans, which produce axial or cross-sectional views of an area not seen on regular X-rays, and magnetic resonance imaging (MRI).

Soft-Tissue Trauma

If a soft-tissue injury is suspected, your doctor will use other examination techniques that generally involve stressing structures and noting classic signs of different injuries. These techniques include the following:

- *Knee stress exams.* These test the integrity of the knee's supporting ligaments by pushing on the knee in different directions. They include *McMurray's test,* which produces a pop when the knee joint is twisted in a wringing fashion, indicating torn cartilage (meniscus), and the *Lachman test*, in which the partially bent knee is pulled forward and backward to help assess the integrity of the ligaments inside the knee.

- *Shoulder ROM (range of motion).* This tests all areas of motion to check for restrictions caused by injury or scarring.
- *Impingement test.* This tests the shoulder joint against resistance. Pain may indicate a muscle imbalance, which causes the shoulder bones to grind against each other.
- *Muscle strength function tests.* In such a test, resistance applied to an area while you contract the muscle may reveal a hole in the muscle—the gap between torn muscle ends.

Beyond physical tests, certain diagnostic procedures offer excellent images to diagnose soft-tissue trauma. X-rays are excellent for diagnosing bone problems and are considerably less expensive than scanning procedures, but they can't distinguish between bone and soft tissue—it all appears to be the same density in an X-ray picture. MRI is the imaging test most commonly used in the United States to diagnose soft-tissue injuries. Ultrasound is less stressful and less expensive than MRI, but is used less often because it requires special skill in analysis. It can, however, provide an accurate picture adequate for diagnosis if the examining physician is experienced in ultrasound interpretation.

Some tests involve equipment in a sports laboratory. For example, a procedure called the KT-1000 uses a machine that tests injured knee ligaments with the application of force. The knee joint is moved back and forth while its motion is analyzed and compared with that of the normal knee joint. Other sports lab tests include the Kincom test for muscle strength and a video analysis of the gait to determine if a change in running style will prevent future stress fractures.

Under certain circumstances, a more invasive procedure may be necessary to confirm diagnosis of a soft-tissue injury. In cases such as internal shoulder joint abnormalities, diagnosis necessitates arthrography—an X-ray of the area using an injection of contrast dye (sometimes used with a CT scan). This invasive technique is less expensive than MRI. Synovial fluid aspiration, during which a needle is inserted into the joint and fluid removed, may be used to relieve pressure and/or test the fluid to check for infection or arthritis.

The most recent advance in diagnosing soft-tissue trauma is office arthroscopy, wherein a tiny scope (arthroscope) introduced into a joint allows a direct view of the internal structures. With the use of portable equipment and disposable arthroscopes, this procedure can be performed in some doctors' offices under local anesthetic. Before undergoing arthroscopy, however, make sure your physician has adequate training in this procedure and performs it regularly.

The following list of common sports-related injuries may help you recognize a condition that warrants diagnosis and treatment by a doctor.

Muscle Injuries

Muscles are bundles of cells or fibers that contract and expand to produce movement.

Strain or Partial Pull. A tear in muscle fibers (see figure 28.2).

Example: Long-distance runner increases training mileage too drastically.

Cause: Overuse or excessive stress on muscle or improper warm-up or stretching; sudden muscle activity such as sprinting while jogging.

Signs and symptoms: Sudden pain, inability to use muscle, spasm, and accompanying bulge.

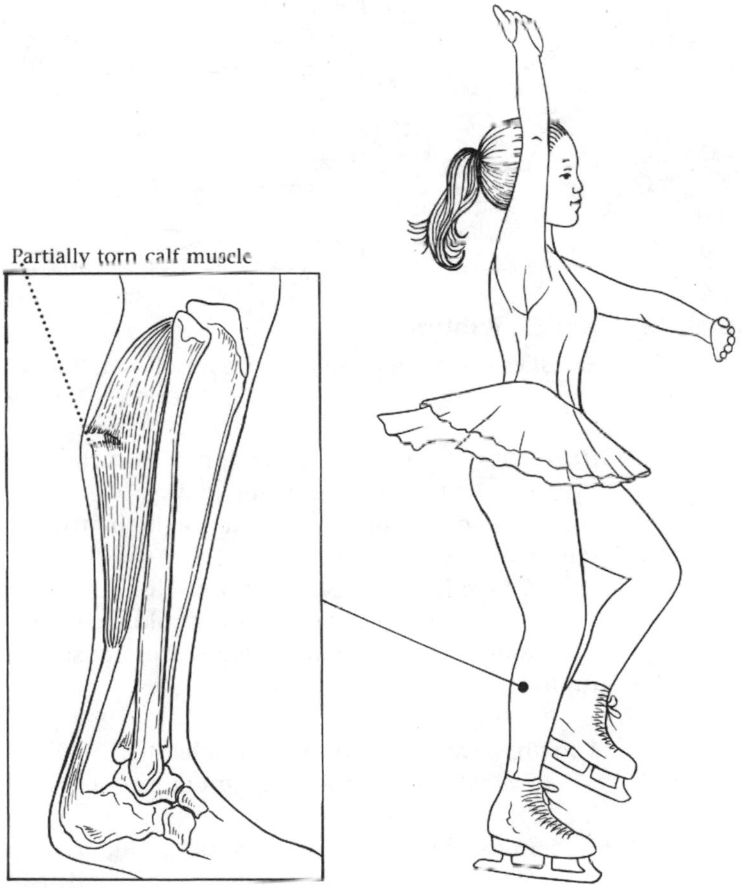

FIGURE 28.2 Muscle Strain

Overuse or excessive stress can result in the partial tear of muscle fibers.

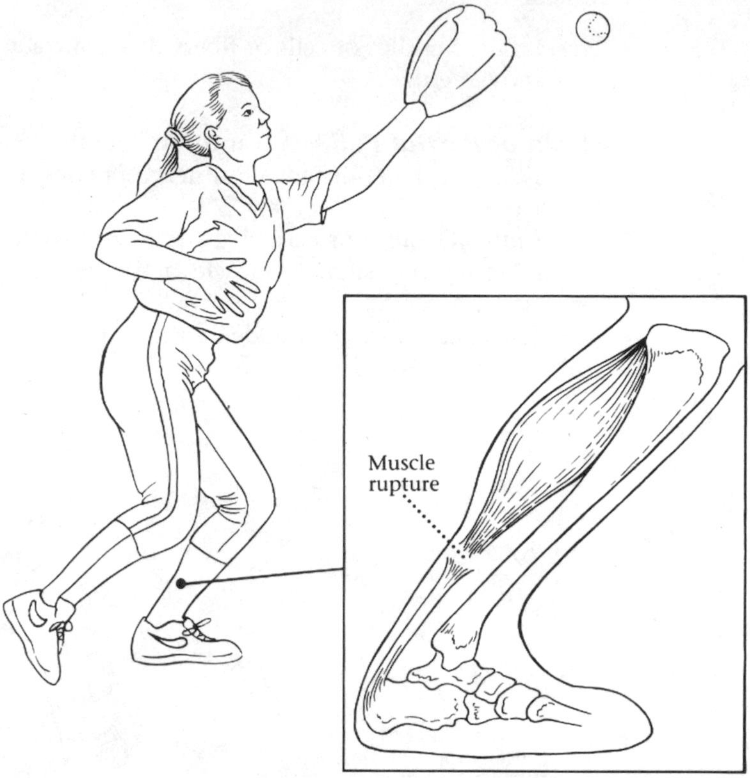

FIGURE 28.3 Muscle Rupture
Excessive stress can cause a muscle to separate from its tendon.

Rupture. A complete separation of muscle at the point where it attaches to its tendon (see figure 28.3).

Example: Rupture of front thigh, hamstring, or calf muscles of tennis player.

Cause: Excessive stress on muscle.

Signs and symptoms: Painful, prolonged clenching of muscle.

Comment: Location differentiates muscle rupture from tendon rupture.

Spasm. Extreme cramp in muscle.

Example: Leg muscle of runner cramps during race on hot summer day.

Cause: Muscle strain, most often due to dehydration.

Signs and symptoms: Swelling, pain, and spasms.

Comment: Best treatment is to stretch cramped muscle.

Contusion. Bruise.

Example: Pitcher hit by batted ball.

Cause: Injurious blow to muscle area, damaging blood vessels in the muscle and forming blood clot.

Signs and symptoms: Subdural hematoma (black and blue mark).

Comment: Best treatment is immediate ice and compression wrap.

Mild Inflammation (Myositis). Soreness.

Example: Sore muscles upon starting an aerobics class after being sedentary.

Cause: Overuse or activity to which the muscle has not accommodated itself.

Signs and symptoms: Sore muscles within 12 to 24 hours of overuse, lasting for three to four days.

Comment: Location (usually affects large muscle groups) distinguishes it from tendinitis.

Scarred Muscle Tissue. Formation of fibrous tissue in the muscle.

Example: Scar tissue formed when a sprinter's torn leg muscle heals.

Cause: Aftermath of a torn muscle, area is less elastic and easier to reinjure.

Signs and symptoms: Pain that occurs at site of old injury, or lump in tissue.

Atrophy. Muscle shrinkage.

Example: Leg in a cast, or immobilization due to nerve damage from slipped disc.

Cause: Disuse; damaged nerves.

Signs and symptoms: Decrease in muscle size, and weakness.

Calcium Deposits (Myositis Ossificans). Formation of calcified tissue in the muscle.

Example: Single or multiple blows to a body area during a contact sport results in deposit of calcium.

Cause: Unclear, but sometimes occurs as a contused muscle heals.

Signs and symptoms: Pain, tenderness, and warmth.

Comment: X-ray shows calcium deposits in the muscle.

Tendon Injuries

Tendons are sinewy connective tissue that attaches muscle to bones.

Tendinitis. Tendon inflammation.

Example: Tennis elbow.

Cause: Overuse of or excess stress or tension on a tendon.

Signs and symptoms: Pain, swelling, point tenderness, or grating sensation as tendon moves.

Comment: Swelling of the tendon area and point tenderness distinguish tendinitis from muscle sprains and pulls.

Tear and Rupture. Break in the tendon.

Example: Achilles tendon in the back of the heel tears during racketball, basketball, or other stop-and-go sport.

Cause: Excess stress, especially during exercise that begins without a proper warm-up, giving tendon inadequate time to accommodate itself to stressful activity.

Signs and symptoms: Pain in tendon area, especially when stretched; sharp immediate pain and spasm with accompanying bulge (in cases of rupture).

Comment: Can also be due to use of an anabolic steroid such as a local cortisone injection.

Ligament Injuries

Ligaments are flexible, fibrous tissue that binds joints, bones, and cartilage.

Sprain. Partial or complete tear of the ligaments supporting a joint (see figure 28.4).

Example: Sprained ankle after stepping in a hole on a grass playing field.

Cause: Usually caused by hyperextension, or turning over, of the ankle.

Signs and symptoms: Immediate pain and swelling around the joint.

Comment: Can often be prevented by checking playing areas for holes, rocks, and so on, and by wearing good supportive shoes.

Dislocation. Loss of joint position; separation of bone ends that comprise the joint.

Example: Shoulder dislocation while rock climbing.

Cause: Excessive stress on a joint that causes separation of the bones that make up the joint.

Signs and symptoms: Severe pain and deformity of the joint.

Comment: Often this problem can recur because of permanent loosening of the joint.

Connective Tissue Injuries

Connective tissue joins and supports other tissues and body parts.

Partial Tear (Fasciitis). Connective tissue separates under the skin or between the muscles.

Example: Plantar fasciitis—inflammation of the fascia (fibrous connective tissue) on the bottom of the foot.

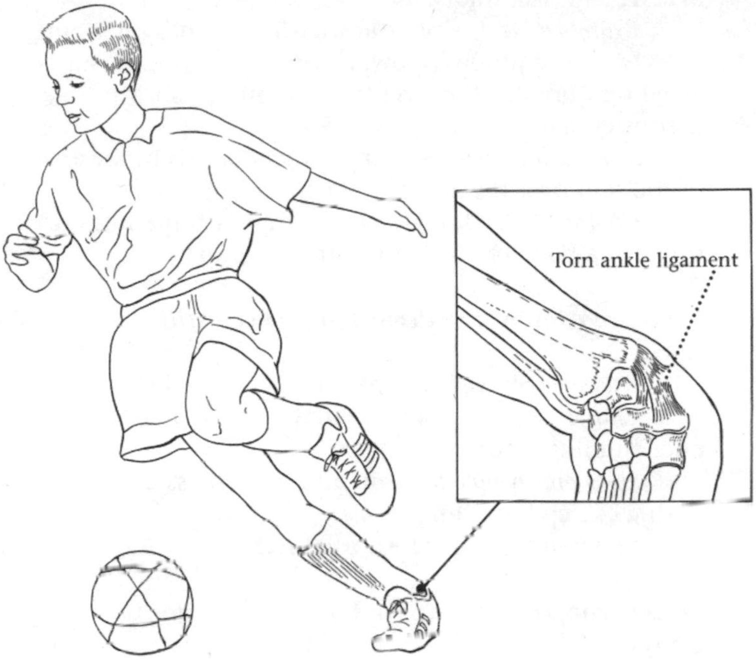

FIGURE 28.4 Sprain
A tearing of the ankle ligaments results in the familiar painful, swollen sprained ankle.

Cause: Overuse or excessive stress, often as a result of ill-supporting footwear.

Signs and symptoms: Inflammation.

Comment: Can often be treated with supportive footwear.

Cartilage Injuries

Cartilage joins and supports other tissues and body parts.

Tear. Break in the tissue that most commonly occurs in the knee but can occur in other joints, such as the shoulder or ankle.

Example: Tear of meniscus (knee cartilage) during high-impact aerobics class.

Cause: Wear and tear, or acute traumatic injury.

Signs and symptoms: Acute pain, instability of joint, and inability to put weight on foot if knee or ankle injury.

Comment: Many of these injuries can be diagnosed by a physical exam; confirmation requires MRI or CT scan arthrography.

Bone Injuries

Bone is the hard tissue that forms the skeleton.

Bruise. Impact injury.

Example: Heel bone (calcaneus) bruised by jumping.

Cause: Injurious blow causing damage to surface tissue and bleeding under the vessel-containing sheath over the bone (periosteum).

Signs and symptoms: Pain and tenderness in the area, and bruising of the skin over the affected bone.

Comment: An X-ray or bone scan is sometimes necessary to distinguish a bone bruise from a stress fracture.

Inflammation of the Periosteum (Periostitis). Bone sheath irritation.

Example: Shinsplints (pain in the shins from running).

Cause: Overuse, poor athletic shoes, hard running surface, or poor running technique.

Signs and symptoms: Pain and tenderness in the area that worsens during exercise; swelling.

Comment: Can progress to a stress fracture.

Stress Fracture. Small bone cracks that are not usually visible on X-rays.

Example: Stress fractures in the feet and shinbones of runners.

Cause: Overuse or poor running technique, or repeated impact during activities such as aerobics or dance.

Signs and symptoms: Gradually increasing pain and tenderness that ease upon rest; swelling.

Comment: Stress fractures often occur in women who are underweight and have ceased to menstruate.

Fracture. A break in the bone (see figure 28.5). In a compound fracture, the broken bone sticks out and breaks the skin surface. In a segmental fracture, the bone is broken in more than one place.

Example: Broken collarbone when a rollerblader uses an arm to break a fall or when a skier crashes into a tree.

Cause: Direct blow to area or pressure that occurs when area or limb absorbs force of fall.

Signs and symptoms: Dull or sharp pain, aggravated by motion; grating of bones rubbing together; inability to move affected area; abnormal appearance or contour of bone—swelling of soft tissue surrounding bone, abnormal bend of bone; bruising and bleeding under the skin.

Osteoporosis. Loss of bone calcium. (Also see chapter 26.)

Example: Underweight female runner with brittle bones.

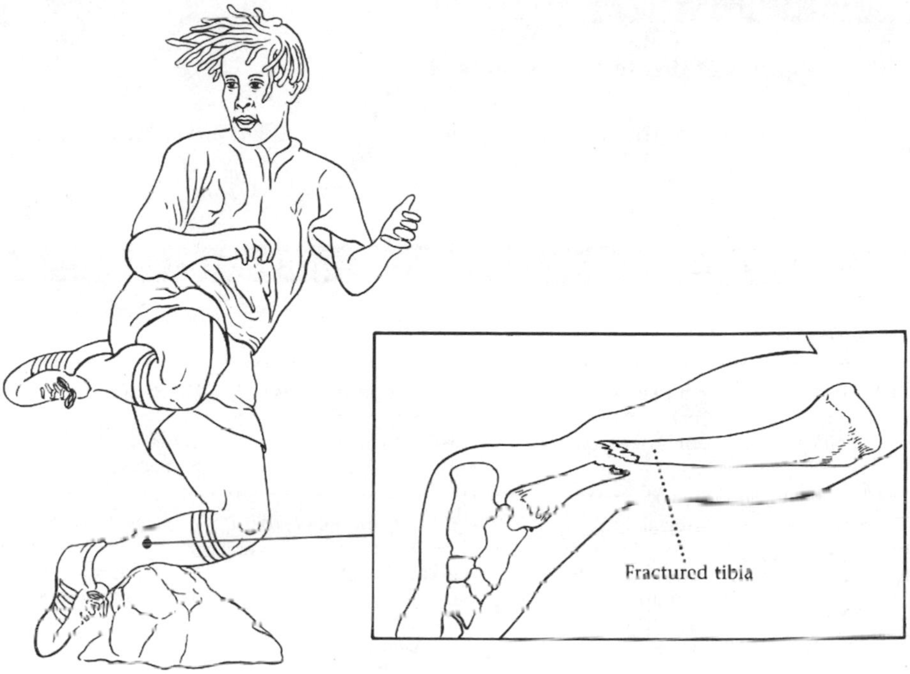

FIGURE 28.5 Fractures
The long bones of the legs and arms are especially vulnerable to fractures.

Cause: Excessive exercise over a long period of time; lack of exercise, loss of estrogen (from menopause or amenorrhea), or lack of dietary calcium.

Signs and symptoms: May be no obvious symptoms until stress fractures appear.

Comment: Most common in postmenopausal women (see chapter 26) and in athletes who are so thin that they cease to menstruate.

Osteomyelitis. Infection of bone tissue. (Also see chapter 22.)

Example: Infected break in the skin after a hurdler's compound leg fracture.

Cause: Bacteria enter the bone tissue and/or blood supply (causing bone infection) through a cut or other injury.

Signs and symptoms: Pain, tenderness, and redness of skin over area; fever; and pus discharge.

OFFICE ARTHROSCOPY

For a full description of this test, see chapter 13.

Purpose To observe the interior of a joint (knee, shoulder, ankle, or elbow).

ARTHROGRAPHY WITH COMPUTED TOMOGRAPHY (CT) SCAN

General information

Where It's Done	Who Does It	How Long It Takes	Discomfort/Pain
Radiologist's office.	Doctor or radiologist.	1–2 hours.	Some, when anesthesia is injected.
Results Ready When	**Special Equipment**	**Risks/Complications**	**Average Cost**
1–2 days.	Special needles, CT scanning machine, and contrast dye.	Risk of infection, possible allergic reaction to contrast fluid, and radiation exposure.	$$ (varies according to joint being studied).

Other names Joint study.

Purpose To evaluate damage to cartilage, ligaments, and bony structures of the ankle, elbow, hip, knee, shoulder, wrist, and other joints.

How it works With the help of a contrast dye, a CT scan creates an image of the injured joint.

Preparation

- You undress and don a hospital gown.
- You receive local anesthesia in the affected joint area.

Test procedure

- A small needle is inserted into the knee joint, and any fluid is withdrawn and sent for analysis.
- Contrast dye and some air are inserted into the joint space.
- A CT scan records images of the joint.

After the test

- The area is bandaged.
- You must wear loose clothing that won't constrict the affected joint.
- You receive instructions concerning use of the joint. Usually 24 hours of rest for the joint is recommended.

Factors affecting results

- Bleeding abnormalities.
- Excess fluid in the joint.
- Inability to inject contrast fluid into the joint because of scarring or other tissue abnormalities.

Interpretation A radiologist evaluates images of the joint. Multiple images are interpreted by a radiologist trained in musculoskeletal imaging.

Advantages

- It's usually less expensive than MRI.
- It allows three-dimensional imaging of the affected joint and effective preoperative planning.
- Unlike X-rays, which show only bone, CT scans can show details of soft tissues such as cartilage.

Disadvantages

- It's invasive.
- It involves significant radiation exposure.

The next step No other testing is required. Surgery or other treatment can begin.

LIGAMENT TEST

General information

Where It's Done	Who Does It	How Long It Takes	Discomfort/Pain
Doctor's office.	Specially trained physician.	5 minutes.	None.
Results Ready When	**Special Equipment**	**Risks/Complications**	**Average Cost**
Immediately.	Ligament tester and KT-1000 machine.	None.	$

Other names Stryker test.

Purpose To test the strength of knee ligaments.

How it works The test isolates and compares the normal joint to the abnormal joint.

Preparation You lie on an examining table and remain totally relaxed.

Test procedure You are strapped onto a machine called a ligament tester that applies stress to the knees by moving them back and forth.

After the test You may return to normal activities.

Factors affecting results

- Not relaxing.
- Pain that makes the test too uncomfortable.

Interpretation A doctor examines the results printed on a graph and compares them to normal results.

Advantages

- The test accurately documents physical strength of the knee and ligaments, and injury to the cruciate ligaments of the knee.
- It provides quantitative numbers to use for documentation (as required for workmen's compensation.

Disadvantages It's expensive.

The next step Exercises are prescribed to strengthen knee ligaments. No other tests are required.

KINCOM TEST

General information

Where It's Done	Who Does It	How Long It Takes	Discomfort/Pain
Doctor's office or physical therapist's office.	Physical therapist or technician.	30–40 minutes.	Some muscle pain or burning sensation.
Results Ready When	**Special Equipment**	**Risks/Complications**	**Average Cost**
Immediately.	Machines made by Kincom, Cybex, Biodex, etc.	Muscle pain and fatigue.	$$

Other names Cybex or Biodex.

Purpose

- To measure muscle function and strength at different rates of exercise.
- Can train muscle.

How it works A hydraulic or electromagnetic machine measures muscle strength by applying constant resistance over a range of motion and speed.

Preparation You complete trial runs to get used to the equipment.

Test procedure You move your muscles in repetitive motions quickly and as powerfully as possible, and resistance is applied by a machine.

After the test You may return to normal activities.

Factors affecting results

- Your motivation. If you don't work hard, the results will be inaccurate.
- Familiarity with the machine may improve your performance.

Interpretation A doctor evaluates the graphed results, often with the help of a computer.

Advantages It accurately measures muscle function.

Disadvantages It's expensive.

The next step Based on test results, strengthening exercises may be prescribed. The test may be repeated periodically to monitor progress.

DYNAMIC GAIT ANALYSIS WITH VIDEO RECORDING

General information

Where It's Done	Who Does It	How Long It Takes	Discomfort/Pain
Doctor's office or exercise lab.	Doctor, physical therapist, or technician.	Usually less than 30 minutes.	None, unless done to reproduce pain that occurs during exercise.
Results Ready When	**Special Equipment**	**Risks/Complications**	**Average Cost**
Immediately.	Treadmill or other equipment used during the sport being analyzed, and high-speed video recorder.	None.	$$

Other names None.

Purpose

- To assess how people run or do another sport.
- Used to help elite athletes learn a more efficient style.

How it works You simulate your sports activity while being clinically observed.

Preparation You don an appropriate clothing for the activity being analyzed.

Test procedure	■ You perform the activity that caused discomfort or that needs improvement.
	■ Your activity is recorded on film and observed by trained clinicians.
After the test	You may resume normal activities.
Factors affecting results	Being observed may cause you to exercise differently than usual.
Interpretation	■ A clinician experienced in sports medicine reports on the observations during the test and while viewing the tape.
	■ You may watch the tape.
Advantages	Better than static tests, this test observes what actually happens during exercise.
Disadvantages	It may reproduce pain.
The next step	Strengthening exercises or changes in technique may be recommended. No further testing is necessary.

COMPARTMENT PRESSURE TEST

General information

Where It's Done	Who Does It	How Long It Takes	Discomfort/Pain
Doctor's office.	Doctor.	10–20 minutes.	Needle in muscle may cause pain.

Results Ready When	Special Equipment	Risks/Complications	Average Cost
Immediately.	Compartment pressure monitor.	Bleeding and pain in muscle.	$200–$400.

Other names	None.
Purpose	To measure muscle pressure within its containing compartment during activity (see figure 28.6).
How it works	A Stryker compartment pressure machine monitors an array of pressure-measuring devices.
Preparation	You don appropriate clothing for exercise.

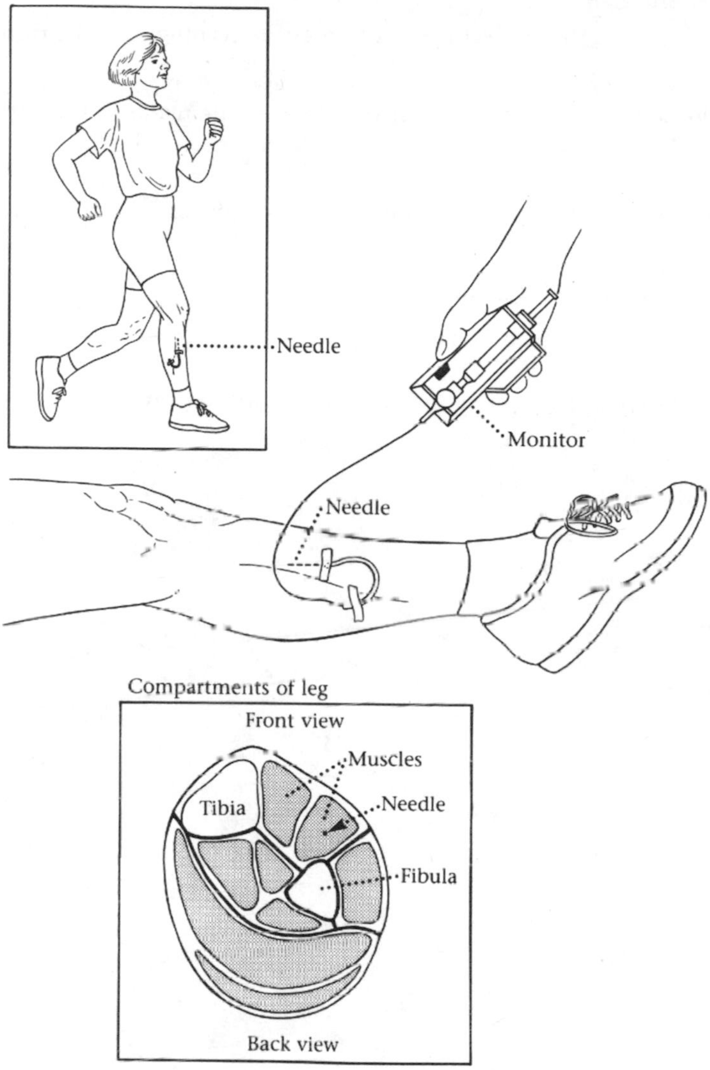

FIGURE 28.6 Compartment Pressure Test

A special monitor is inserted into a muscle bundle (compartment) to measure pressure during various activities.

Test procedure

- As you begin to run or perform other exercise, the normal pressure within your pain-free limb is checked.
- You continue exercising until the muscle discomfort occurs.
- A needle placed inside the painful muscle is hooked to a pressure-measuring machine. (The pressure can be monitored constantly, but this requires additional expense.)

After the test

After the needle insertion point is bandaged, you may return to normal activities.

Factors affecting results If you feel tense, the pressure readings may be distorted.

Interpretation A clinician compares the pressure readings from the painful muscle with those of a normal muscle.

Advantages It allows for an immediate diagnosis.

Disadvantages

- It's painful.
- It may cause bleeding.

The next step Depending on the results, further testing or treatment may be recommended.

29

Petrie M. Rainey, MD, PhD ■ *David J. Schonfeld, MD*

Toxicology, Monitoring of Drug Therapy, and Testing for Substance Abuse

Tests Covered in This Chapter

The case of 1-year-old Mercedes G., as recounted by her mother, Mary:

> *We had recently moved to a new apartment when I took my three youngest children for a routine physical checkup, which includes a lead test. Although their previous tests had been negative, this time my 2-year-old twins had higher-than-normal levels of lead in their blood. And my 1-year-old, Mercedes, had a very high result. I was shocked because she seemed like a normal, healthy baby.*
>
> *After a follow-up test four months later, the doctor immediately put her on pills to help her get rid of the lead and admitted her to the hospital for the weekend. He explained that in order to begin the drug, she needed to be in a lead-free environment.*
>
> *The landlord had the paint removed but, unfortunately, the job wasn't done properly. They let paint chips from the windowsills fall to the ground outside, where the kids play. Within three months, Mercedes's lead level went even higher, and she had to go on medication for another three weeks and be tested weekly.*

The Tests Blood lead levels are measured in micrograms per deciliter (μg/dL). In children, any test result higher than 9 μg/dL is cause for concern and more-frequent-than-usual retesting. A child who tests over 44, as Mercedes did, would require drug treatments, called chelation, to accelerate the removal of lead from the body. Some children with lower levels (that is, 20 to 44) may receive this treatment as well. But unless the child is relocated to a lead-free environment, the medication is ineffective (see figure 29.1).

To gauge the length of exposure and to monitor for reexposure to lead, doctors analyze the blood for an iron-free hemoglobin derivative called erythrocyte protoporphyrin (EP). The higher the initial EP level, the longer the exposure. The EP level rises and falls more

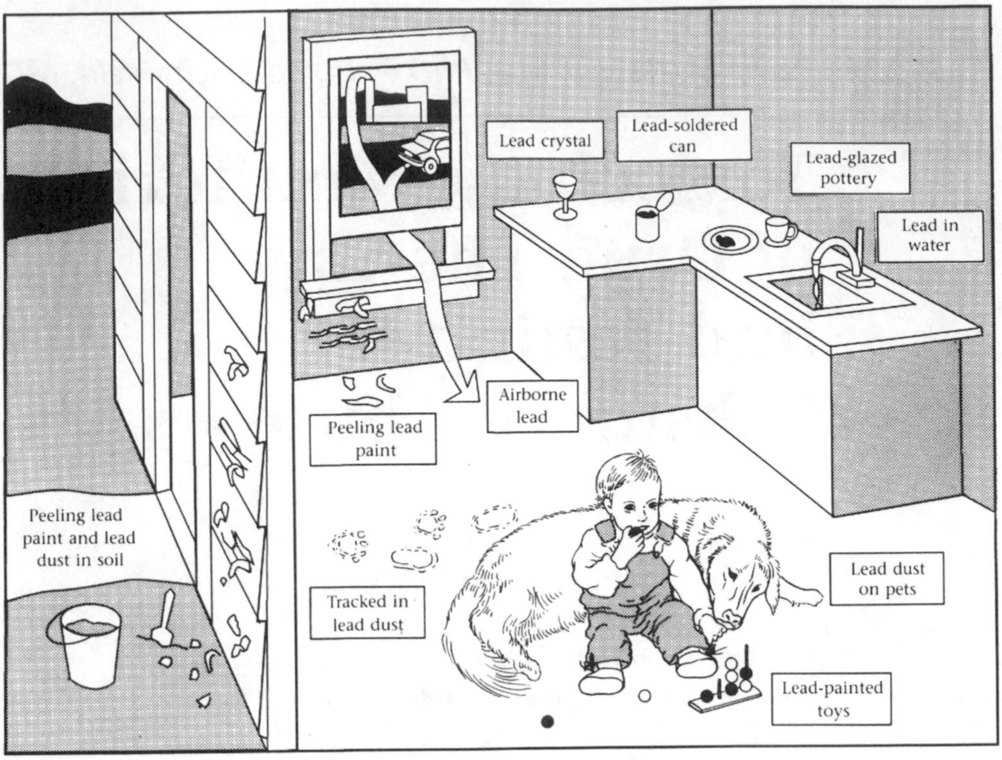

FIGURE 29.1 Environmental Lead

Although lead is no longer added to gasoline and household paints, many other sources remain in our environment. This drawing illustrates some of the more common ones.

slowly than the lead level, making it a valuable tool for assessing whether or not the patient has been reexposed to lead during and shortly after chelation.

The Outcome The family ended up moving to another apartment. Ever since, Mercedes's lead levels have been getting better. She and the twins all go for testing every two to three months. And Mercedes's mother keeps a closer eye on Mercedes now, to make sure she doesn't put her hands in her mouth.

INTRODUCTION

Lead is only one of the potentially toxic substances that abound in our world. More than 65,000 manufactured chemicals have been introduced into our environment, joining an impressive number of naturally occurring toxins. Virtually everything is harmful if taken in large enough amounts.

We can be exposed to small amounts of many of these substances daily without any ill effects. However, when we take drugs, either therapeutically or recreationally, or work in hazardous occupations, or live in certain environments, we risk being overexposed. Toxicologists have developed tests to identify these risks (see table 29.1). These tests are commonly used for the following purposes:

- To monitor drug therapy, in order to ensure proper dosages.
- To determine the agent involved in an accidental or intentional overdose of a therapeutic or recreational drug or poisonous substance.
- To detect hazardous levels of environmental or occupational exposure to toxic substances.
- To screen for illicit drug use in the workplace.

DID YOU KNOW?

Toxicology is the study of potentially dangerous substances, their detection, their biological effects, and how people who are overexposed to them can be effectively treated. Humans have studied poisons since ancient times. In fact, the word toxicology developed from the roots *toxicon*—the poison used on arrowheads—and *toxikos*—the bow that delivered them. Now, however, the aim of toxicology is to limit exposure to toxic substances.

Although occasionally samples of hair or fingernails might be tested to detect levels of certain toxic substances, the majority of toxicological tests are performed on blood taken from a finger (finger stick) or vein (venipuncture) or on urine (see chapter 4 for general descriptions of blood and urine tests).

HOW YOUR DOCTOR EVALUATES A TOXIC EXPOSURE

Overdoses and Poisonings

Overdoses and poisonings have been a common cause of death, both accidental and intentional, throughout the history of mankind. It was 2,400 years ago that the famous philosopher Socrates was condemned to die by drinking the poison hemlock. Even drugs you might consider fairly harmless can cause serious health problems if you take too much of them. Classic examples involve the adolescent who overdoses on acetaminophen (Tylenol, Datril, and others) to get attention, only to find that it has caused severe and permanent liver damage, or the party-goer who on a dare drinks a large quantity of liquor in a short time and ends up with alcohol poisoning.

Children are the most common victims of household poisonings. Sources include medications, various cosmetic products, certain house and garden plants, leaded paint, gasoline and other solvents, swimming pool chemicals, weed killers, pesticides, rodenticides, cleaning products, and carbon monoxide from faulty heating devices. Most acute poisonings in adults are the result of either an

DID YOU KNOW?

Not all poisons are man-made chemicals. Many are natural toxins, poisonous substances that are produced by a plant or animal, usually as a defense mechanism. Dumb cane, philodendrons, holly, poke weed, rhubarb leaves, and rhododendrons are among the more common sources of plant poisonings.

overdose of a medication or an accidental exposure to a toxic substance used in the workplace.

Testing to Identify the Toxin. In any case of suspected poisoning, your doctor will take a careful history whenever possible. You will be asked to identify the poison if you can, as well as the amount or duration of exposure, time elapsed since exposure, symptoms, and any medications currently being used. (Always bring to the hospital or doctor's office the container in which the toxic substance came.) Other clues may come from the following:

- Examining the skin for temperature, color, and perspiration.
- Evaluating movement of the eyes and their reaction to light.
- Listening to the abdomen for activity.
- Evaluating brain and nervous system function.

The doctor may then order tests to measure poisons in the blood or urine and to determine their effects on body functions. A toxicological screen ("tox screen")—one or more tests for drugs and poisons frequently involved in overdoses—may be ordered if the substance is still unknown. Tests for toxins commonly involved in overdoses, such as aspirin, are available in most hospitals, but screens for less common ones may be done only in larger hospitals, or the specimen may be sent to a specialized lab. (For many uncommon substances, no tests are available.)

Emergency Treatment. If the overdose was recent, the doctor may insert a tube into the stomach and try to wash out the unabsorbed drug. This is often referred to as "pumping the stomach," although no pump is involved. Powdered charcoal may be given because it combines with many poisons and prevents them from being absorbed from the stomach and intestine. If there is a specific antidote for a drug, it will be given once a toxic level of the drug has been found or is strongly suspected. Some drugs can be removed directly from the blood, while for others there is no specific treatment. Serious overdoses require hospitalization for monitoring and supportive care until symptoms cease and drug levels fall into the nontoxic range. Medical treatment for intentional overdoses will be followed by psychiatric care.

Monitoring of Drug Therapy

The effectiveness of a drug depends on its ability to affect the body powerfully. As a result, almost all drugs are also poisons if taken in excess. As Paracelsus, a Swiss physician and alchemist, wrote in the sixteenth century, "The right dose differentiates a poison from a remedy."

When your doctor prescribes a medication, he or she must not only determine the best drug for your illness but also the correct dose for your particular size, age, and physical condition. Blood tests may be necessary to establish the dose initially and to monitor for adjustments as therapy progresses. This is called therapeutic drug monitoring.

Some drugs may produce toxic effects—side effects—even at proper doses, so your doctor will aim for the lowest possible effective dose. These drugs include heart medications such as procainamide, digoxin, quinidine, amiodarone, and other antiarrhythmics; drugs used to treat seizures, such as phenytoin, phenobarbital, carbamazepine, and valproic acid; asthma drugs such as theophylline; and drugs used to suppress the immune system, such as cyclosporine.

In addition, certain people have unusual reactions to normal doses of drugs. The doctor must decide whether the dose can be adjusted to limit or eliminate a reaction or whether an alternative drug would be better.

A type of toxic reaction that is becoming more common, especially in older people, is the effect of interaction between different medications. The potential is greatest when a person has several doctors and fails to inform each of them about the drugs the others have prescribed.

Caution: It is extremely important to notify each physician you see about *all* drugs you take on a regular basis. It is also wise to fill all of your prescriptions at the same pharmacy, because the pharmacist can recognize combinations of drugs that may cause problems. Sometimes these interactions are unavoidable; in these cases, therapeutic drug monitoring may help in adjusting the doses to minimize the effects of the interaction.

DID YOU KNOW?

The number of possible interactions between drugs increases much faster than the number of drugs taken. For example, one interaction is possible with two drugs, three interactions with three drugs, six with four drugs, and ten with five drugs.

Testing. How frequently the drug levels in your blood are monitored will depend on how long you have been taking the drug, whether the dose has to be altered, and whether you have any conditions that make you more susceptible to the toxic potential of the drug. For example, someone with decreased kidney function who takes the powerful heart medication digoxin would be tested more often than someone who is otherwise healthy.

Unless you are currently hospitalized, you will go to your doctor's office or a laboratory to have your drug level measured. Ask your doctor when you should take your medication on the day you are scheduled for testing, as timing can affect the outcome. Results are usually available within a day or two; if they are too high or too low, your physician may change your prescription over the phone or may ask you to come in for a consultation.

Substance Abuse

Testing for illicit drugs and alcohol is required for certain jobs, particularly those that involve public health and safety, and in criminal proceedings, such as those involving charges of driving while intoxicated.

Alcohol Testing. Depending on the state, intoxication is usually defined as an alcohol concentration in whole blood (which includes red blood cells) greater than 0.08% or 0.10%. Tests for legal purposes are usually made in forensic or police laboratories but are sometimes done in a hospital lab. When a person injured in a motor vehicle accident is brought to an emergency room, an alcohol test may be ordered to help determine whether any neurological impairment is due to head injury or intoxication. Alcohol measurements for medical purposes are usually made on serum (the liquid portion left after blood clots) and are not the same as whole blood alcohol levels. This can cause interpretation problems if the serum levels are later subpoenaed for legal purposes. (For more information on legal considerations, see chapter 1.)

Substance Abuse Testing. Workplace screening tests usually test for the following substances:

- Opiates (including morphine, codeine, and heroin).
- Cocaine.
- Tetrahydrocannabinol (THC, the active ingredient in marijuana).
- Amphetamines.
- Phencyclidine (PCP).
- Benzodiazepines and/or barbiturates (sometimes).

Because these substances are either illegal or available only by prescription, *any* drug finding is significant. Since the amount is not as important as it is in alcohol testing, testing is done on urine, which is simpler and, because the drugs are concentrated in the urine, more sensitive than a blood test.

Because of the serious consequences of a positive finding, drug testing is done very carefully, and positive results are not reported until they have been confirmed by a second, completely different test. In many cases, the results will also be reviewed by a physician (the medical review officer). While it is true that a urine specimen provided shortly after eating poppy seeds may give a positive test for opiates, it is highly unlikely that passive inhalation of marijuana smoke at a party will result in a positive test for THC.

If you are asked to take a drug test, be sure that the following conditions are met:

- The testing is done in a laboratory certified in forensic urine drug testing by a recognized agency. Such agencies include the Substance Abuse and Mental Health Services Administration (formerly the National Institute on Drug Abuse), various state departments of health, and the College of American Pathologists. This will ensure against a false-positive test.
- The specimen container is closed with a tamper-proof seal that you sign to ensure against mix-ups.
- You provide the names of any medications you may be taking, because some of these may give a false-positive result. (This information should be available only to the medical review officer, not your employer.)

PATIENT TIP

Avoid eating poppy seeds or drinking exotic herbal teas before a drug screening test. Poppy seeds contain small amounts of opiates and can produce a positive test for opium. Small amounts of cocainelike or amphetaminelike substances can be found in some herbal teas (the herbal teas commonly found in supermarkets should not cause a problem).

While the levels of drugs found in these foods are too small to cause intoxication, they can cause positive drug screening results if they are ingested shortly before a test. These are technically not false-positives, because the drugs are actually in the urine. They can, however, lead to a false conclusion of illicit drug use.

A large number of prescription and over-the-counter cold and allergy medications contain decongestants that may react with screening tests for amphetamines. These substances are generally identified during confirmatory testing with a technique known as gas chromatography/mass spectroscopy. If screening is done without confirmatory testing, false-positive results can occur. (Certified laboratories will always perform confirmatory testing.)

Because of the care with which testing is currently done, a person with a positive test will find it very difficult to challenge the result successfully. The only certain way to pass a drug screening test is not to have used drugs recently. Specimens that have been diluted or adulterated can be readily identified.

Tests for most drugs will be positive for two to three days after occasional use and longer after heavy use. Tests for benzodiazepines and barbiturates may be positive for one or more weeks, and tests for THC may be positive for a month or more.

TESTING FOR OCCUPATIONAL AND ENVIRONMENTAL EXPOSURE

Although the number of potentially hazardous substances found in various occupational settings is vast, information about what constitutes a toxic level of exposure is skimpy. Where information is available, exposure is usually regulated by measuring the levels in the work environment rather than in the worker. In general, workers are monitored only when government regulations specify testing frequency and acceptable levels.

Heightened awareness of environmental pollutants such as mercury and polychlorinated biphenyl compounds (PCBs) has led some people to request testing, but frequently this is not helpful. Even when tests are available, interpreting their results is often difficult. Many of these substances persist in the body, just as they do in the environment. Levels considered safe for long-term exposure may be much lower than levels that cause immediate symptoms. Where the risks associated with the levels are unknown, as is often the case, there is little point in measuring the levels. The best advice is to take reasonable steps to minimize unnecessary exposure, regardless of what the safe level is thought to be.

Lead Testing. Lead is one of the oldest known environmental poisons and one of the best studied. The symptoms of acute lead poisoning were well described by Greek physicians 25 centuries ago. However, only in the past 25 years have we begun to recognize that lead can have harmful effects at levels well below those required to cause symptoms (see the accompanying box on monitoring and treatment guidelines for lead poisoning).

Before the full toxicity of lead was appreciated, it was widely used in paint, gasoline, and solder. Because it is not biodegradable, all

Monitoring and Treatment Guidelines for Lead Poisoning

In 1991, the Centers for Disease Control and Prevention made the following recommendations:

- Children should receive blood lead testing between ages 1 and 6. (Opinions vary among health care providers as to when testing should be done. The American Academy of Pediatrics recommends testing at 12 and 24 months; however, for children at high risk, such as those who live in older, poorly maintained housing, the AAP recommends that testing begin at 6 months and be repeated more frequently.)
- The test can be obtained from your doctor, a nurse-practitioner, or the local department of health. Either a finger stick test or one using blood from a vein is acceptable. A finger stick is less traumatic for the child and less expensive but more likely to be contaminated by lead dust. Thus, any elevated reading on a finger stick test should be confirmed by a venipuncture test.
- The desirable level for children is less than 10 mg/dL. Levels between 10 and 20 mg/dL call for efforts to decrease exposure and may require more frequent testing.
- Levels of 20 mg/dL or greater in children call for medical evaluation and investigation of the home to identify sources of exposure that can be eliminated.
- Children with 45 to 69 mg/dL require chelation therapy within 48 hours. This must be done in a lead-controlled environment.
- A level of 70 mg/dL or above in children requires immediate hospitalization and chelation therapy.

Comment

A lead level of less than 10 mg/dL is desirable for adults as well as children, although the Occupational Safety and Health Administration (OSHA) guidelines suggest that levels less than 40 mg/dL are acceptable in adults who are occupationally exposed.

Although lead levels between 10 and 20 mg/dL in children are cause for concern, parents should keep them in perspective. Most parents, who grew up when lead was still widely used in gasoline, had lead levels in this range throughout their childhood. Yet their generation did just as well in school as their children, most of whom have levels of less than 5 mg/dL.

Some physicians believe that chelation therapy is helpful for children with lead levels between 20 and 44 mg/d L, but this has never been proved in medical studies. Other physicians believe that preventing further exposure is the critical therapy, and that chelation adds little additional benefit at these lead levels. There is general agreement, however, that chelation therapy is needed for levels of 45 mg/dL or greater.

P. M. Rainey, MD

the lead used in these products remains in the environment. However, the last 20 years have seen lead levels drop significantly—due in large part to the federal ban on lead-based paints for residential use and the phaseout of leaded gasoline.

Young children are more affected by environmental lead than adults. Their intestines absorb much more of the lead dust that they swallow than do those of adults, and their developing nervous systems are more susceptible to any given level of lead. Contrary to popular belief, children don't have to eat paint chips in order to get lead poisoning. They can get enough exposure through the hand-to-mouth behavior that is normal for toddlers: playing in lead-contaminated dirt, then putting their fingers in their mouths; or chewing on or mouthing toys and other objects that may be coated with lead-contaminated dust. Improperly removing or otherwise disturbing lead-based paint during renovation can generate huge amounts of lead dust (or fumes, if a heat gun is used) that can cause massive exposures in children (see the accompanying box on minimizing exposure to lead).

Minimizing Exposure to Lead

- If you suspect your home is contaminated with lead, contact your local or state health department for the names of certified or licensed lead-abatement inspectors and contractors.
- Do not try to remove lead-based paint by sanding, scraping, or burning, which send lead dust and fumes into the air.
- Supervise your children's play to keep them from swallowing paint chips or lead-contaminated dirt. Do not let them play in soil near the foundation of your home where paint chips may have fallen.
- Wash or wet-mop hard surfaces in your home with a high-phosphate cleaner.
- Use only cold water for drinking and cooking. Run tap water for a few minutes to let it reach its coldest temperature before using it. As hot water lingers in the pipes, the high temperature dissolves greater quantities of lead.
- Wash youngsters' toys with mild soap and water, then dry them thoroughly; dampness is a magnet for dust, which may contain fine particles of lead.
- Rinse pacifiers regularly.
- Encourage children to wash their hands with soap and water before eating and after outdoor play.
- Avoid serving fatty or fried foods, which promote lead absorption in the body.
- Be sure that children get sufficient iron in their diet, or ask your doctor about supplements. In children, absorption of lead from the intestines into the bloodstream may be increased by iron deficiency.
- Do not serve food on imported earthenware unless you test it first (test kits are available). Souvenir folk art pottery is especially likely to contain lead. Reserve it instead for decoration.
- Do not use lead-based insecticides.
- Any family member whose work involves lead (eg, radiator repair, mining, or brass and copper manufacturing) should change all clothing and shoes before entering the home.

TABLE 29.1 Common Toxicologic Blood and Urine Tests

Test	Use	What Measurement Means	Additional Information
Blood test for lead level	To test exposure to lead.	Levels of 10 micrograms per deciliter (µg/dL) or more may be harmful to young children. Levels of 20 µg/dL or higher in children call for medical evaluation. The Occupational Safety and Health Administration (OSHA) requires medical monitoring for adult workers with levels of 40 µg/dL or more.	Initial testing in children is usually by a finger stick. False-positive results may occur if lead dust sticks to the finger, so confirmatory test is on venous blood. Screening begins at 6 months of age for children in older homes with lead-based paint, and at 1 year of age for other children.
Blood test for therapeutic drug level	To assure a proper dosage or to assist in adjusting it.	If concentration in blood falls within the target range for the drug, the dosage will usually be enough to achieve the desired effect without unacceptable side effects.	Individual tests are available for a wide variety of drugs, including antiarrhythmic drugs, anticonvulsants, some antibiotics, antidepressants, cyclosporine, digoxin, lithium, and theophylline.
Blood test for toxicity (drugs)	To determine cause of drug poisoning.	Concentrations greater than toxic thresholds indicate a high probability of serious toxicity.	Substances detected may vary with the laboratory used, but the test often includes screening for acetaminophen, barbituates, benzodiazepines, salicylates (aspirin), and tricyclic antidepressants. It may be used after an overdose of a known drug to identify other drugs that may also have been taken. Sometimes both blood and urine will be tested.
Urine test for toxic drugs (drug screen)	To indicate the presence of various poisons in cases of overdose.	A positive finding confirms the presence of the substance but does not indicate whether the amount is toxic.	Used to document or rule out exposure to toxic drugs or drugs of abuse but not to determine amounts. More economical than blood test.
Urine test for workplace drug screening	To test for the use of illicit or abused drugs.	A positive finding indicates recent use but not necessarily intoxication at the time the specimen was provided.	Screen usually includes tests for amphetamines, cocaine, opiates, PCP, and THC (marijuana). Barbiturates, benzo-diazepines, and alcohol may also be included.

A

An Overview of Home Tests

A number of tests that were once done only in a doctor's office or other medical setting can now be done at home. Not only are home tests more convenient, but they are also less expensive. When properly done, they can help patients monitor the results of medical treatments, such as whether blood pressure is being kept under control. Even so, home tests should not be considered as alternatives to seeing a doctor. In general, home tests are not as reliable as those done by a medical professional, so a positive result should be confirmed by a doctor. Even if a home test is negative and symptoms persist, you should see a doctor; false-negative results are fairly common with some home tests.

Many home tests, such as taking one's temperature or pulse, are so commonplace that most people don't regard them as tests. Others require special equipment, such as blood pressure or blood glucose monitors. Following are descriptions of some of the most common home medical tests.

Temperature. The "normal" body temperature of 98.6°F (37°C), based on a 19th century survey in Germany, has been superseded by results obtained in the United States with modern, more accurate thermometers. Doctors agree that normal temperature is not a single number but a range. The average temperature is closer to 98.2°F, and 98.9°F is now considered the upper limit of the normal range for temperatures measured by mouth.

Glass-bulb thermometers. Once found in almost every home, glass bulbs use mercury or alcohol to register temperature in the mouth or rectum. Mercury registers temperature with a silver streak; the alcohol is tinted red to make it easier to read.

Electronic thermometers. When the heat-sensitive tip of the wand is placed in the mouth or ear, a computer chip records the temperature and displays it in digital form. These thermometers are expensive but accurate and easy to use.

Pharmacies and stores stock many different types of disposable thermometers, including some in the form of pacifiers for taking babies' temperatures.

Pulse and Fitness. With the aid of a device about the size of a paperback book, a person can measure fitness indicators including heart rate, oxygen use, caloric expenditure, and duration of exercise. This self-monitoring device can be used to calculate target heart rate as well as a fitness index based on age, gender, weight, and oxygen use. Useful for those following exercise and fitness programs, the device may have special value for people with cardiac disorders who need to keep their physicians informed about changes in their condition. Smaller devices, the size of a wristwatch, may be used for heart-rate monitoring. Other monitoring devices to be used during exercise include earlobe- and fingerclips and a small device strapped across the chest.

Blood Pressure. When blood pressure is monitored in the doctor's office, tension sometimes affects the reading and the true figure may be difficult to determine. Indeed, a condition called "white-coat hypertension" causes some people's blood pressure to rise when they see the doctor, nurse, or physician's assistant, whereas their pressure may be close to normal at other times. One-time readings in pharmacies and stalls may also give an inaccurate picture. The advantage of home blood pressure monitoring is that a person can take several stress-free readings over the course of a day or week, average them to arrive at the true pressure, and thereby better evaluate the effects of diet and medical treatment. The manually pumped blood pressure cuff (sphygmomanometer) is still used but is increasingly being replaced by the electronic model. This computerized device automatically records the pressure and displays the diastolic and systolic values digitally.

Cholesterol. An electronic device can measure blood cholesterol levels from a finger stick (like the systems available to diabetics for blood sugar measurements). While home cholesterol testing shows the overall lipid level, however, it is not capable of determining the critical ratio of high-density lipoprotein (HDL) to low-density lipoprotein (LDL). Since HDL is the "good" lipid that prevents heart attacks, and LDL the "bad" lipid that promotes heart disease, the overall reading may not be particularly useful, except for those whose doctors have advised them to decrease their total cholesterol.

Home Diabetes Monitoring. Doctors generally recommend that all patients with insulin-dependent (Type I) diabetes learn how to monitor their own blood sugar (glucose). Several different types of home monitors are available, but all entail using a small lancet to obtain a drop of blood, typically from a fingertip. The blood is smeared onto a chemically treated strip, which is then inserted into an automated device that determines the blood glucose level, which is displayed digitally. An alternative method involves observing the chemical strip for a change in color, which is compared to a chart that gives an approximate range of glucose levels.

Some patients are also instructed to test their urine for the presence of glucose. This involves placing a chemically treated strip into a sample of urine and observing it for a change in color. Urine tests have largely been replaced by the more accurate and timely glucose monitoring but are still useful in some circumstances.

Respiratory Function. For a quick evaluation of lung function, the match test requires no special equipment. A person who can blow out a lighted match from about 6 inches away is unlikely to have any serious lung disorder.

Children and adults with asthma must learn to use a peak flow meter to calculate the amount of air they exhale. Treatment decisions are based on this important reading. Asthmatics and those with other lung disorders also use a spirometer to measure the maximum volume of air they can inhale and exhale in one minute, as well as to determine the amount of air they can expel with force after taking a deep breath.

Vision. Many forms of vision testing can be done at home by means of eye charts similar to those used in doctors' offices. Home vision kits are available for testing overall visual acuity, astigmatism, color blindness, and macular degeneration, which causes loss of central vision.

Visual acuity. The Snellen alphabetical chart, with letters graduated from large to small, is designed to let people judge how well they see. A person who can read the lowest line (letters ⅜ of an inch high) from 20 feet away is described as having 20/20 vision.

Astigmatism. The eyes' ability to focus can be gauged with a chart resembling a clock face.

Color blindness. Charts are designed to detect the most common forms of color blindness, namely red/green and yellow/blue.

Macular degeneration. The Amsler grid uses a geometric pattern to detect blurring of the central vision due to macular degeneration. This is one of the most common causes of vision loss, particularly afflicting older people. Anyone who perceives lines in the Amsler grid as wavy or indistinct should consult an eye care professional; treatment can help the condition and, in many cases, prevent the loss of sight. Most people with macular degeneration are able to remain independent even if they are legally blind, because although the central vision may be lost, the outer vision field remains intact.

Ears. Parents whose children are prone to ear infections may gain peace of mind by learning to use the otoscope to detect signs of infection in the ear canal and eardrum. The otoscope—the same instrument doctors use—permits examination of the ear by means of a powerful light, a magnifying lens, and a viewer. Using the otoscope is a skill easily acquired. The results of the examination are not useful, however, unless the person using the scope knows how to recognize signs of inflammation or typical symptoms of bacterial and viral infections, including pressure behind the eardrum. To recognize disease, it is essential to be thoroughly familiar with the normal appearance and anatomy of the ear.

Urinary Tract. A variety of dipstick tests can be used to test for urinary infections. Some reveal the presence of white blood cells drawn to fight infecting microorganisms, and others show the presence of nitrites produced by bacteria. If there is any suspicion of a urinary tract infection, a doctor should be consulted and antibiotic treatment started.

Ovulation and Pregnancy. Ovulation test kits allow women to calculate their periods of maximum fertility and either plan conception efforts or take contraceptive measures accordingly. Pregnancy testing uses a color change in a urine sample to indicate if a woman is pregnant. False-negative results are more common than false-positive ones; a woman who obtains a negative result should repeat the test, taking care to follow the recommended procedure exactly.

Bowel Cancer. Home screening tests allow people to test stool specimens for the presence of occult (hidden) blood, which may be an early sign of bowel cancer. Test kits are widely available; some doctors provide them at the time of an annual checkup. As with many other cancers, the earlier bowel cancer is detected, the better the prospects for treatment and recovery. (See occult blood in stool, chapter 8.)

Breast Self-Examination. The American Cancer Society recommends that premenopausal women examine their breasts every month in the week following their menstrual periods, when their breasts are least likely to be swollen or tender. Postmenopausal women, as well as younger women who do not have regular periods, should nevertheless examine their breasts on the same day each month so that testing conditions will be reasonably similar. Most breast lumps are found by women during self-examination and, fortunately, most lumps are not cancer. At any sign of an unusual lump, however, a woman should seek a doctor's attention.

Testicular Cancer. Men should examine themselves for testicular lumps each month, just as women check for breast lumps. Despite the high malignancy and rapid growth rate of testicular cancers, the outlook for these tumors is good: the recovery rate is approximately 90% provided the cancer is detected early. The presence of any lump or irregularity should prompt a call to the doctor.

Home HIV Tests. As of this writing, two home tests for HIV, the virus that causes AIDS, have been approved for nonprescription use, and several more are being tested. The test kits, which cost $30 to $50, allow people to take a blood sample at home, mail it to a laboratory, and then call a few days later to get the results. These tests have generated considerable controversy. Their defenders argue that being able to test for HIV in the privacy of one's home, without having to go to a doctor or clinic, might encourage more people at high risk of developing AIDS to get tested. Anonymity is assured because the tests are coded with a personal identification number, rather than a name. Opponents of home HIV testing counter that the tests are not always accurate, and a positive result still needs to be confirmed by medical testing (see chapter 21). Also, when a person goes to a doctor or clinic for HIV testing, counselors are available to help a person deal with a positive result. One of the home tests gives negative results by way of a recorded phone message and has trained personnel talk to patients whose results are positive. Still, even this type of telephone counseling tends to be rather impersonal and is unlikely to be sufficient to help a person handle the emotional shock of a positive HIV test.

Index